AF332961

# 1998
## YEAR BOOK OF
## OTOLARYNGOLOGY–
## HEAD AND NECK SURGERY®

# Statement of Purpose

## The YEAR BOOK Service

The YEAR BOOK series was devised in 1901 by practicing health professionals who observed that the literature of medicine and related disciplines had become so voluminous that no one individual could read and place in perspective every potential advance in a major specialty. In the final decade of the 20th century, this recognition is more acutely true than it was in 1901.

More than merely a series of books, YEAR BOOK volumes are the tangible results of a unique service designed to accomplish the following:

- to *survey* a wide range of journals of proven value
- to *select* from those journals papers representing significant advances and statements of important clinical principles
- to provide *abstracts* of those articles that are readable, convenient summaries of their key points
- to provide *commentary* about those articles to place them in perspective

These publications grow out of a unique process that calls on the talents of outstanding authorities in clinical and fundamental disciplines, trained literature specialists, and professional writers, all supported by the resources of Mosby, the world's preeminent publisher for the health professions.

## The Literature Base

Mosby and its editors survey more than 1,000 journals published worldwide, covering the full range of the health professions. On an annual basis, the publisher examines usage patterns and polls its expert authorities to add new journals to the literature base and to delete journals that are no longer useful as potential YEAR BOOK sources.

## The Literature Survey

The publisher's team of literature specialists, all of whom are trained and experienced health professionals, examines every original, peer-reviewed article in each journal issue. More than 250,000 articles per year are scanned systematically, including title, text, illustrations, tables, and references. Each scan is compared, article by article, to the search strategies that the publisher has developed in consultation with the 270 outside experts who form the pool of YEAR BOOK editors. A given article may be reviewed by any number of editors, from one to a dozen or more, regardless of the discipline for which the paper was originally published. In turn, each editor who receives the article reviews it to determine whether the article should be included in the YEAR BOOK. This decision is based on the article's inherent quality, its probable usefulness to readers of that YEAR BOOK, and the editor's goal to represent a balanced picture of a given field in each volume of the YEAR BOOK. In addition, the editor indicates when to include figures and tables from the article to help the YEAR BOOK reader better understand the information.

Of the quarter million articles scanned each year, only 5% are selected for detailed analysis within the YEAR BOOK series, thereby assuring readers of the high value of every selection.

## The Abstract

The publisher's abstracting staff is headed by a seasoned medical professional and includes individuals with training in the life sciences, medicine, and other areas, plus extensive experience in writing for the health professions and related industries. Each selected article is assigned to a specific writer on this abstracting staff. The abstracter, guided in many cases by notations supplied by the expert editor, writes a structured, condensed summary designed so that the reader can rapidly acquire the essential information contained in the article.

## The Commentary

The YEAR BOOK editorial boards, sometimes assisted by guest commentators, write comments that place each article in perspective for the reader. This provides the reader with the equivalent of a personal consultation with a leading international authority—an opportunity to better understand the value of the article and to benefit from the authority's thought processes in assessing the article.

## Additional Editorial Features

The editorial boards of each YEAR BOOK organize the abstracts and comments to provide a logical and satisfying sequence of information. To enhance the organization, editors also provide introductions to sections or individual chapters, comments linking a number of abstracts, citations to additional literature, and other features.

The published YEAR BOOK contains enhanced bibliographic citations for each selected article, including extended listings of multiple authors and identification of author affiliations. Each YEAR BOOK contains a Table of Contents specific to that year's volume. From year to year, the Table of Contents for a given YEAR BOOK will vary depending on developments within the field.

Every YEAR BOOK contains a list of the journals from which papers have been selected. This list represents a subset of the more than 1,000 journals surveyed by the publisher and occasionally reflects a particularly pertinent article from a journal that is not surveyed on a routine basis.

Finally, each volume contains a comprehensive subject index and an index to authors of each selected paper.

# The 1998 Year Book Series

**Year Book of Allergy, Asthma, and Clinical Immunology:** Drs. Rosenwasser, Borish, Boguniewicz, Nelson, Routes, and Spahn

**Year Book of Anesthesiology and Pain Management®:** Drs. Tinker, Abram, Chestnut, Roizen, Rothenberg, and Wood

**Year Book of Cardiology®:** Drs. Schlant, Collins, Gersh, Graham, Kaplan, and Waldo

**Year Book of Chiropractic®:** Dr. Lawrence

**Year Book of Critical Care Medicine®:** Drs. Parrillo, Balk, Calvin, Franklin, and Shapiro

**Year Book of Dentistry®:** Drs. Meskin, Berry, Jeffcoat, Leinfelder, Roser, Summitt, and Zakariasen

**Year Book of Dermatologic Surgery®:** Drs. Greenway, Barrett, Papadopoulos, and Whitaker

**Year Book of Dermatology®:** Dr. Thiers

**Year Book of Diagnostic Radiology®:** Drs. Osborn, Groskin, Dalinka, Maynard, Pentecost, Rebner, Ros, Smirniotopoulos, and Young

**Year Book of Drug Therapy®:** Drs. Lasagna and Weintraub

**Year Book of Emergency Medicine®:** Drs. Wagner, Dronen, Davidson, King, Niemann, and Roberts

**Year Book of Endocrinology®:** Drs. Bagdade, Braverman, Horton, Kannan, Landsberg, Molitch, Morley, Nathan, Odell, Poehlman, Rogol, and Ryan

**Year Book of Family Practice®:** Drs. Berg, Bowman, Davidson, Dexter, and Scherger

**Year Book of Gastroenterology®:** Drs. Aliperti and Fleshman

**Year Book of Geriatrics and Gerontology®:** Drs. Burton, Beck, Ostwald, Rabins, Reuben, Roth, Shapiro, and Whitehouse

**Year Book of Hand Surgery®:** Drs. Amadio and Hentz

**Year Book of Hematology®:** Drs. Spivak, Bell, Ness, Quesenberry, Wiernik, and Horowitz

**Year Book of Infectious Diseases:** Drs. Keusch, Barza, Bennish, Poutsiaka, Skolnik, and Snydman

**Year Book of Medicine®:** Drs. Cline, Frishman, Jett, Klahr, Malawista, Mandell, McCallum, and Utiger

**Year Book of Neonatal and Perinatal Medicine®:** Drs. Fanaroff, Maisels, and Stevenson

**Year Book of Nephrology, Hypertension, and Mineral Metabolism:** Drs. Schwab, Bennett, Emmett, Hostetter, Kumar, and Toto

**Year Book of Neurology and Neurosurgery®:** Drs. Bradley and Gibbs

**Year Book of Nuclear Medicine®:** Drs. Gottschalk, Blaufox, Neumann, Strauss, and Zubal

**Year Book of Obstetrics, Gynecology, and Women's Health:** Drs. Mishell, Herbst, and Kirschbaum

**Year Book of Occupational and Environmental Medicine®:** Drs. Emmett, Frank, Gochfeld, and Hessl

**Year Book of Oncology®:** Drs. Ozols, Eisenberg, Glatstein, Loehrer, and Tallman

**Year Book of Ophthalmology®:** Drs. Wilson, Augsburger, Cohen, Eagle, Grossman, Laibson, Maguire, Nelson, Penne, Rapuano, Sergott, Spaeth, Tipperman, Ms. Gosfield, and Ms. Salmon

**Year Book of Orthopedics®:** Drs. Morrey, Beauchamp, Currier, Tolo, Trigg, and Swiontkowski

**Year Book of Otolaryngology–Head and Neck Surgery®:** Drs. Paparella and Holt

**Year Book of Pathology and Laboratory Medicine®:** Drs. Raab, Cohen, Olson, Sirgi, and Stanley

**Year Book of Pediatrics®:** Dr. Stockman

**Year Book of Plastic, Reconstructive, and Aesthetic Surgery®:** Drs. Miller, Bartlett, Garner, McKinney, Ruberg, Salisbury, and Smith

**Year Book of Psychiatry and Applied Mental Health®:** Drs. Talbott, Ballenger, Frances, Lydiard, Meltzer, Schowalter, and Tasman

**Year Book of Pulmonary Disease®:** Drs. Jett, Maurer, Ryu, Strollo, and Wenzel

**Year Book of Rheumatology®:** Drs. Panush, Hadler, LeRoy, Liang, Reichlin, Simon, and Weinblatt

**Year Book of Sports Medicine®:** Drs. Shephard, Drinkwater, Eichner, Torg, Alexander, and Mr. George

**Year Book of Surgery®:** Drs. Copeland, Bland, Deitch, Eberlein, Howard, Luce, Seeger, Souba, and Sugarbaker

**Year Book of Thoracic and Cardiovascular Surgery®:** Drs. Ginsberg, Wechsler, and Williams

**Year Book of Urology®:** Drs. Andriole and Coplen

**Year Book of Vascular Surgery®:** Dr. Porter

1998

# The Year Book of OTOLARYNGOLOGY–HEAD AND NECK SURGERY®

## Otology

**Editor**

**Michael M. Paparella, M.D.**

*Clinical Professor and Chairman Emeritus, Department of Otolaryngology, University of Minnesota; Director of Otopathology Laboratory; President, Minnesota Ear, Head, and Neck Clinic; Secretary, International Hearing Foundation*

## Head and Neck Surgery

**Editor**

**G. Richard Holt, M.D., M.S.E., M.P.H.**

*Clinical Professor of Otolaryngology–Head and Neck Surgery, The University of Texas Health Science Center at San Antonio, The University of Texas Health Science Center at Houston; Adjunct Institute Scientist, Southwest Research Institute, San Antonio*

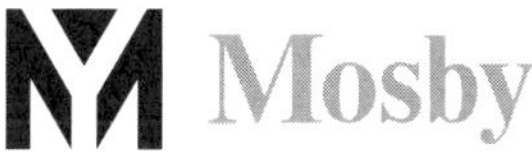

St. Louis  Baltimore  Boston  Carlsbad  Naples  New York  Philadelphia  Portland  London  Madrid  Mexico City  Singapore  Sydney  Tokyo  Toronto  Wiesbaden

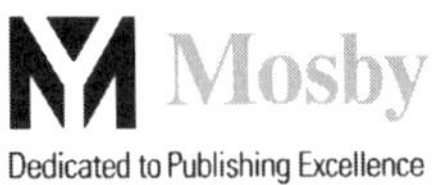 Mosby

Dedicated to Publishing Excellence

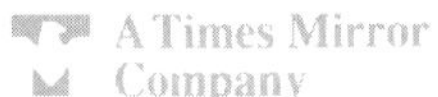 A Times Mirror
Company

*Publisher:* Theresa Van Schaik
*Developmental Editor:* Gary O'Brien
*Manager, Periodicals Editing:* Kirk Swearingen
*Manuscript Editor:* Amanda Maguire
*Project Supervisor, Production:* Joy Moore
*Production Assistant:* Karie House
*Manager, Literature Services:* Idelle L. Winer
*Illustrations and Permissions Coordinator:* Phyllis K. Thompson

**1998 EDITION**
**Copyright © July 1998 by Mosby, Inc.**



Printed in the United States of America
Composition by Reed Technology and Information Services, Inc.
Printing/binding by Maple-Vail

Editorial Office:
Mosby, Inc.
11830 Westline Industrial Drive
St. Louis, MO 63146
Customer Service: customer.support@mosby.com
            www.mosby.com/Mosby/CustomerSupport/index.html

International Standard Serial Number: 1041-892X
International Standard Book Number: 0-8151-9718-7

# Table of Contents

# Journals Represented

Mosby and its editors survey more than 1,000 journals for its abstract and commentary publications. From these journals, the editors select the articles to be abstracted. Journals represented in this YEAR BOOK are listed below.

Acta Oto-Laryngologica
Acta Radiologica
Allergy
American Journal of Epidemiology
American Journal of Human Genetics
American Journal of Industrial Medicine
American Journal of Otolaryngology
American Journal of Otology
American Journal of Physiology
American Journal of Respiratory and Critical Care Medicine
American Journal of Roentgenology
American Journal of Surgery
Anesthesia and Analgesia
Annals of Internal Medicine
Annals of Neurology
Annals of Oncology
Annals of Otology, Rhinology, and Laryngology
Annals of Plastic Surgery
Annals of the Royal College of Surgeons of England
Archives of Disease in Childhood
Archives of Neurology
Archives of Ophthalmology
Archives of Otolaryngology—Head and Neck Surgery
Cancer
Cephalalgia
Chest
Dermatologic Surgery
European Respiratory Journal
Head and Neck
International Journal of Oral and Maxillofacial Implants
International Journal of Radiation, Oncology, Biology, and Physics
Journal of Acquired Immune Deficiency Syndromes and Human Retrovirology
Journal of Allergy and Clinical Immunology
Journal of Clinical Oncology
Journal of Computer Assisted Tomography
Journal of Cranio-Maxillo-Facial Surgery
Journal of Epidemiology and Community Health
Journal of Laryngology and Otology
Journal of Oral and Maxillofacial Surgery
Journal of Otolaryngology
Journal of Pediatrics
Journal of the American Medical Association
Journal of the National Cancer Institute
Medical Problems of Performing Artists
Neurosurgery
ORL (Journal for Oto-Rhino-Laryngology)
Otolaryngology—Head and Neck Surgery

Pediatric Infectious Disease Journal
Pediatrics
Plastic and Reconstructive Surgery
Psychotherapy and Psychosomatics
Radiology
S.A.M.J./S.A.M.T—South African Medical Journal
Scandinavian Journal of Rehabilitation Medicine
Southern Medical Journal
Surgery
Surgical Neurology
The Laryngoscope Journal

## STANDARD ABBREVIATIONS

The following terms are abbreviated in this edition: acquired immunodeficiency syndrome (AIDS), cardiopulmonary resuscitation (CPR), central nervous system (CNS), cerebrospinal fluid (CSF), computed tomography (CT), deoxyribonucleic acid (DNA), electrocardiography (ECG), health maintenance organization (HMO), human immunodeficiency virus (HIV), intensive care unit (ICU), intramuscular (IM), intravenous (IV), magnetic resonance (MR) imaging (MRI), and ribonucleic acid (RNA).

## NOTE

The YEAR BOOK OF OTOLARYNGOLOGY–HEAD AND NECK SURGERY is a literature survey service providing abstracts of articles published in the professional literature. Every effort is made to ensure the accuracy of the information presented in these pages. Neither the editors nor the publisher of the YEAR BOOK OF OTOLARYNGOLOGY–HEAD AND NECK SURGERY can be responsible for errors in the original materials. The editors' comments are their own opinions. Mention of specific products within this publication does not constitute endorsement.

To facilitate the use of the YEAR BOOK OF OTOLARYNGOLOGY–HEAD AND NECK SURGERY as a reference tool, all illustrations and tables included in this publication are now identified as they appear in the original article. This change is meant to help the reader recognize that any illustration or table appearing in the YEAR BOOK OF OTOLARYNGOLOGY–HEAD AND NECK SURGERY may be only one of many in the original article. For this reason, figure and table numbers will often appear to be out of sequence within the YEAR BOOK OF OTOLARYNGOLOGY–HEAD AND NECK SURGERY.

# OTOLOGY

MICHAEL PAPARELLA, M.D.

# Introduction

## Hearing Aids and the Otolaryngologist (Otologist)

The otolaryngologist, otologist-neurotologist has every reason to be interested in hearing aids. His or her role is to make a medical diagnosis (preferably based on pathogenesis) of the disease or disorder that underlies each hearing loss, then to consider and apply therapeutic methods of medical or surgical care as indicated, and finally to direct and oversee the process of rehabilitation, which predominantly includes the use of hearing aids. The specialist in hearing aids or the audiologist actively participates in the prescription and fitting of the hearing aid. These patients then require follow-up both by the specialist in hearing aids or the audiologist, to obtain and learn to use the hearing aid, and by the otolaryngologist (otologist) for medical evaluation. Hearing aids are increasingly being fitted in otolaryngologist's (otologist's) offices for good medical care and care of the hearing aid, as well as for other reasons.

I thought it would be of interest to the readers of the 1998 YEAR BOOK OF OTOLARYNGOLOGY–HEAD AND NECK SURGERY to peruse an update on hearing aids written by an expert and leader in the field. I am pleased that my friend and colleague William Austin, chairman and CEO of Starkey Laboratories Inc., agreed to contribute to this introduction his perspectives on the current status in hearing aids. Under Austinable leadership, Starkey Laboratories has become the world leader in dollar-volume sales and #1 in sales overall in North America. He and Starkey pioneered the successful utilization of in-the-ear hearing aids, which now constitute 80% of the market; this percentage was a miniscule fraction of the market when he started out.

Michael M. Paparella, M.D.

## Perspectives on Hearing Aids

WILLIAM AUSTIN
*Chairman and CEO, Starkey Laboratories Inc., Eden Prairie, Minnesota*

### Advances in Technology of Hearing Aids

Modern hearing aids have come a long way from the days when users strapped wet-cell batteries to their legs and ran wiring under their clothing to obtain noisy and tinny amplification of sounds they hoped to hear better. Even large button-shaped receivers plugged into the ear and connected to hearing aids worn on the body, which were state of the art less than 40 years ago, have evolved into a new generation of virtually invisible devices for the amplification of hearing. Today's state-of-the-art hearing aids are tiny, self-contained plastic earpieces, comfortably custom fitted to the individual user, that contain all the components necessary to optimize sound delivered to the ear. Fitting strategies are available to compensate for a variety of hearing losses, to a degree far beyond the early days of limited amplification for conductive losses. Modern techniques for fitting aids for sensorineural and mixed hearing losses are well proven and effective.

## Continued Miniaturization

Today's completely-in-the-canal (CIC) hearing aids are virtually invisible; they are powered by a battery smaller than a tablet of aspirin and can provide a degree of improvement in hearing not even thinkable for previous generations of hearing aid users. Several factors help to explain this success. One is the placement of the microphone at the entrance to the ear-canal, which enhances sounds in high frequencies by taking advantage of naturally occurring concha-related resonances. Another is the termination of the canalward tip of the hearing aid beyond the second bend of the ear canal. This effectively reduces the residual volume in front of the tympanic membrane and, thus, correspondingly reduces the amount of gain required in the hearing aid to produce a given level of sound pressure at the eardrum. An associated benefit is that there is a progressive effective increase in amplification of the high frequencies over the low frequencies, because the middle ear cavity has a more pronounced acoustic effect compared to the diminishing residual volume in front of the tympanic membrane as the insertion of the hearing aid becomes deeper. This combination of acoustic factors creates a high-frequency emphasis that allows less gain to be prescribed in the hearing aid, which decreases the probability of acoustic feedback.

The recessed position of the microphone in the ear canal often leads to a decrease in complaints about noise from windy conditions. The relative position of the canalward tip of the hearing aid in the ear also reduces complaints of occlusion, often described by the user as an echoing, hollow, unnatural sound. Termination of the hearing aid in the bony (osseous) portion of the ear canal reduces or eliminates those low-frequency effects of occlusion. Reduced complaints of occlusion make it possible to fit CIC hearing aids even for users with mild hearing losses in the high frequencies. These potential users may have previously rejected amplification, even though their hearing loss created difficulty in understanding speech in adverse, noisy situations.

Modern methods of making impressions of the ear and molding the shell of the hearing aid provide a better and more comfortable fit for the user. Factory training and support in techniques for modifying the physical characteristics of the hearing aid, such as for fit and appropriate venting, allow the dispenser superior flexibility in the final fitting, to create a satisfied user. Users are often motivated by the cosmetic advantage of the small size of CIC hearing aids and the enhanced acoustic benefits. Although CIC hearing aids are fitted primarily for adults, this configuration of hearing aids is easily accepted by users of all ages, due to the small, inconspicuous size of the case. Individual manufacture of customized earpieces allows a comfortable and accurate fit, even for ears with unusual morphology or for those that have undergone radical surgical procedures.

## Improvements in Quality of Sound

The days when a hearing aid sounded like listening to a noisy, distorted echo in a barrel have gone. Modern hearing aids have wide bandwidths, smooth frequency responses, and low levels of distortion. Improvements in microphones and earphones, coupled with advances in electronic circuitry, have removed the peaky quality of sound that often generated complaints from users. The scratchy sound quality of carbon microphones has been replaced with modern electret technology that can rival the sound quality of recording microphones.

Improvements in the reduction of distortion during processing through the hearing aid have led to substantial improvements in the quality of the sound delivered to the listener. This improvement in sound quality by the removal of non-linear distortion components has also led to a reduction of undesired masking and other interference, with desired sounds being amplified. The reduction of audible distortion has led to a corresponding reduction in the amount of fatigue often experienced by users listening to the distorted sounds of poor-quality hearing aids.

## Advanced Methods for Fitting

Although a well-fitting, correctly prescribed hearing aid is a key to improved hearing, enhancement of hearing does not involve merely the hearing aids; it includes a whole armamentarium of new techniques and technology for fitting them. Because of the complexity of sound-processing algorithms in use today, computer-based fitting systems are often used to assist the dispenser in selecting the correct fitting strategy for a particular individual. Computer-based analysis of audiologic data and the use of sophisticated fitting formulas can help in arriving rapidly at the optimum recommendations of hearing aid and fitting for a particular individual.

## Digital Technology

Just as advancing technology had made high-tech improvements in everyday living, such as through digital cellular telephones, compact audio discs, and programmable appliances, so also these new technological advances have started to be incorporated into hearing aids. Although still a long way from providing flexible, computer-based processing in the ear comparable to the revolution in home computers, emerging audio-processing using digital signal-processing (DSP) technology in hearing aids holds promise for the future. The first generation of products with DSP available today provide only a limited version of what they will do in the future. Until then, today's analog hearing aids offer a full spectrum of fitting solutions. The functions of today's analog hearing aids can be implemented with either analog or digital circuitry, and the user cannot perceive the difference. The real power of DSP for the future will lie in the ability to perform complex processing-functions and compensations for hearing loss in ways that cannot be implemented easily in current analog hearing aids.

## Conclusion

The hearing aids of today have evolved from the heavy, bulky amplifiers of yesterday into tiny, highly sophisticated electronic devices that offer the promise of solutions for almost any hearing loss. Improvements in the technology of modern hearing aids and in the techniques for fitting have increased the potential spectrum of persons who may be helped. While early hearing aids with their limited processing power and flexibility allowed successful fitting primarily for only relatively straightforward hearing losses, modern hearing aids can be fitted successfully for hearing losses that range from very mild to profound, over an expanded range of frequencies, and with a wide variety of sophisticated signal-processing techniques.

# 1 Vestibular Function

**Nonspecific Vertigo With Normal Otoneurological Examination: The Role of Vestibular Laboratory Tests**
Gordon CR, Shupak A, Spitzer O, et al (Israel Naval Medicine Inst, Haifa; Meir Gen Hosp, Kfar Saba, Israel; Tel Aviv Univ, Israel; et al)
*J Laryngol Otol* 110:1133–1137, 1996                    1–1

*Introduction.*—Some patients who complain of vertigo have a normal otoneurologic workup and no unusual findings on audiological or neuroimaging examinations. Such patients are described as having "nonspecific dizziness or vertigo" and constitute a diagnostic challenge. A group of 52 patients with nonspecific vertigo and normal otoneurologic findings were studied to assess the diagnostic value of vestibular laboratory tests.

*Methods.*—The patients, 32 men and 20 women, had a mean age of 40.4 years. All had protracted (>3 weeks) or recurrent episodes of nonspecific vertigo, with an ill-defined illusion of movement but no clear spinning sensation. None had associated CNS symptoms. Their medical history and CT findings were unremarkable, although 9 had a history of head trauma and 13 reported ear disorders or hearing loss. The vestibular laboratory tests included a standard electronystagmography (ENG) examination and the sinusoidal harmonic acceleration (SHA) test.

*Results.*—Vestibular test results showed abnormalities in 35 (67%) patients; 22 finally received a diagnosis of a unilateral peripheral vestibular lesion (UPVL), and 13 had benign positional vertigo (BPV) diagnosed. Twenty of the 22 patients with UPVL had abnormal SHA test results. Five of the 13 patients with BPV exhibited unilateral canal paresis on caloric stimulation, and 3 also had asymmetry on the SHA test. Eight of the 22 patients with a history of trauma or otological disorders had normal vestibular tests, 5 had BPV, and 9 had UPVL.

*Conclusions.*—A high percentage of these patients with nonspecific vertigo and a normal otoneurologic workup had a peripheral vestibular dysfunction that could be documented objectively by vestibular laboratory tests. The ENG examination and SHA tests allow such patients to receive a definite diagnosis and provide the physician with direction for a therapeutic approach.

▶ This study is of interest because we see many patients, for example, who have classic, incapacitating, intractable Ménière's disease and yet an ENG

"

shows normal caloric test results. These authors have found when patients have nonspecific vertigo, a normal otoneurologic examination sometimes can demonstrate objective documentation by ENG testing. Thus, an ENG test may demonstrate abnormal findings in a patient with little or no vestibular symptomatology, or as mentioned above, a patient with incapacitating vertigo may have essentially normal findings on ENG. In fact, approximately half of our patients with Ménière's disease would fall into this latter category.

**M.M. Paparella, M.D.**

## Vestibular Abnormalities in CHARGE Association

Murofushi T, Ouvrier RA, Parker GD, et al (Royal Prince Alfred Hosp, Sydney, Australia; Royal Alexandra Hosp for Children, Sydney, Australia)
*Ann Otol Rhinol Laryngol* 106:129–134, 1997                    1–2

*Introduction.*—Anomalies of the external, middle, and inner ear are common in patients with CHARGE association (Coloboma, Heart disease, Atresia of choanae, Retarded growth and development and/or CNS anomalies, Genital hypoplasia, and Ear anomalies). Vestibular abnormalities have not been well described in this population of patients. Vestibular abnormalities are reported in 5 patients with CHARGE association.

*Methods.*—Four women and 1 man with CHARGE association whose ages ranged from 3 to 23 years had histories taken and underwent CT scans, temporal bone and neurologic and neurotologic examinations that included tests of stance and gait with and without blindfolds and tests of proprioception, impulse-tests of horizontal and vertical vestibulo-ocular reflexes, and a test of postrotatory nystagmus using Frenzel glasses after 10 revolutions.

*Results.*—All patients had delayed motor development and absent vestibular function, as determined by absent vestibulo-ocular reflexes and severe imbalance on simultaneous deprivation of proprioception and vision. All 6 semicircular canals were aplastic in all 5 patients. Cochlear function was severely decreased in 6 of 10 ears, absent in 3 ears, and intact below 3 kHz in 1 ear. Bony cochleas were observed on CT of all 10 ears (Fig 2). Of these, 7 appeared abnormal and 3 appeared normal.

*Conclusion.*—The absence of bony semicircular canals and the presence of a bony cochlea is typically observed in patients with CHARGE association. These disproportionate structural abnormalities are manifested in their functional abnormalities (absent vestibular function with preservation of some cochlear function).

▶ These authors describe the syndrome of Coloboma, Heart disease, Atresia of choanae, Retarded growth and development and/or anomalies of the CNS, Genital hypoplasia, and Ear anomalies—the so-called CHARGE association or syndrome. This unusual combination of findings occurred in 5 patients, all of whom had absent vestibular function. All the semicircular canals were absent, according to the study, which would account for the

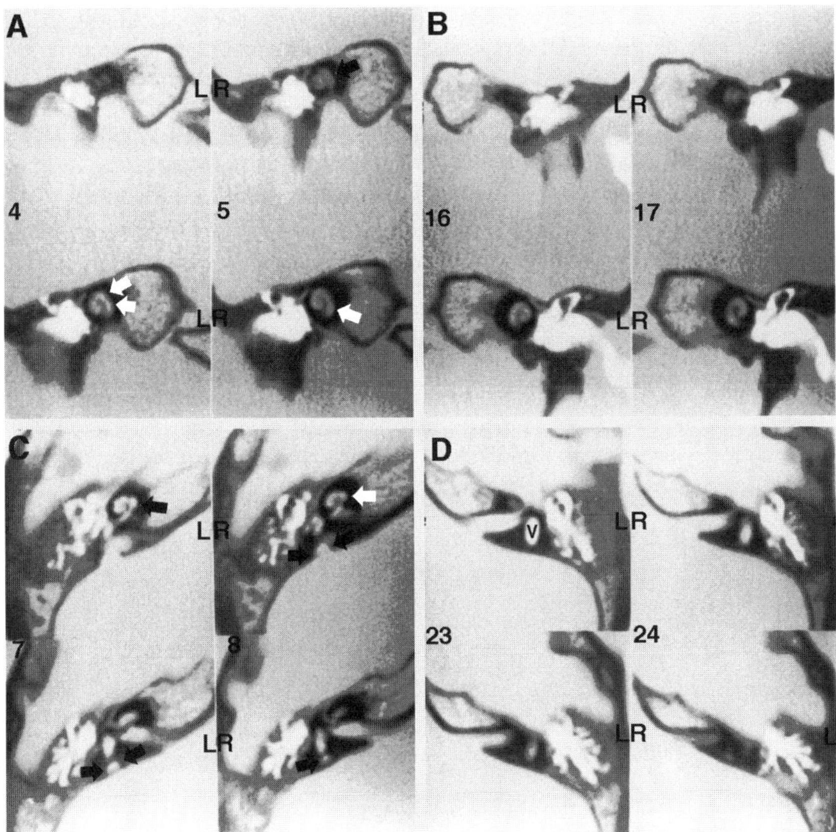

FIGURE 2.—(Patient 1) **A,B,** coronal and **C,D,** axial video-reversed temporal bone CT scans. Semi-circular canals are bilaterally absent, vestibule (*V*) is dilated on left (**B,D**), and vestibular aqueduct is dilated on right (**A,C**; *black arrows*). Bony cochlea is bilaterally present and appears normal, apart from basal turn on right (**A,C**), which appears to be slightly dilated (*white arrows*). (Courtesy of Murofushi T, Ouvrier RA, Parker GD, et al: Vestibular abnormalities in CHARGE association. *Ann Otol Rhinol Laryngol* 106:129–134, 1997.

absent vestibular response. We will be more alert for this curious combination of findings in the future, even though this certainly is a very rare disease.

**M.M. Paparella, M.D.**

## Benign Paroxysmal Positional Vertigo

Hughes CA, Proctor L (Georgetown Univ, Washington, DC; Johns Hopkins Univ, Baltimore, Md)
*Laryngoscope* 107:607–613, 1997

1–3

*Background.*—Many different causes of benign paroxysmal positional vertigo (BPPV) have been proposed, including cerebellar, cervical, vascular, and labyrinthine causes, the latter being the most accepted. This condition may be associated with various labyrinthine disorders, including head trauma, viral labyrinthitis, previous surgery, and suppurative otitis media, but most cases are idiopathic. The results of otologic vestibular testing in patients with a diagnosis of BPPV were analyzed.

*Methods.*—The retrospective study included 781 patients tested in an otologic vestibular laboratory on 2 or more occasions over a 16-year period. Of those, 187 (24%) had clinical evidence of BPPV. Most of these patients had torsional or vertical nystagmus and vertigo during head-hanging positional tests with Frenzel's glasses. The patients' records were reviewed in detail, including vestibular tests and eye-movement reports, audiograms, questionnaires, and hospital charts.

*Results.*—After review, 36 patients with an initial diagnosis of BPPV were reclassified as having nystagmus resulting from another disease-process. This left 151 patients, 52 0f whom had no significant preceding disorder. Thus, 34% of this group was regarded as having primary BPPV. The other 99 patients had other disorders, such as Ménière's disease, head trauma, previous ear surgery, vestibular neuronitis, and migraine. In 31% of the 151 patients, the associated disease was Ménière's disease.

*Conclusions.*—Many patients with diagnosed BPPV have associated or coexisting disorders. The possibility of such disorders, particularly Ménière's disease, should be entertained whenever BPPV is considered. The mechanism of this association could involve hydropic injury to the otolithic apparatus, injury to the otolithic apparatus by a common underlying disorder, or hydropic distention resulting from obstruction by otolithic debris. Further clinical and histopathologic studies are needed to determine the significance of these associations.

▶ These authors describe a finding that we have observed for a long period of time—that patients with so-called "benign paroxysmal positional vertigo" may have other diseases such as Ménière's disease. In fact, in a previous study of its natural history, we found that more than 70% of patients will have positional vertigo along with their attacks of Ménière's disease, which can occur during and/or between attacks. Thus, I think this article is of interest, and it is true indeed that patients with positional vertigo may or may not have another disease process co-existing and/or predisposing to it, such as Ménière's disease. Naturally, when we have positional vertigo in a patient with Ménière's disease, we are dealing with hydrops of the saccule, which in turn may explain stimulation of the ampullae, and this certainly might require a modification of the cupulolithiasis theory.

**M.M. Paparella, M.D.**

## Comparison of Effectiveness of Maneuvers and Medication in the Treatment of Benign Paroxysmal Positional Vertigo

Itaya T, Yamamoto E, Kitano H, et al (Kobe City Gen Hosp, Japan; Shiga Univ, Japan)
*ORL J Otorhinolaryngol Relat Spec* 59:155–158, 1997                    1–4

*Introduction.*—New maneuvers have been discovered for treating benign paroxysmal positional vertigo (BPPV), the pathophysiology of which has been labeled canalithiasis. The newest hypothesis assumes that debris floats freely within the endolymph of the canal and the viscosity and hydrodynamic drag of the particle induce an endolymph current that induces nystagmus and vertigo. These maneuvers, called the "particle repositioning maneuver" and the "liberatory maneuver," cause debris floating in the canal to be excreted from the posterior semicircular canal to the utricle. Conventional medication alone was compared with the use of these maneuvers in treating patients with BPPV.

*Methods.*—There were 31 patients with BPPV. Fifteen were treated with the particle repositioning maneuver and 16 were treated with the liberatory maneuver. Both groups also had standard drugs administered for vertigo and inner-ear disease, including vitamin B12, antivertigo drugs, and a minor tranquilizer. A retrospective comparison was conducted between 26 patients treated with medication only and the patients given the maneuvers and the drugs. After the maneuvers, the patients were evaluated at 3, 7, and 14 days.

*Results.*—After 2 weeks, 11 of 14 patients (78.6%) treated with the liberatory maneuver and 14 of 15 patients (93.3%) treated with the particle repositioning maneuver experienced improvement. In the medication group, 8 of 26 patients (30.8%) improved after 2 weeks. After 3 months, the improvement rate in the medication group reached 96.2%.

*Conclusion.*—These maneuvers resulted in a speedier recovery than that with medication alone. After 3 months, there was no significant difference in the late success rate between medication alone and the maneuvers. High success rates were demonstrated with these maneuvers, with no significant differences in outcomes between the maneuvers.

▶ The authors compare maneuvers and medication in the treatment of BPPV. We use medication first and, if medication fails, we resort to these maneuvers and positioning procedures. Our experience is that many patients who have had a canalith repositioning procedure continue to have problems, even after the positional maneuvers—a much lower incidence than these authors show in this comparative study.

**M.M. Paparella, M.D.**

## Illness Behaviour, Personality Traits, Anxiety, and Depression in Patients With Ménière's, Disease

Savastano M, Maron MB, Mangialaio M, et al (Padua Univ, Padova, Italy)
*J Otolaryngol* 25:329–333, 1996                                               1–5

*Background.*—The psychological distress that is common in patients with Ménière's disease has led some authors to suggest that the condition may have a psychosomatic basis. The vertigo of Ménière's disease affects the patient's psychosocial balance, including their psychologic bearing, interpersonal relations, and subjective interpretations of their signs and symptoms. The last of these, defined as illness behavior (IB), has important implications for therapy, including the quality of the physician-patient relationship. Illness behavior, personality traits, and anxiety and depression were evaluated among patients with Ménière's disease.

*Methods.*—Fifty patients with Ménière's disease seen at 1 ENT department were prospectively studied. All were evaluated on 4 psychometric questionnaires: the Illness Behavior Questionnaire (IBQ), the Eysenck Personality Inventory, the State Trait Anxiety Inventory, and the Zung Self-Rating Depression Scale. Illness behavior was assessed in terms of personality and psychological distress.

*Results.*—Compared with established norms, the Ménière's disease patients had higher scores for neuroticism, a stronger psychological perception of disease, and a lower level of affective inhibition. Cluster analysis of the IBQ scores suggested that a subgroup of patients had severe psychological distress, high levels of neuroticism and psychoticism, and abnormal IB. These patients were older, had a longer history of Ménière's disease, and more hospitalizations. Time since the last attack of vertigo was significantly correlated with the dysphoria score on the IBQ.

*Conclusions.*—Some patients with Ménière's disease may have a combination of predisposing personality and anxiety traits and disease-related psychological effects that lead to abnormal IB. No specific association between the psychological aspects and clinical disease is apparent, however. The IBQ may be a useful tool for identifying patients with abnormal IB. The overall psychological stress that can accompany Ménière's disease must be considered in treatment programs.

▶ These authors have conducted a very careful study of patients, prospectively, as well as having reviewed the literature very carefully. They find in their conclusion and final analysis that the data suggest there is no specific link between psychological aspects and the clinical disease process. It would seem that any of us—if we were to have episodic, unannounced, severe vertigo—would be anxious and might have a nervous or psychoneurotic trait because of this severe problem. Thus, a psychological aberration can result from the disease. Certainly, anxiety can exacerbate the disease as well, and that is true of any disease, not only Ménière's disease. But the cause of this disease is certainly not a psychological one but a physiologic one.

**M.M. Paparella, M.D.**

**Migraine-associated Vertigo**
Savundra PA, Carroll JD, Davies RA, et al (Natl Hosp for Neurology & Neurosurgery, London)
*Cephalalgia* 17:505–510, 1997                                             1–6

*Introduction.*—The association between migraine and vertigo is not well defined, partly because of the lack of standardized definitions of both disorders. A retrospective analysis of 363 patients who sought treatment for vertigo examined the prevalence of migraine and compared the prevalence of vestibular disturbances in migraineurs and nonmigraineurs.

*Methods.*—The group studied was drawn from a database at the National Hospital for Neurology and Neurosurgery in London. Eligible patients had symptoms that included an illusion of movement. Excluded were patients with alternobaric vertigo, Tullio's phenomenon, and hyperventilation. Migraine was defined according to the Classification and Diagnostic Criteria for the Diagnosis of Migraine, with modifications to allow for vertigo as an aura of migraine and an extension of the duration of aura. All patients had a standardized neurologic assessment, a full medical history and examination, audiovestibular investigations, electrooculographic assessment, bithermal caloric testing, and blood tests.

*Results.*—There were 116 (32%) migraineurs among the 363 patients with vertigo. Migraine with aura had a prevalence of 24.5%. Other identifiable pathologic conditions were present in 17 of the 116 migraineurs and in 122 of the 247 nonmigraineurs. Idiopathic vertigo was present significantly more often in migraineurs (85%) than in nonmigraineurs (51%). Migraineurs and nonmigraineurs also differed significantly in the proportion without a demonstrable vestibular disturbance (47% versus 6%, respectively); in the proportion with an idiopathic central vestibular disturbance (6% versus 0.8%); in the proportion with an idiopathic combined central and peripheral vestibular disturbance (9% versus 0%); and in the proportion with an idiopathic peripheral vestibular disturbance (37% versus 94%).

*Discussion.*—Although there have been many reports of an association and a possible pathophysiologic relationship between vertigo and migraine, the issue remains controversial. Approximately one third of these patients with vertigo also had migraine, indicating a definite association between the 2 disorders. The combination of central and peripheral vestibular signs was a feature of migraine with aura.

▶ This study is of interest because it describes how patients with migraine headaches can have dizziness including vertigo. Many patients who have migraine headache diagnosed are referred to my vestibular clinic, and indeed

I find that some of these patients have Ménière's disease. I have had the opposite experience in a subgroup of patients with intractable, classic Ménière's disease who were treated by, in some instances, multiple neurologists over a prolonged period for migraine headache.

After successful treatment of their disease, either with medication or conservative surgery, such as endolymphatic sac enhancement, or both, I have had a significant number of these patients in whom the "migraine headaches" mysteriously disappeared, suggesting the possibility that so-called migraine headaches may be concomitant with Ménière's disease. We know that patients with Ménière's disease will have a variety of cochlear symptoms, a variety of vestibular symptoms, and a variety of symptoms related to pressure-headache, some of which may mimic migraine.

**M.M. Paparella, M.D.**

---

## Long-term Effects of Ménière's Disease on Hearing and Quality of Life

Kinney SE, Sandridge SA, Newman CW (Cleveland Clinic Found, Ohio)
*Am J Otol* 18:67–73, 1997
1–7

---

*Introduction.*—Characterized by aural fullness, tinnitus, fluctuating hearing loss, and episodic vertigo, Ménière's disease is a non–life-threatening inner ear process. Throughout the natural history of the disease, there is a continuum of change. The disease can be considered life-altering as it impacts the quality of life, resulting in communication and psycho-social handicaps. Surgery has resulted in a success rate that ranges from 10% to 56%. A group of patients with unilateral Ménière's disease were evaluated to determine long-term change in hearing, a difference in hearing status between medically and surgically treated patients, and long-term handicaps.

*Methods.*—There were 31 medically treated patients and 20 surgically treated patients with a mean age of 48±10.3 years. Medical treatment usually consisted of a salt-restricted diet, diuretics, and labyrinthine sedatives with treatment time varying from 3 months to 15 years. Surgical treatment included sac decompression, shunt, and vestibular nerve section. They all received audiometric testing, the Hearing Handicap Inventory, the Dizziness Handicap Inventory, the Tinnitus Handicap Inventory, and the SF-36 Health Survey.

*Results.*—In long-term hearing results, there were no statistically significant differences detected from natural history in surgically or medical treated patients with Ménière's disease. Patients were heterogenous regarding dizziness, self-perceived hearing, and tinnitus disability or handicap. More than three fourths of the patients indicated that dizziness, hearing loss, and/or tinnitus affected their quality of life to some degree. There was a greater global health handicap for emotional disability than for physical disability.

*Conclusion.*—In Ménière's disease, medical and surgical treatment does not significantly influence hearing results. There is a greater emotional disability than a physical disability among patients with Ménière's disease.

▶ The subject of this study, long-term effects of Ménière's disease on hearing and quality of life, certainly is an important question to be addressed by those who treat patients with Ménière's disease. The conclusions of these authors are of interest and seem reasonable. For the variety of procedures done, for example, sac decompression, shunt, vestibular nerve section, the numbers were rather small; there were 5 decompressions, 1 vestibular nerve section, and 15 shunts. The question is whether these numbers are sizable enough to draw long-term conclusions, with the many variables that relate not only to the disease but also to its management. Nevertheless, this is an important question that should be addressed—the long-term quality of life is important in these patients, as well as quality of labyrinthine preservation.

**M.M. Paparella, M.D.**

---

**Impact of Vestibular Disorders on Fitness to Drive: A Census of the American Neurotology Society**
Parnes LS, Sindwani R (Univ of Western Ontario, London, Canada)
*Am J Otol* 18:79–85, 1997                                                  1–8

---

*Background.*—Legislation mandating physician reporting of patients unfit to drive varies substantially among the United States and Canadian provinces. The impact of vestibular disorders on fitness to drive was determined via a survey.

*Methods.*—An anonymous questionnaire was mailed to all members of the American Neurotology Society (ANS). The response rate was 69.4%.

*Findings.*—Most respondents were aware of the potential risk of driving by patients with vestibular diseases, especially patients with Tumarkin's attacks. Although 94% of the clinicians said they counseled their patients and 75% have considered reporting these patients, only 14% of the respondents have actually reported them. No consensus was apparent on the best method for reporting patients unfit to drive. Mandatory physician reporting was supported by only 18.9% of the respondents. Those living in states where reporting is not mandatory were more likely to be satisfied with their state's legislation and less likely to report patients unfit to drive.

*Conclusions.*—At this time, the authors do not advocate mandatory reporting of patients with vestibular disorders. There is no general consensus among ANS members responding to the current survey, and the safety risk appears to be relatively low compared with that of other disorders.

▶ This survey by Parnes and Sindwani is a practical one because we face these questions each day in our clinic. Is it safe for the patient to drive? As we do with every patient, we need to individualize; certain patients with vestibular problems, including Ménière's disease, are so incapacitated or disabled that it would be unsafe to them and others if they did drive. At the same time, most of my patients are able to drive, if they have these problems. Once again, individualization, relating to the individual disease process and its relative or absolute incapacitation, will be the determinating factor.

**M.M. Paparella, M.D.**

## The Diagnostic Value of Imaging the Patient With Dizziness: A Bayesian Approach

Gizzi M, Riley E, Molinari S (Seton Hall Univ, Edison, NJ)
*Arch Neurol* 53:1299–1304, 1996                                                    1–9

*Purpose.*—In evaluating the patient with dizziness, an important task is to rule out the possibility of a mass in the cerebellopontine angle (CPA). This exclusion may be done using imaging studies. However, the rate of CPA masses among patients with dizziness is low, calling into question the value of performing imaging studies in this group. A Bayesian approach was used to figure the likelihood that a patient with dizziness will have a CPA mass.

*Methods.*—A meta-analysis was performed of epidemiologic data on CPA masses and the incidence of dizziness and hearing loss. Also, in a consecutive series of patients with dizziness, the frequency of asymmetric hearing loss was determined. Bayes' theorem was applied to the combined data to calculate the probability of a CPA mass in a patient with dizziness.

*Results.*—Calculations suggested that the probability of a patient with dizziness having a CPA mass was 0.0004. Thus, a total of 2,500 imaging studies would have to be performed in patients with dizziness to identify 1 patient with a CPA mass. For patients with isolated dizziness but subjectively normal hearing, the probability fell to 0.000107. In this group, it would take 9,307 scans to identify 1 CPA mass. The probability increased to 0.00156 for patients with dizziness and asymmetric hearing loss, 638 of whom would have to be scanned to identify 1 CPA mass.

*Conclusions.*—In patients with dizziness—even those with asymmetric hearing loss—the probability of detecting a CPA mass is too low to warrant imaging studies. If CNS or invasive otologic disease is suspected on neurologic and otologic examination, then imaging studies may be considered. Imaging is probably indicated for patients with acute vertigo who are at high risk for cerebrovascular disease. Otherwise, if the hearing loss is not progressive, imaging studies are not indicated. Patients with progressive hearing loss and abnormal speech reception thresholds should be considered for MRI scanning of the internal auditory canals.

▶ This article comes from the *Archives of Neurology*, and it is interesting that these authors describe what seems logical and prudent—namely that it is not always necessary to get an MRI for every patient who has dizziness. They indicate, appropriately, that the odds of finding a mass in the CPA are extremely low, even in the presence of asymmetrical hearing loss. They describe an appropriate workup; however, a test of auditory brain stem response is part of our workup to help screen for or rule out a mass in the CPA, if the patient has sufficient vertigo, especially with asymmetry. Certainly, MRI is indicated in selected patients but not in every patient who has dizziness and, as these authors indicate, not in every patient who has a hearing loss. If, however, progression of hearing loss continues and is documented, then an appropriate imaging study is indicated. Also, any adult who has progressive unilateral hearing loss and is considered to be at high risk of having a lesion in the CPA, such as a vestibular schwannoma, should be considered for an MRI.

**M.M. Paparella, M.D.**

---

## The Possible Effect of Pregnancy on Ménière's Disease

Uchide K, Suzuki N, Takiguchi T, et al (Kanazawa Univ, Japan)
*ORL J Otorhinolaryngol Relat Spec* 59:292–295, 1997          1–10

---

*Purpose.*—Various otolaryngologic problems are believed to get worse during pregnancy. However, little is known about the possible effects of pregnancy on Ménière's disease. A case report of Ménière's disease during pregnancy is reported.

> *Case.*—Ménière's disease was diagnosed in a 28-year-old woman. With regular treatment with mecobalamine, difenidol hydrochloride, betahistine mesilate, and isosorbide, the number of vertigo attacks decreased. After the patient became pregnant, she started having vertigo attacks again, along with general malaise. Liver dysfunction was diagnosed on the basis of elevated transaminase levels. The patient underwent therapeutic abortion, and the vertigo attacks stopped. Several months later, when the patient became pregnant again, she developed frequent vertigo attacks with severe appetite loss and emesis, requiring hospitalization. The patient was treated with reduction in dietary salt intake, 5 g/day; oral isosorbide, 90 mL/day; and IV fluid therapy. The frequency of vertigo attacks decreased with isosorbide and occasional IM injections of diazepam. During hospitalization, results of all laboratory tests were normal, except for hyponatremia and serum osmolality as low as 268 mOsm/kg.
>
> After hospital discharge, the pregnancy proceeded uneventfully, although the patient continued to have 1 to 3 vertigo attacks per month. A healthy baby was delivered by cesarean section at 38 weeks. The patient had frequent vertigo attacks in the months after delivery. Fluctuating hearing loss was present, and electrocorticography showed negative dominant SP ($-$SP/AP $=$ 41%). After sur-

gery for endolymphatic shunt, the number of vertigo attacks gradually decreased to 0. The average number of vertigo attacks was 0.8/month when the patient was pregnant vs. 3.0 when she was not, with a peak of 10 attacks during the third month.

*Discussion.*—This case shows an increased rate of vertigo attacks during pregnancy in a patient with Ménière's disease, particularly during early pregnancy. The attacks seem to be related to declining serum osmolality. As pregnancy proceeds and serum osmolality normalizes, attacks become less frequent. Conservative management is indicated; most patients will respond to reduced salt intake and diuretic treatment.

▶ It is well known that pregnancy has an effect on patients with otosclerosis. It is not so well known that pregnancy can sometimes influence patients with Ménière's disease. We have seen this in a small subset of patients, but not as commonly as we would see otosclerosis exacerbated during pregnancy. I believe these authors are correct in that it is most likely a fluid imbalance relating to hormonal changes that might in fact help trigger an existing condition of Ménière's disease. Attention to diuretics plus an attempt to balance hormonal changes would be helpful in managing these patients from a general point of view.

**M.M. Paparella, M.D.**

---

## The Effect of Surgical Removal of the Extraosseous Portion of the Endolymphatic Sac in Patients Suffering From Ménière's Disease

Gibson WPR (Univ of Sydney, Australia)
*J Laryngol Otol* 110:1008–1011, 1996                    1–11

---

*Purpose.*—There is ongoing debate about the performance of endolymphatic sac (ELS) surgery in patients with Ménière's disease. The ELS is a complex structure that appears to function in longitudinal absorption of endolymph, removal of debris and viral particles, secretion of immunoproteins, and secretion of glycoproteins. There are several possible mechanisms by which the ELS may act to cause vertiginous attacks of Ménière's disease. At surgery, it is difficult to define the extraosseous portion of the ELS. The effects of removing the extraosseous portion of the ELS in patients with Ménière's disease were analyzed.

*Methods.*—Forty-three patients who underwent surgical removal of the ELS and were followed up for at least 2 years were studied. All had unilateral Ménière's disease with hearing loss of at least 30 dBHL. The extraosseous part of the ELS was removed without any drainage procedure. In the latter part of the experience, the duct of the ELS was avulsed.

*Results.*—None of the patients showed any increase in the frequency or severity of vertigo attacks. During follow-up, just 19% of patients had more than 2 recurrent attacks of vertigo lasting more than 2 minutes. For 3 of the 8 patients in this group, the frequency of vertigo attacks was substantially reduced. Fifty-six percent of ears showed hearing deterioration of at least 10 dBHL across 5 audiometric frequencies. When vertigo ceased, so did tinnitus. There was no increase in the sensation of fullness in the operated ear.

*Conclusions.*—Surgical removal of the ELS in patients with Ménière's disease seems to provide better relief of vertigo than a simple drainage procedure. The mechanism of this effect may be reduction in glycoprotein secretion, reducing the movement of endolymph toward the ELS. With ELS removal, the vertigo is less likely to recur during follow-up. The results show no apparent difference between removal of the extraosseous portion of the ELS and ELS drainage procedures.

▶ Dr. Gibson is a lovable academic iconoclast. He describes how removing the extraosseous portion of the ELS helps his patients with Ménière's disease. I am convinced that his patients are benefited, that is those who have vertigo. As he indicates, however, the long-term effects in hearing are probably going to be less than desirable. We know, from animal studies, that complete and careful destruction of the osseous and extraosseous portion of the sac leads to hydrops; therefore, it is hard to imagine that complete destruction would benefit patients.

What is, I believe, happening in these patients is that he is not removing or destroying the total sac. To do so, one would have to remove the medial wall of the sac, which requires putting a large hole in the dura. No one would want to do this because a profuse flow of spinal fluid would occur. Thus, I do not believe the total sac is being destroyed, but rather the procedure is providing some enhancement of function in these patients. Of course, if one were specifically to attempt enhancement, I think this would be to the patient's long-term benefit. Nevertheless, it is of interest to hear these theories, which have interest and some validity, and I do think that we would agree that a more physiologic approach to treating Ménière's disease is suitable in the first place, before we consider destroying the ear and/or its attachments to the brain.

**M.M. Paparella, M.D.**

---

**Outcome-based Assessment of Endolymphatic Sac Surgery for Ménière's Disease**
Smith DR, Pyle GM (Univ of Wisconsin, Madison)
*Laryngoscope* 107:1210–1216, 1997                    1–12

---

*Introduction.* The question of whether endolymphatic sac decompression (ELSD) is an effective intervention for patients with Ménière's disease remains controversial. In the first published report using outcome-based assessment, investigators evaluated quality of life in 33 patients who underwent ELSD for disabling and medically intractable vertigo.

*Methods.*—The patients were treated between 1990 and 1996. All had failed to respond to diet, diuretics, vestibular suppressants, vasodilators, or calcium channel blockers and selected ELSD over other surgical options. Results were reported using the American Academy of Otolaryngology—Head and Neck Surgery (AAO–HNS) 1995 guidelines. Functional and quality of life issues were assessed with the medical outcomes survey's 36–item, short-form health survey (SF-36).

*Results.*—Postoperative data were available for 29 of 33 patients. Twenty-two had positive outcomes (class A, B, or C of the AAO–HNS reporting guidelines) with improvement of vertigo. Outcome in the remaining 7 patients was judged as class D in 1 patient, class E in 1, and class F in 5, all negative outcomes. Thus, 76% of patients had positive outcomes. Those with class A or B outcomes did not differ significantly from population norms on the SF-36. Patients in classes C to E, however, scored significantly below norms. The SF-36 scores correlated well with the AAO–HNS classification.

*Discussion.*—Many otolaryngologists employ ELSD because the procedure is nondestructive and associated with relatively low morbidity. Previous studies, however, have not determined conclusively that ELSD is effective for disabling Ménière's disease. This first published study using an outcomes approach to analyze ELSD, and the first to report data using the 1995 AAO–HNS guidelines, found a 76% improvement of vertigo in the most difficult population of patients with Ménière's disease. The SF-36 was a good measure of functional impairment and quality of life and correlated well with AAO–HNS guidelines.

▶ As we live under the present aegis of "managed care," there are many who encourage studies of outcome. These studies are, of course, at best difficult to do and have many variables. Nevertheless, these authors attempt such an outcome-based assessment of endolymphatic sac surgery for Ménière's disease. Their observations, although somewhat preliminary, are of interest and do describe that the procedure is efficacious in general for these patients. Other studies of outcome, I am certain, will evolve, and they too will need to be controlled in order to provide meaningful interpretive conclusions.

**M.M. Paparella, M.D.**

# 2 Hearing and Tests of Hearing

**Inherited Nonsyndromic Hearing Loss: An Audiovestibular Study in a Large Family With Autosomal Dominant Progressive Hearing Loss Related to DFNA2**
Marres H, van Ewijk M, Huygen P, et al (Univ Hosp Nijmegen, The Netherlands; Univ of Antwerp, Belgium)
*Arch Otolaryngol Head Neck Surg* 123:573–577, 1997                     2–1

*Introduction.*—Eight autosomal dominant nonsyndromic forms of sensorineural hearing loss (SNHL) have been distinguished clinically, and 11 genes responsible for autosomal dominant hearing loss have been localized. In a large, 6-generation Dutch family, investigators examined nonsyndromic progressive SNHL with significant linkage to the *DFNA2* locus on chromosome 1p.

*Methods.*—The family had 194 living members, 109 of whom were examined for the study. Audiograms were obtained to evaluate hearing loss and progression in 43 individuals, and 37 underwent vestibulo-ocular examination. Participants provided venous blood samples for gene-linkage studies.

*Results.*—Hearing impairment was found in 59 of the 109 participating family members, but 16 cases of hearing loss may not have been the result of genetic defect. The remaining 43 individuals showed strong evidence of having a hereditary form of hearing impairment. Most of the audiograms were classified as the sharply sloping, high-frequency sensorineural type. There was significant and equal linear progression in SNHL with age, close to 1 dB per year, at all frequencies. Vestibulo-ocular examinations revealed vestibular hyperreactivity in 13 (35%) patients; only 3 had significant unilateral caloric hyporeflexia. Significant linkage to the 1p locus appeared in 41 affected family members.

*Conclusion.*—Members of this Dutch family exhibited a hearing loss that can be defined as a progressive high-frequency SNHL. Audiologic data demonstrated a progression of 1 dB per octave per year. Gene linkage analysis showed a positive linkage to the *DFNA2* locus, which is expected to play an important role in gene identification in inherited, nonsyndromal

21

autosomal dominant hearing loss. In addition to the family studied here, 3 other families have been reported to show linkage to chromosome 1p.

▶ Indeed, in my practice, I see many patients whom I diagnose as having hearing loss caused by genetic factors, which can be present at birth or can be delayed. Most of the hearing losses I see in fact are *not* associated with an identifiable syndrome. Thus, it is helpful to have these articles appear in our refereed journals so that we can better diagnose specific diseases that cause these hearing losses. Some of these genetically induced losses may have progression, as is discussed in this article. A clear-cut pathologic correlate, which has been found in patients who have delayed-onset genetically induced hearing losses, is atrophy of the stria vascularis. In these patients, however, one sees a flat audiometric configuration, usually with good measurable scores in discrimination of speech.

**M.M. Paparella, M.D.**

---

**Nonsyndromic Hearing Impairment: Unparalleled Heterogeneity**
van Camp G, Willems PJ, Smith RJH (Univ of Antwerp, Belgium; Univ of Iowa, Iowa City)
*Am J Hum Genet* 60:758–764, 1997                                    2–2

---

*Introduction.*—Until recently, there were only 3 identified loci for nonsyndromic hearing impairment (NSHI). In the last 3 years, however, many genes for recessive and dominant hearing impairment—both prelingual and postlingual—have been localized and mapped. Current knowledge of the genetic bases of NSHI is reviewed.

*Autosomal and X-linked Loci.*—There are currently 13 known autosomal recessive and 13 known autosomal dominant gene localizations for NSHI. The prefix DFNA is used for dominant loci, and DFNB is used for recessive loci. Most families with recessive loci had profound, prelingual hearing impairment, whereas those with dominant NSHI had postlingual impairment. More than 1 linked family has been reported for 7 recessive and 2 dominant loci. Several NSHI loci have been mapped to overlapping chromosomal regions, including 3 genes in the dominant group that map to 11q. The finding that recessive and dominant loci sometimes both map to the same chromosomal region suggests that different phenotypes may result from different mutations in the same gene.

Several X-linked NSHI loci, which have the prefix DFN, have been reported. Five have been fully reported: 3 cause a stable, prelingual hearing loss and 2 cause a progressive, postlingual hearing loss. Further research has suggested that hearing loss associated with DFN1 is actually syndromic and does not belong in the category of NSHI.

*Genes and Mutations.*—Only 2 nuclear genes for NSHI have been cloned. These are POU3F4, mutations of which have been found in unrelated DFN3 patients, and myosin-VIIa, an unconventional myosin responsible for DNFB2. In addition to causing hearing impairment in syndromic deafness, mitochondrial DNA mutations can cause hearing impairment as a sole feature. Penetrance resulting from these mutations is very low, which suggests involvement of unknown genetic or environmental factors.

*Discussion.*—With the recent surge in research, 30 chromosomal loci for NSHI have been mapped. Although only 2 nuclear genes have been identified, several additional NSHI genes are expected to be cloned during the next few years. This information will open new pathways to understanding the molecular mechanisms of auditory function. The Hereditary Hearing Loss Homepage (http://dnalab-www.uia.ac.be/dnalab/hhh) offers continuously updated genetic information on NSHI.

▶ Those patients who have hearing impairments, sensorineural hearing losses, or, for that matter, conductive hearing losses do not have a particular syndrome. Thus, this article is relevant in assessing NSHI and questions of heterogeneity. This article was abstracted from the *American Journal of Human Genetics* and will be of interest to otolaryngologists as we start to, again, sort our way through the many genetic aspects of hearing loss in our patients.

**M.M. Paparella, M.D.**

## Genetic and Clinical Features of Sensorineural Hearing Loss Associated With the 1555 Mitochondrial Mutation

Usami S-I, Abe S, Kasai M, et al (Hirosaki Univ, Japan; Boys Town Natl Research Hosp, Omaha, Neb)
*Laryngoscope* 107:483–490, 1997                                                    2–3

*Background.*—Studies of familial aggregation of aminoglycoside-induced hearing loss suggest that some families have a constitutional susceptibility for cochlear damage from aminoglycoside antibiotics. The genetic and clinical features of sensorineural hearing loss associated with the 1555 mitochondrial mutation were investigated.

*Methods and Findings.*—Thirty-two members of 5 Japanese families with aminoglycoside-induced hearing loss were studied clinically and genetically. Twenty-eight research subjects with and without bilateral sensorineural hearing loss had a mitochondrial mutation at nucleotide 1555. In 100 American control research subjects, no evidence of mutation of this nucleotide was found, which suggested that the 1555 A→G (A1555G) mitochondrial mutation may be more common among Asian populations (Figs 4 and 5).

*Conclusions.*—These data confirm the A1555G mitochondrial mutation involvement in susceptibility to aminoglycoside antibiotics. Individuals with this mutation have a mild, high-frequency, progressive hearing loss even without aminoglycoside injection, which suggests that the A1555G mutation may play a more general role in the pathogenesis of hearing loss. This mutation seems to be limited to Asian populations.

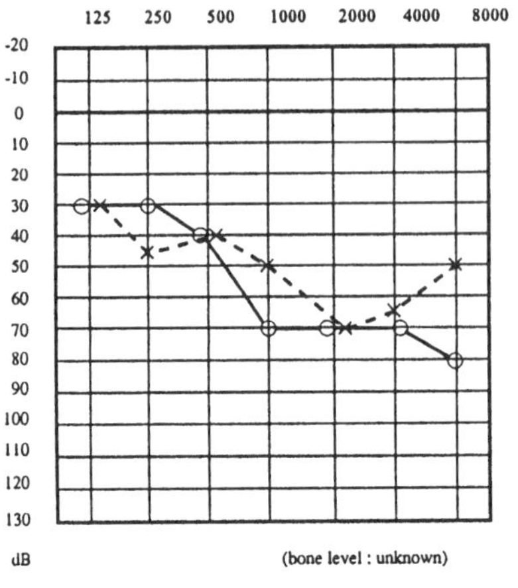

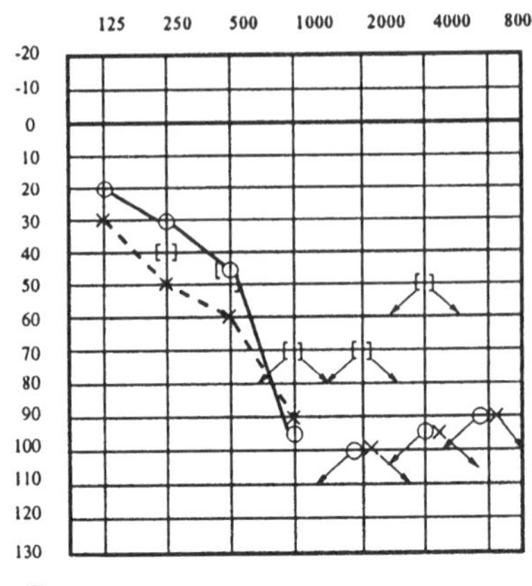

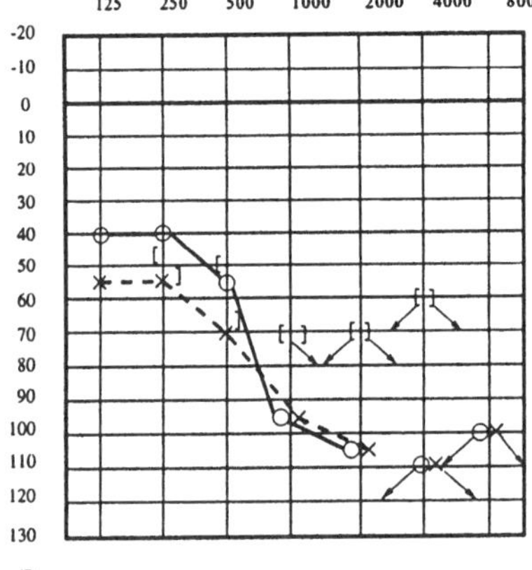

FIGURE 4.—A collection of audiograms at ages 5, 13, and 33 years showing progressive hearing loss in 1 individual with A1555G mutation and aminoglycoside injection history. (Courtesy of Usami S-I, Abe S, Kasai M, et al: Genetic and clinical features of sensorineural hearing loss associated with the 1555 mitochondrial mutation. *Laryngoscope* 107:483–490, 1997. Copyright Triological Society.)

▶ Five Japanese families showing aminoglycoside-induced hearing loss were genetically as well as clinically investigated. This mitochondrial mutation, the authors indicate, may be found more frequently in Asians and not in Americans. Many exhibited a high-frequency progressive hearing loss, with or without aminoglycoside injection. It was hypothesized that this A1555G mutation may play a more general role in causing hearing loss. There will be many specific gene mapping–encoding studies like this 1 that will result in the literature, which will contribute to our understanding of genetically induced hearing loss. We are becoming more and more aware of the fact that genetically induced hearing losses, or even multifactorial inheritance, play a role in many, if not most, of the otologic problems that we encounter.

**M.M. Paparella, M.D.**

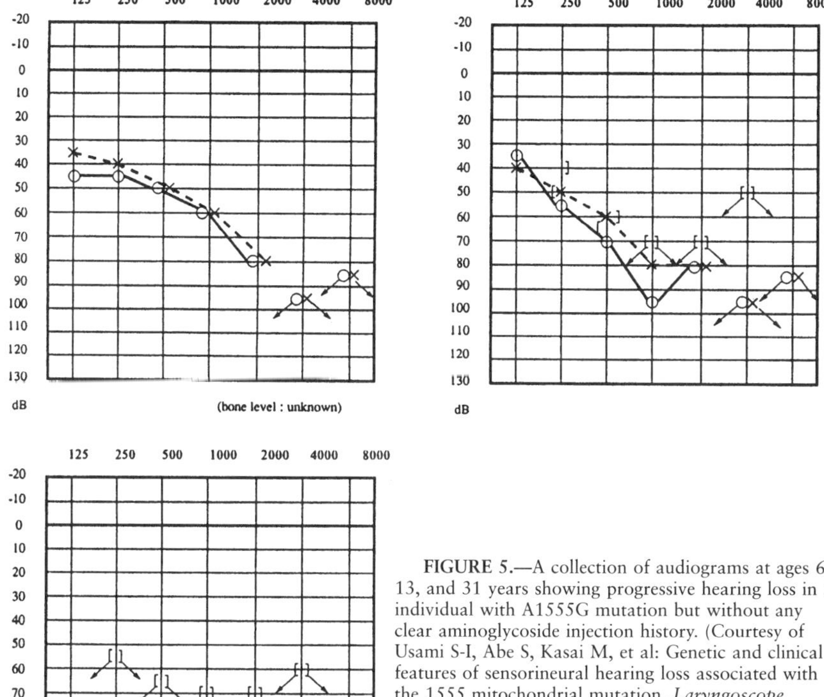

FIGURE 5.—A collection of audiograms at ages 6, 13, and 31 years showing progressive hearing loss in 1 individual with A1555G mutation but without any clear aminoglycoside injection history. (Courtesy of Usami S-I, Abe S, Kasai M, et al: Genetic and clinical features of sensorineural hearing loss associated with the 1555 mitochondrial mutation. *Laryngoscope* 107:483–490, 1997. Copyright Triological Society.)

## Ribonucleases May Limit Recovery of Ribonucleic Acids From Archival Human Temporal Bones

Lee KH, McKenna MJ, Sewell WF, et al (Harvard Med School, Boston)
*Laryngoscope* 107:1228–1234, 1997                                    2–4

*Objective.*—The authors use the reverse transcription polymerase chain reaction (RT-PCR) to detect specific RNA sequences in archival specimens of human temporal bone. Only about 10% of specimens showed detectable actin messenger ribonucleic acid (mRNA). This low detection rate could arise partly because of enzymatic degradation of mRNA by exogenously introduced ribonucleases (RNases). Potential sources of RNase contamination in the process of temporal bone processing were analyzed. The effects of minimizing RNase contamination on the retrieval of intact RNA were determined as well.

*Findings.*—First, the steps of the temporal bone processing protocol were analyzed to discover where RNases could be introduced into the specimens. Active RNases were identified in the 80% ethanol solutions used to store temporal bones, with higher levels of RNases found in older storage jars. Further analysis demonstrated that the RNases were not present in the reagents to begin with; rather, they were introduced later, possibly during processing or handling stages. The finding of RNase on electrophoresis was related to the ability to detect actin mRNA on RT-PCR.

Next, the investigators looked at modified processing specimens to prevent RNase contamination. In the modified protocol, gloves were worn at all stages of processing and analysis, RNase-free reagents were used, and all equipment and containers were cleaned with RNase Erase. This protocol improved recovery of intact RNA from bone specimens. Storage conditions appeared to have a critical influence on RNA integrity.

*Conclusions.*—Enzymatic RNA degradation can affect mRNA analysis of archival human temporal bone specimens. However, relatively simple steps to prevent RNase contamination may improve RNA recovery. Modified, RNase-free protocols should be followed in the preparation of temporal bones intended for RNA analysis.

▶ The potential for analyzing gene expression in archival human temporal bones remains a great promise for the future. These authors identify a small speed-bump in the road: that m-RNA is affected in celloidin-embedded archival human temporal bones. They identify a possible reason as enzymatic degradation of RNA by exogenously introduced RNases. A simple modification in the processing protocol can improve the data from such studies, as described by these authors: a useful contribution for those involved in temporal bone processing.

**M.M. Paparella, M.D.**

---

**Risk Factors Associated With Hearing Loss in Neonates**
Kountakis SE, Psifidis A, Chang CJ, et al (Univ of Texas, Houston; Aristotle Univ of Thessaloniki, Greece)
*Am J Otolaryngol* 18:90–93, 1997                                                    2–5

---

*Introduction.*—In order to identify newborns who should undergo screening for hearing loss, the Joint Committee on Infant Hearing (JCIH) compiled a list of risk factors associated with greatest risk for hearing impairment. Although the JCIH criteria seem comprehensive, there are reports that additional risk factors should be included in the list. The medical records of 100 infants were reviewed to determine those variables most strongly associated with hearing loss in neonates.

*Methods.*—Fifty consecutive infants had hearing impairment by auditory brainstem response (ABR) audiometry; the other 50 were randomly selected and had normal hearing. Complete records were available for 95 infants, 52 boys (26 with abnormal ABR findings) and 43 girls (20 with hearing impairment). The 18 variables evaluated for their association with hearing loss included those listed by the JCIH and others identified in the literature. Hearing loss was diagnosed if a repeatable response was not obtained at an intensity of 35 Db nHL.

*Results.*—Only 5 of the 18 variables were found to be significantly associated with infant hearing impairment: hyperbilirubinemia, craniofacial anomalies, length of stay in the ICU, respiratory distress syndrome, and retrolental fibroplasia. The last 3 of these 5 variables are not included in the JCIH list of risk factors. Respiratory distress syndrome was the most strongly statistically significant variable. Surprisingly, low birth weight and earlier gestational age at birth were more common in the infants with normal hearing than in the hearing-impaired infants.

*Discussion.*—Only 2 variables listed by the JCIH, craniofacial anomalies and hyperbilirubinemia, were found to be associated with hearing impairment in this infant population. Three additional variables had a statistically significant correlation with hearing loss: respiratory distress syndrome, retrolental fibroplasia, and ICU length of stay. Although a family history of hearing loss may be relevant, this factor could not be documented in most cases.

▶ This study is of interest because it specifically looks for risk-factors associated with hearing loss in a neonatal patient population compared to the factors listed by the Joint Committee on Infant Hearing. This study, out of 18 variables, found only 5 associated with hearing impairment, including hyperbilirubinemia, craniofacial anomalies, length of stay in the intensive care unit, respiratory distress syndrome, and retrolental fibroplasia, the last three of which are not listed in the register published by the Joint Committee on Infant Hearing. The population studied might, of course, reveal dissimilar results and might indicate that the variables are more numerous in that particular study. Nevertheless, this study is of interest in that it provides a comparative study in 50 consecutive infants with hearing impairment assessed by auditory brainstem response (ABR).

**M.M. Paparella, M.D.**

---

**Profound Permanent Hearing Impairment in Childhood: Causative Factors in Two European Countries**
Parving A, Stephens D (Bispebjerg Hosp, Copenhagen; Univ Hosp of Wales, Cardiff)
*Acta Otolaryngol (Stockh)* 117:158–160, 1997                                      2–6

---

*Introduction.*—Two 6-year birth cohorts from Denmark and Wales were examined for differences between countries in factors causing permanent childhood hearing impairment (PCHI). A lack of information about this rare disorder has limited the possibility of comparative studies both within and between countries.

*Methods.*—Included in the analysis were 2 identical birth cohorts from 1975 through 1980. At the time of collection of these data, members of the cohorts were living in 2 Danish health authority districts and 8 Welsh counties. Those eligible for evaluation had a permanent hearing loss of 90 or more dB in the better hearing ear, averaged across 0.5–4 kHz. The overall prevalence of children with PCHI was 0.45 per 1,000 live births in Denmark (34 children) and 0.41 per 1,000 live births in Wales (59 children). Differences in prevalence between the 2 countries were not significant. Both cohorts were investigated according to a protocol consisting of a thorough history; ophthalmologic, radiologic (CT), pediatric, and genetic evaluations; electrocardiography, and urinalysis.

*Results.*—In both countries, the most common cause of PCHI was genetic. Fourteen cases in Wales and 13 in Denmark were classified as nonsyndromal. Syndromal cases numbered 14 and 4, respectively. Overall, 7 cases were attributed to fetal rubella, 8 to perinatal complications, 7 to meningitis, and 1 to mumps encephalitis. The cause of PCHI was unknown in 20 cases from Wales and in 5 from Denmark.

*Discussion.*—Using identical birth cohorts and uniform criteria for PCHI, investigators found no significant differences between countries in the proportion of hearing impairment caused by various factors. Denmark had a somewhat higher proportion of children affected by fetal rubella infection and, among those with a genetic cause, a higher proportion of nonsyndromal inheritance (76%), compared with Wales (50%). Overall, however, the proportion of inherited loss was 47%–50% in both countries. The high proportion of both genetic and unknown factors indicates the need for further investigation of PCHI.

▶ It is very interesting to find these epidemiologic studies and to include 2 separate countries. This helps take into account racially genetic as well as individually genetic and environmental factors. Thus, this is a very interesting approach, and I would hope that other studies would take place that would reflect a similar protocol. Interestingly, this multidisciplinary effort showed no significant differences between the countries in the proportion of hearing impairment caused by these factors. Genetic hearing loss was found in approximately half of the subjects studied in the 2 countries. One assumes that these children in both countries would have had proper otologic diagnoses and tests applied, but this is not clearly stated in the article. The authors identify the ophthalmologic, pediatric, and genetic evaluations but do not specify that a careful otologic workup was carried out. Every hearing loss is caused by an otologic disease, whether it is congenital or acquired, genetic or nongenetic. It would be assumed that this was incorporated in the study, and if not, it certainly should have been.

**M.M. Paparella, M.D.**

**Investigation of the 4,000–Hertz Dip by Detailed Audiometry**
Murai K (Iwate Med Univ, Morioka, Japan)
*Ann Otol Rhinol Laryngol* 106:408–413, 1997                                  2–7

*Introduction.*—The 4,000 Hz dip, or c5 dip, is hearing loss localized at 4,000 Hz on an octave audiogram. This dip is most commonly observed in the first stages of noise-induced hearing loss and acoustic trauma. However, these causes are not always present, and sometimes the cause is unknown. Although the pure-tone audiogram gives the impression that the damage is localized at 4,000 Hz, there is reason to believe that it is merely centered at that location, and extends to surrounding frequencies. A detailed audiometric examination was performed to clarify the phenomenon of the 4,000 Hz dip.

*Methods.*—The analysis included 159 patients: 76 with noise-induced hearing loss, 62 with hearing loss of unknown cause, and 21 with familial hearing loss. All had a 4,000 Hz dip on their pure-tone audiogram. The detailed audiometic technique described by Tsuiki et al. was used to measure hearing thresholds of the 2 octaves from 2,000 to 8,000 Hz. This permits a more precise recording of hearing threshold than using the Bekesy audiometry conditioned method.

*Results.*—Eleven main types of 4,000 Hz dip were identified on the detailed audiograms, but the 3 most basic were the cone, bowl, and dish types, which depict the smooth line of the hearing threshold. The other types oadip showed a narrow, wedgelike area of deterioration in hearing threshold superimposed on some portions of the 3 basic types. Patients with various causes of hearing loss had similar configurations in the dips on their audiograms.

*Conclusions.*—A detailed audiometric study of 4,000 Hz dips identified the basic configurations of these dips as the cone, bowl, and dish types, the others consisting of "microdips" superimposed on the basic configurations. The configurations of these dips appear similar regardless of the cause of hearing loss. Future studies may offer insight into lesions of the inner ear that rise to these clinical audiologic findings.

▶ This article was selected and is of interest because, indeed, we see many patients without the characteristic audiometric configuration of a dip and a rise at 8,000 cps and a dip of course occurring at 4,000 Hz. This author is quite correct in that some patients will be seen with these findings who demonstrate no history of exposure to acoustic trauma or any other noises. Thus, there may be some patients (albeit in our experience they have been the minority) who have this audiometric configuration who may have genetic and other factors in terms of the underlying etiologic agencies or pathogenesis of the 4,000–cycle elevation of threshold.

**M.M. Paparella, M.D.**

## Noise-related Ailments of Performing Musicians: A Review

Behroozi KB, Luz J (Loewenstein Hosp, Raanana, Israel; Occupational Health and Rehabilitation Inst, Raanana, Israel)
*Med Probl Perform Art* 12:19–22, 1997                    2–8

*Objective.*—Intensity of sound is known to affect hearing; hearing loss among industrial workers exposed to high levels of noise is well documented, but less is known about the effects of noise on hearing in musicians. There is also little information on how noise affects the cardiovascular system and cardiovascular risk factors, and their interaction with stress factors. Noise-related disorders in musicians, both auditory and nonauditory, are reviewed.

*Exposure to Sound and Hearing Loss.*—Loud jazz or rock music has well-known adverse effects on hearing. Less well recognized is the fact that classical musicians are also prone to this type of hearing loss. Studies of orchestra conductors find that hearing loss or discomfort on exposure to intense levels of sound is common. Very high intensities of sound—even higher than industrial exposures—have been measured in an opera orchestra. Musicians spend a large percentage of their time exposed to levels of sound that are over the accepted safe limit of 85 dB. Personal dosimetry studies show that hearing loss is affected by proximity of the instrument to the ear: players of the violin, viola, and cello show greater loss in the left ear. Hearing loss was found in 15% of musicians in a German study and 58% of those in a Danish study. The results suggest that classical musicians have the potential for occupational hearing loss that can interfere with their profession.

*Occupational Noise and the Cardiovascular System.*—Research in industrial populations and in musicians shows that noise can affect cardiovascular risk factors such as blood pressure and heart rate. Relationships between hearing loss and cardiovascular disease have been documented as well, although it is unclear which precedes the other. The cardiovascular effects of noise may involve the "arousal" or "stress" responses, which are difficult to distinguish from emotional responses. In addition to heart rate and blood pressure, noise can affect other factors such as cholesterol level and changes in the ambulatory ECG. In addition to intensity of the noise, its type and source, also to be considered are the effects of age, sex, and previous hearing acuity.

*Discussion.*—In musicians as in industrial workers, exposure to high levels of noise has considerable auditory and nonauditory effects. Musicians should be made aware of and protected against the deleterious effects of habitual noise and stress. Preventive measures, such as steps to reduce the dose of mechanical vibration absorbed, may help to reduce the ill effects of noise. Further epidemiologic studies of hearing loss among musicians are warranted.

▶ These authors well document a real problem of professional musicians who perform with orchestras or bands frequently or continuously. I have had occasion to examine individual members of the Minnesota Orchestra. One orchestra member who played contrabassoon sat in front of the trumpet section for many years and, indeed, had severe acoustic trauma and ringing tinnitus that was very disabling. Music is lovely and to be appreciated, but if the level of intensity is too high and if the human ear is the recipient of such damaging thresholds, then, indeed, music becomes traumatic, as documented in this article. The position of an individual within a band or orchestra will also determine, to a significant extent, the amount of acoustic trauma received from colleagues playing other instruments with intensity elsewhere in the ensemble.

**M.M. Paparella, M.D.**

---

**Hearing Loss During Bacterial Meningitis**
Richardson MP, Reid A, Tarlow MJ, et al (Royal United Hosp, Bath; Birmingham Heartlands Hosp)
*Arch Dis Child* 76:134–138, 1997                                                         2–9

---

*Introduction.*—A prospective study done in several medical centers investigated the pathophysiology and natural history of hearing loss in children with acute bacterial meningitis. Although both permanent sensorineural hearing loss and transient impairments are thought to develop during the first few days of the illness, the site of the causal lesions has not been identified.

*Methods.*—Children were recruited from 21 hospitals between November 1993 and April 1995. Those eligible were between the ages of 4 weeks and 16 years. Investigators asked to be informed of all cases of bacterial meningitis within 1 hour of diagnosis. Recordings of transient evoked otoacoustic emissions (OAEs), minute sounds produced by the cochlea, were attempted as soon as possible after diagnosis, 3 times over the following 48 hours and at discharge from the hospital. Auditory brainstem responses were also recorded. Children with hearing loss at discharge were tested again at 1, 3, and 9 months after diagnosis.

*Results.*—The study group included 124 children with a median age of 2.1 years. All survived their illness. A total of 92 (74%) children received a diagnosis of meningococcal meningitis, and 18 (15%) had pneumococcal meningitis. Three (2.4%) children had permanent sensorineural hearing loss, and 13 (10.5%) experienced transient hearing loss. All cases of hearing loss were apparent at the initial assessment. Of 13 children with transient impairment, 9 had normal hearing assessments within 48 hours of diagnosis. The absence of OAEs in the 3 permanently impaired children indicates cochlear damage. Children with reversible hearing loss had absent OAEs and normal tympanograms, indicating cochlear dysfunction. There was a trend toward a higher incidence of deafness in children who had been ill for more than 24 hours before diagnosis.

*Conclusion.*—Findings in this study confirm that hearing loss develops early in the course of bacterial meningitis. Three children complained of deafness at admission, and most of those with hearing loss had been ill for 24–48 hours at the time of diagnosis. The inner ear is the site of the auditory lesions. Early diagnosis and prompt treatment may reduce the incidence of hearing loss.

▶ This is a remarkable study including 21 hospitals in England and South Wales. Researchers were able to identify 124 children between the ages of 4 weeks and 16 years with newly diagnosed bacterial meningitis. Of interest is that the majority of these children (74%) had meningococcal meningitis, whereas 15% had pneumococcal meningitis. It is a surprise that some of these children did not have *Haemophilus influenzae* meningitis because it continues to be a problem in the United States.

In this study, 13 children had reversible hearing loss, and this is not surprising. Just as when one has tympanogenic labyrinthitis, one can have meningogenic labyrinthitis, and this may be serious or toxic labyrinthitis, which can be followed by suppurative labyrinthitis. If indeed the child has serous or toxic labyrinthitis subsequent to meningococcal meningitis, and if the primary disease is treated properly and swiftly, there can be a return of function or reversible hearing loss as indicated in this article. If, however, there is a sustainable loss (and sometimes there can be, in fact, progression often related to hydrops, which can occur in subsequent years), this of course indicates that the bacteria have invaded the inner ear, causing permanent damage.

**M.M. Paparella, M.D.**

---

**Mumps Labyrinthitis, Endolymphatic Hydrops and Sudden Deafness in Succession in the Same Ear**
Hydén D (Linköping Univ, Sweden)
*ORL J Otorhinolaryngol Relat Spec* 58:338–342, 1996                   2–10

---

*Objective.*—Acute sensorineural hearing loss can occur in patients with mumps. This complication is usually reversible and in 1 ear only. Few reports have described secondary endolymphatic hydrops (Ménière's syndrome) associated with previous mumps infection. Such a case was reported.

> *Case.*—Woman, 39, was evaluated for recurrent audiovestibular symptoms. She had been seen 12 years earlier with unilateral hearing loss, vestibular symptoms, and caloric depression associated with mumps. All of these symptoms cleared up within a few months. The recurrent symptoms included vertigo with hearing deterioration, a feeling of fullness, and basal-tone loss in the same ear as before. A slight caloric depression was again noted. Despite treatment, she had continued symptoms of Ménière's syndrome for 2 years. Suddenly, hearing in the affected ear deteriorated in the course of a single day. This sensorineural hearing loss, like the

original mumps-associated episode, was localized to the middle- and high-tone area. There was no nystagmus or abnormal caloric reaction. Tests for brain lesions and epidemic parotitis virus were negative. At most recent follow-up, the patient was left with non-fluctuating hearing loss and slight tinnitus in the affected ear, with no balance problems.

*Conclusions.*—A patient with secondary Ménière's syndrome developing 12 years after mumps-related sensorineural hearing loss was described. In this case, hydrops most likely resulted from viral damage to the resorptive structures of the inner ear. Weakening of the neuronal structures of the ear seems to have become overt after repeated pathologic pressure changes.

▶ This case report is of interest because this patient had mumps and then, 12 years later, had Ménière's symptoms in the same ear. This has been termed "delayed hydrops" by some; but of course, all patients with Ménière's disease have so-called "delayed" hydrops. That means that it takes a long time for symptoms to evolve after the etiologic agent initiates the process. What is of interest to me in this study is that this patient has a variety of conditions present in 1 ear. Indeed, we do see this in patients, and indeed we see this in our collection of temporal bones also. There can be multiple diseases in a given temporal bone, sometimes 1, sometimes 2, sometimes 3, and sometimes 4. In fact, 1 of our patients had 5 separate otologic diseases occuring concurrently in the same temporal bone.

**M.M. Paparella, M.D.**

## Sudden Bilateral Sensorineural Hearing Loss

Fetterman BL, Luxford WM, Saunders JE (House Ear Clinic and Inst, Los Angeles; Saints Hearing and Balance Ctr, Oklahoma City, Okla)
*Laryngoscope* 106:1347–1350, 1996                                     2–11

*Introduction.*—Sudden bilateral sensorineural hearing loss (BSHL) is a frightening condition with many possible causes. As in unilateral sudden sensorineural hearing loss (USHL), the specific cause is usually unknown. Few studies have focused on sudden BSHL, which is less common than sudden USHL. Patients with sudden BSHL were retrospectively studied.

*Methods.*—The charts of 823 patients with sudden sensorineural hearing loss seen during a 5-year period were reviewed. This group included 14 patients with sudden BSHL, representing 1.7% of the total. The characteristics of patients with sudden USHL and BSHL were compared.

*Findings.*—The mean age was 64 years in the patients with BSHL vs. 52 years in those with USHL. The patients with BSHL were more likely to have associated cardiovascular disease and more likely to have a positive antinuclear antibody titer. Audiologic tests showed that BSHL was usually asymmetric. Patients with BSHL most often received a combination of steroid and vasodilator treatment, whereas those with USHL were more likely to receive only 1 of these treatments. Audiologic improvement occurred in 67% of patients with BSHL and 52% of those with USHL, a nonsignificant difference. When improvement occurred in BSHL, it occurred in both ears.

*Conclusions.*—About 2% of patients with sudden sensorineural hearing loss have BSHL. Some differences between patients with BSHL and USHL were elucidated, which will be useful in patient counseling. No cause can be identified in most patients with BSHL. However, other causes should be ruled out, including autoimmune inner ear disease, intracranial infection or tumor, and stroke.

▶ These authors studied a large number of patients who had sudden BSHL. The number of patients they were able to identify represents 1.7% of patients with sudden hearing loss, or 14 patients. I have seen patients with sudden deafness, a very disturbing entity for both the patient as well as for otologist, to say the least. Of course one needs to be careful how sudden deafness is defined. One can have a sudden (rapid) hearing loss bilaterally as a part of Ménière's disease; but here we are talking about patients who have a profound loss after perfectly normal hearing, and indeed one assumes the etiologic agent to be viral endolymphatic labyrinthitis. Nevertheless, active treatment with steroids, as these authors indicate, is clearly indicated. It is reassuring to note that 67% of the bilateral cases improved, a higher percentage than for the unilateral cases; this, I think, might be expected. Sudden sensorineural hearing loss is a tragedy when it occurs, especially when it leads to complete deafness and when it is bilateral. Fortunately, the vast majority of cases of sudden deafness are unilateral, as also indicated by this study.

**M.M. Paparella, M.D.**

## Sudden Sensorineural Hearing Loss Following Nonotologic, Noncardiopulmonary Bypass Surgery

Cox AJ III, Sargent EW (St Louis Univ, Mo)
*Arch Otolaryngol Head Neck Surg* 123:994–998, 1997                    2–12

*Introduction.*—Sudden sensorineural hearing loss (SSHL) is defined as a loss of more than 30 dB in 3 contiguous frequencies that occurs in less than 3 days. Most cases of SSHL are idiopathic, but a variety of causes have been identified, including neoplastic, infectious, inflammatory, and traumatic. In addition, a number of cases have been reported after cardiopulmonary bypass (CPB) surgery. The 3 cases of SSHL described here occurred after nonotologic surgery performed without CPB.

*Methods and Results.*—After they encountered these cases of SSHL, the authors used clinical records and MEDLINE and Health-star databases to identify similar reports in the world literature. The 3 patients who experienced SSHL after nonotologic and non-CPB surgery were a 50-year-old woman (revision of a nasal fracture), a 64-year-old woman (lumbar spine surgery), and a 72-year-old man (decompression of the lumbar spine for spinal stenosis). None appeared to have had previous otologic problems; all complained of hearing loss shortly after the surgical procedure. The loss was unilateral and profound in 2 patients and bilateral and moderate in 1. Despite diuretic and prednisone therapy, their hearing loss persisted after up to 2 years of follow-up.

*Discussion.*—Including these 3 patients, there have been 21 reported cases to date of SSHL after nonotologic, non-CPB surgery. General anesthesia was used in all cases but 1, a patient who had a urologic procedure performed under spinal anesthesia. Overall, approximately 30% of patients subsequently experienced significant improvement. In contrast, patients with sporadic SSHL are reported to have a 50% to 70% rate of improvement. Because of the scarcity of reported cases and a lack of detail in many of the cases, no conclusions can be made on the apparent connection between surgery and SSHL.

▶ I have observed sporadic cases as described by these authors in this article. They discuss 3 patients who developed sudden sensorineural deafness after nonotologic, noncardiopulmonary bypass surgery; they conclude that the possibility of this apparent association may be "spurious." One can argue that, indeed, such sporadic cases may not be spurious but might have some cause-and-effect relationship. One can conceptualize a cause and effect such as dispersed microemboli, other vascular phenomena, and indeed other phenomena that might relate either to the surgical procedure or the anesthesia that accompanies the surgery. The authors are correct in that this relationship is not established, but I do think there is a sufficient number of cases in the literature, prior to this article reported to date, which suggest a possible cause-and-effect relationship.

**M.M. Paparella, M.D.**

---

**Comparison of Carbogen Inhalation and Intravenous Heparin Infusion Therapies in Idiopathic Sudden Sensorineural Hearing Loss**
Rahko T, Kotti V (Tampere Univ, Finland)
*Acta Otolaryngol (Stockh)* Suppl 52:86–87, 1997                    2–13

---

*Introduction.*—Various methods have been used to treat patients with idiopathic sudden sensorineural hearing loss (ISSNHL). The reported recovery rate with anticoagulants is 69.6%, compared with 66% for spontaneous recovery. An alternative therapy consists of a carbon dioxide and oxygen mixture for inhalation. A review of 43 patients treated with heparin infusion and 44 with carbogen (5% carbon dioxide, 95% oxygen) inhalation compared the effectiveness of these 2 treatments.

*Methods.*—The unselected patients were all treated as inpatients. Those receiving heparin were seen before 1990, and the carbogen group was seen during a corresponding period thereafter. Patients were examined by means of conventional audiograms and speech audiometry in the acute stage, after 5 days of treatment, at 1 month, and at 6 months.

*Results.*—During the acute stage of the hearing loss, PTA was 62 Db in the heparin group and 55 in the carbogen group. After 5 days of treatment, PTA was 46 dB in the heparin group and 38 Db in the carbogen group; corresponding figures at 1 month were 34 and 32 Db, not a significant difference. Too few patients returned at 6 months for statistical analysis.

*Discussion.*—Neither heparin nor carbogen was found to be superior to the other in the treatment of ISSNHL, and recovery of hearing loss in this patient series did not markedly differ from previous reports of natural recovery. There is a risk of hemorrhagic complications, however, with heparin.

▶ There have been many methods described to treat sudden deafness, including the two described in this article: inhalation of carbogen and intravenous infusion of heparin. Neither of these methods proved superior in the treatment of sudden hearing loss, the major reason being that approximately half of sudden losses will spontaneously resolve. Sudden hearing loss usually results from endolymphatic viral labyrinthitis, or secondarily it can result from middle ear/inner ear interactive difficulties as well as other possible causes. Nevertheless, it is interesting to see this comparative study and its results.

**M.M. Paparella, M.D.**

---

**Sudden Deafness: A Comparison of Anticoagulant Therapy and Carbogen Inhalation Therapy**
Kallinen J, Laurikainen E, Laippala P, et al (Turku Univ, Finland; Univ of Tampere, Finland)
*Ann Otol Rhinol Laryngol* 106:22–26, 1997                      2–14

---

*Background.*—Sudden deafness (SD) is defined as a sudden or rapidly progressive, partial or complete, typically unilateral sensorineural hearing impairment with no known cause. The effects of anticoagulant treatment and carbogen inhalation therapy were compared in 1 group of patients with SD.

*Methods and Findings.*—One hundred sixty-eight consecutive patients with SD were studied. They were 91 males and 77 females, aged 12–78 years. Group 1 received anticoagulant therapy; group 2, anticoagulant therapy plus carbogen inhalation therapy; and group 3, only carbogen inhalation treatment. The configuration of the audiogram of SD was found to be a prognostic indicator. Anticoagulant treatment was most effective in low-sloping hearing losses, and carbogen inhalation appeared to be more effective for high-sloping hearing losses. Patients with low-frequency–sloping hearing impairment had a better prognosis than those with a high-sloping loss.

*Conclusions.*—The configuration of the audiogram of patients with SD has prognostic value. Anticoagulant treatment appears to be more effective for patients with low-sloping hearing loss, whereas carbogen inhalation appears more effective in high-sloping hearing losses.

▶ These authors, as we all do, continue to search for a medical therapy for SD. They compare anticoagulant therapy with carbogen-inhalation therapy and find that anticoagulant treatment was most effective for low-frequency losses. One wonders whether some of these low-frequency losses represent Ménière's disease and not what we would usually term SD. The term "sudden deafness" ought to be reserved for patients who have rather profound sudden hearing loss, usually caused by a virus, but it can result from vascular problems and other lesions as well.

**M.M. Paparella, M.D.**

## Otoneurologic and Audiologic Findings in Fibromyalgia

Rosenhall U, Johansson G, Örndahl G (Karolinska Inst, Stockholm; Sahlgren's Univ, Göteborg, Sweden; Östra Hosp, Göteborg, Sweden)
*Scand J Rehabil Med* 28:225–232, 1996                    2–15

*Background.*—Fibromyalgia, a syndrome of unknown cause and pathophysiology, is characterized by widespread, chronic muscular pain. Fatigue and symptoms of autonomic dysfunction are also common. Otoneurologic and audiologic results in patients with fibromyalgia were reported.

*Methods.*—One hundred sixty-eight patients underwent otoneurologic and audiologic testing. One hundred forty-one of these patients were women. Seventy-two percent reported vertigo and dizziness. Fifteen percent had sensorineural hearing loss. Findings on auditory brainstem response (ABR) and oculomotor assessment were compared with those in a control group. Differences in the absolute latency of wave V and in the I–V and III–V interpeak latencies were significant, indicating brainstem dysfunction in the patients. Thirty percent of the patients had abnormal ABR recordings. Patients and control research subjects also differed significantly in the mean velocity gain for smooth pursuits and in the mean saccadic latency on oculomotor assessment. Twenty-eight percent of the patients had abnormal saccades, and 58% had pathologic smooth pursuit eye movements. Electronystagmography was abnormal in 45% of the patients.

*Conclusions.*—Central nervous system dysfunction often occurs in patients with fibromyalgia. Proprioceptive disturbances may also explain some of the abnormalities documented in this study.

▶ In my practice, I am increasingly finding patients who have coexisting diagnoses of fibromyalgia. These authors find that vertigo or dizziness was reported in 72% of their patients, whereas sensorineural hearing loss was found in only 15%. This suggests that CNS dysfunction frequently occurs in patients with fibromyalgia. The electronystagmographic result was abnormal in 45% of cases. We need, once again, to ask whether labyrinthine symptoms in these patients are coincidental or in some way linked to fibromyalgia. I am not aware of any pathologic or causative linkage that could connect labyrinthine symptoms or disease with fibromyalgia. Certainly, CNS symptoms have been described as part of this disease, and further studies will need to be done before we can identify any otologic relationship.

**M.M. Paparella, M.D.**

**Progressive and Fluctuating Sensorineural Hearing Loss In Children With Asymptomatic Congenital Cytomegalovirus Infection**
Fowler KB, McCollister FP, Dahle AJ, et al (Univ of Alabama, Birmingham)
*J Pediatr* 130:624–630, 1997                                    2–16

*Introduction.*—In the United States, the leading cause of congenital infection is cytomegalovirus, with a rate of 40,000 new cases each year. There is limited information on children with symptomatic congenital cytomegalovirus. Serial audiologic examinations were performed in infected children with asymptomatic congenital cytomegalovirus to define the prevalence of hearing impairment and temporal changes in audiologic function.

*Methods.*—There were 307 children who had asymptomatic congenital cytomegalovirus infection and 76 uninfected siblings of children who had asymptomatic congenital cytomegalovirus infection. Audiologic evaluations were conducted for these children to determine their hearing status and were compared with those of 201 children whose neonatal screen for congenital cytomegalovirus infection showed negative results.

*Results.*—Only children with congenital cytomegalovirus infection had sensorineural hearing loss. There were 22 children with asymptomatic congenital cytomegalovirus infection who had sensorineural hearing loss. In 50% of children with hearing loss, further deterioration of hearing occurred, with the median age at first progression being at 18 months. In 18.2% of the children, delayed-onset sensorineural hearing loss was seen, and the median age of detection was 27 months. In 22.7% of children with hearing loss, fluctuating sensorineural hearing loss was documented.

*Conclusion.*—A leading cause of sensorineural hearing loss in young children is asymptomatic congenital cytomegalovirus infection. The need for continued monitoring of hearing status is emphasized by the continued deterioration of hearing and delayed onset of sensorineural hearing loss in these children. These children should be identified in the newborn period when infection can be documented.

▶ These authors have a large series with very interesting results. Congenital hearing loss, they conclude, occurred only in children with congenital cytomegalovirus (CMV) infection. Of the children with asymptomatic CMV infections, 22 (7.2%) had sensorineural hearing loss. Of those children with hearing loss, further deterioration of hearing occurred in half of them. Thus the importance of delayed-onset sensorineural hearing loss in asymptomatic congenital CMV infections is stressed in considering the deterioration of hearing and delayed onset of sensorineural hearing loss in children.

**M.M. Paparella, M.D.**

### Hearing Loss in the Sjögren Syndrome

Tumiati B, Casoli P, Parmeggiani A (Ospedale Santa Maria Nuova, Reggio Emilia, Italy)
*Ann Intern Med* 126:450–453, 1997                                    2–17

*Background.*—Autoimmune diseases can involve hearing impairment. However, the association between hearing loss and Sjögren's syndrome has not been studied thoroughly.

*Methods.*—Thirty women with Sjögren's syndrome were included in the cross-sectional study, which was conducted in a secondary referral center in Italy. The results of their assessment for audiovestibular disorder were compared with those of 40 age-matched healthy women.

*Findings.*—Forty-six percent of the patients with Sjögren's syndrome were found to have sensorineural hearing loss compared with only 2.5% of the healthy group. Sixty-four percent of the patients with sensorineural hearing loss had anticardiolipin antibodies compared with 18% of the control research subjects.

*Conclusions.*—The prevalence of hearing loss in patients with Sjögren's syndrome is high. Audiometric studies should be done before excluding cranial nerve involvement in this disease. Further research is needed to investigate the correlation of sensorinueral hearing loss with anticardiolipin antibodies.

▶ The incidence of hearing loss in Sjögren's syndrome, as this study indicates, is approximately 46% and involved 14 patients in this study. These patients all had sensorineural hearing loss. Of course, the question, as always, would be "Is the sensorineural hearing loss connected to or a result of Sjögren's syndrome? Or is it coincidental and unrelated?" Certainly, there may be a relationship or, in some patients, there may not be. Thus, we are not certain that the 46% really represents a causative rather than a coincidontal relationship. Nevertheless, this high prevalence (and I agree with these authors) does suggest that we should consider the patients' hearing if they have Sjögren's syndrome, then proper diagnosis and therapy can be instituted.

**M.M. Paparella, M.D.**

## Asymmetric Hearing Loss: Toward Cost-effective Diagnosis

Raber E, Dort JC, Sevick R, et al (Univ of Calgary, Alta, Canada)
*J Otolaryngol* 26:88–91, 1997

2–18

*Background.*—Clinicians often consider the possibility of retrocochlear disease in patients with unilateral audiovestibular symptoms, which prompts a lengthy, costly assessment process. The diagnostic yield of the various tests done to establish the diagnosis of retrocochlear disease was studied.

*Methods.*—Three hundred ten patients with unilateral audiovestibular symptoms had complete auditory assessments, and 144 had auditory-evoked potential testing (ABR). A total of 258 contrast-enhanced CT (CECT) scans and 86 gadolinium-enhanced MRI (Gd-MRI) scans were obtained.

*Findings.*—Twelve tumors were diagnosed (3.9%). The initial assessment selected by the referring physicians was CECT in 59% of the patients, ABR in 34%, and Gd-MRI in 7%. All patients with tumors eventually underwent Gd-MRI to confirm the diagnosis and for further evaluation. Compared with Gd-MRI, the sensitivity of ABR was 75%, and the specificity was 57%. The sensitivity of CECT was 80%, and the specificity was 24%. Positive predictive values were 26% for ABR and 15% for CECT. The diagnostic yield was not improved by combining ABR and CECT. The percentages of budgets spent on the different diagnostic tests were calculated.

*Conclusions.*—These findings have prompted a change in the authors' diagnostic approach to patients with unilateral audiovestibular symptoms. Patients now undergo MRI or are screened initially with ABR based on clinical suspicion. The assessment of patients with asymmetric sensory neural hearing loss no longer includes CECT.

▶ In this day of managed care and cost curtailment in the United States, it is very timely to see articles in which cost considerations and how they fit into our process of diagnosis become part of the literature. These authors describe, appropriately, that MRI is the diagnostic tool of choice in patients with asymmetric hearing loss. Perhaps it is a semantic misconception, but they are not creating a diagnosis, because the purpose of MRI is to rule out an intracranial tumor rather than to make a specific otologic diagnosis. The diagnosis, as always, will rest on the history and appropriate tests. Certainly, they are correct in stating that MRI is most useful for this reason, but it does not create a diagnosis of hearing loss. Also they find, as we do, that ABR is still useful as a screening device; it is far less costly than MRI and, I think, should be used more often in a physician's office because, in most cases, MRI and its comparatively excessive cost can be obviated.

**M.M. Paparella, M.D.**

**Comparing Implants With Hearing Aids in Profoundly Deaf Children**
Geers AE (Central Inst for the Deaf, St Louis)
*Otolaryngol Head Neck Surg* 117:150–154, 1997                    2–19

*Background.*—Whether cochlear implants are adequately effective in comparison with powerful hearing aids was determined to warrant their expense and invasiveness in certain groups of users.

*Methods.*—Research subjects between the ages of 5½ and 13½ years, enrolled in the Central Institute for the Deaf (CID) oral education program, were divided into 3 groups: (1) CI—those who had Nucleus multichannel implants for 3 years, (2) HA—those who used hearing aids and had a group mean pure-tone average (PTA) threshold of 110 dB, and (3) HA+—those who used hearing aids but who had slightly better PTA thresholds of 90–100 dB but without open-set speech recognition. These students were tested in 3 areas: (1) auditory speech perception and visual enhancement, (2) speech production, and (3) spoken language acquisition.

*Results.*—In the category of auditory speech perception skill, the CI and HA+ groups scored nearly the same. The HA group scored significantly lower. Thus, after 3 years of training, the implant group (with losses in excess of 100) had an advantage over the hearing aid group. After 5 years, the CI group still had an advantage over the HA+ group but not by a significant amount. After 3 years, the lip-reading enhancement results were as follows: HA+ (22%) was better than CI (15%), which was better than HA (4%). After 5 years, the CI group became more adept than the HA+ group; CI scores were 30% and HAT scores were 18%. For the speech production test, after 3 years, the HA+ group scored 75% for recognition and 52% for spontaneous phoneme production. Using the same test after 5 years, the CI and HA+ groups scored the same—80%. For the spoken language skill test, after 3 years, all 3 groups demonstrated the same ability. After 5 years, the CI and HA+ groups were equal, but the CI group seemed to have a better vocabulary.

*Conclusion.*—The cochlear implant may have given a marked advantage in language development to children with PTA thresholds greater than 100 dB. However, those children in the 90–100-dB range may have made nearly as much progress using powerful hearing aids.

▶ This study is of interest and is important because it attempts to compare the use of hearing aids for profoundly deaf or deaf children with the use of cochlear implants. Once again, the pathologic condition will dictate the success of an implant as well as the success of a hearing aid. Interestingly, according to this study, if a child had a hearing loss greater than 100 dB, then receiving an implant resulted in better performance than if the child had received a hearing aid. Children with hearing losses in the 90–100-dB range, however, were able to function with hearing aids on a basis comparable with or equal to those receiving cochlear implantation. Such studies are useful and will encourage us 1 day to understand the role of cochlear implantation in very young children. Certainly, the general policy of most otologists is to use a hearing aid whenever possible and to reserve a cochlear implant only for those children who are absolutely deaf and in whom a hearing aid would not adequately serve the patient.

**M.M. Paparella, M.D.**

**Prior Treatments in a Group of Tinnitus Sufferers Seeking Treatment**
Andersson G (Uppsala Univ, Sweden)
*Psychother Psychosom* 66:107–110, 1997
2–20

*Background.*—Tinnitus is the perception of sound in the absence of external stimulus. It is common, not well understood, and difficult to treat. Although several treatment methods have been attempted, there is little empirical support for their effectiveness. In a descriptive study, the treatment history of patients seeking relief for tinnitus was related to their level of distress.

*Study Design.*—The study group consisted of 69 consecutive patients seen in an audiology clinic with a complaint of tinnitus, 37 men and 32 women, average age 55.3 years. The majority reported hearing impairment. Tinnitus was localized in the right ear in 18%, the left ear in 25%, and in both ears in 57%. Participants completed a questionnaire on background and prior treatment. The results were used to group the patients: group 1, 24 with no prior treatment; group 2, 19 who had received acupuncture; group 3, 13 who had received relaxation therapy from a physiotherapist; and group 4, 13 who received other treatments. There were significantly more women patients in groups 3 and 4. Tinnitus was assessed by the Tinnitus Effect Questionnaire (TEQ), which has 6 subscales: helplessness, capacity for relaxation, acceptability of change, emotional effects, hearing, and ability to ignore.

*Findings.*—Univariate and Tukey's post hoc analysis found only minor differences among these 4 sub groups of patients. The untreated group showed more acceptance of change.

*Conclusions.*—It may be helpful for clinicians to know that many patients with tinnitus have attempted other treatments unsuccessfully before going to an audiologic clinic. Controlled studies are needed to address the distress caused by tinnitus and to avoid the frustration caused by use of nonspecific and ineffective treatments in management of this condition.

▶ This attempt at a controlled study does look at the problem of treatment relative to tinnitus and tinnitus sufferers. Indeed, there are no treatments that I am aware of which are curative, and, therefore, all treatments could be termed palliative, as this study demonstrates. The results indicated minor differences between the groups studied; the untreated group showed more acceptability for change. I believe an explanation of the problem to the patient, that is, what is the problem causing the tinnitus and the pros and cons of management, is helpful. As we tell patients who have tinnitus from disorders of the inner ear, there are no cures, but there are lots of opportunities for help and hope.

**M.M. Paparella, M.D.**

# 3 Interaction of the Middle Ear and Inner Ear

**Perilymphatic Fistula: A Washington, D.C., Experience**
Fitzgerald DC, Getson P, Brasseux CO (Georgetown Univ, Washington, DC)
*Ann Otol Rhinol Laryngol* 106:830–837, 1997                    3–1

*Background.*—The treatment for perilymphatic fistula (PLF) is fairly well established—initial bed rest, followed by surgical repair of the oval window and round window if symptoms persist. However, there are still no accepted guidelines for diagnosis of PLF. A 9-year experience with PLF is reported.

*Patients.*—The review included 197 patients who underwent unilateral PLF repair between 1982 and 1991. The age range was 4 to 75 years; the median duration of symptoms was 3.1 years. Thirty-eight percent of patients had a history of direct trauma to the head or ear, 14% had barotrauma, 13% had an episode of increased intracranial pressure, and 36% had no specific event or incident. The most frequent chief symptom was a combination of vertigo and balance disturbance. Diagnostic tests include air-bone and speech audiometry, with tympanometry if possible. Most patients had standard electronystagmography (ENG), and some had an ENG fistula test. Electrocochleography and platform fistula testing became standard preoperative tests once they became available.

*Outcomes.*—At surgery, just 28% of patients were found to have definite fluid leaks. Of patients whose chief symptom was vertigo or a balance disturbance, 87% had relief of their symptoms after surgery. Forty percent of patients with sudden hearing loss had improved hearing after surgery. The results were similar for patients with various causes, except for those with increased intracranial pressure, who had a lower rate of positive results. Complications included a 2% rate of mild conductive hearing loss and a 3% rate of mild sensorineural hearing loss.

*Conclusions.*—The authors report a high success rate with surgical repair of presumed unilateral PLF. The diagnosis of this condition remains imperfect; however, surgery can be recommended if the clinical picture and test results suggest PLF and other causes have been ruled out. The surgical outcome, as opposed to visual identification of an actual fluid leak during surgery, is the best way of proving the presence of PLF.

▶ These authors have a surprisingly large study of patients who received grafting for perilymphatic fistula. The results are quite impressive in that 87% of those with vestibular symptoms reported complete or near-complete relief of their symptoms. Forty percent of patients had an improvement in their hearing levels. This is somewhat comparable to our own experience, although we do not have the same results with regard to the control of vestibular symptoms. The authors' observations that one need not see an actual fluid leak to achieve a good postoperative outcome is in keeping with our own experience and the experience of many others who have treated similar patients. Of a variety of tests including electrocochleography, MRI, and so forth, the authors are also correct in that the only way to document a pathologic condition in the middle ear and conditions that involve middle ear/inner ear interactions, as in the case here of perilymphatic fistula, is through exploratory tympanotomy.

**M.M. Paparella, M.D.**

---

**Effect of *Pseudomonas Aeruginosa* Exotoxin A on Inner Ear Function**
Stenqvist M, Anniko M, Pettersson Å (Univ Hosp, Uppsala, Sweden)
*Acta Otolaryngol* 117:73–79, 1997                                          3–2

---

*Background.*—*Pseudomonas aeruginosa* is the most commonly cultured microorganism in chronic suppurative otitis media. Auditory brainstem response (ABR) thresholds after middle ear instillation of *P. aeruginosa* exotoxin A in a rat model were studied.

*Methods.*—The exotoxin was instilled into the middle ear cavity through the tympanic membrane of albino rats. Hearing thresholds were determined by a burst-elicited, frequency-specific ABR method before exposure and periodically after exposure.

*Findings.*—One dose of 1 µg/20 µL of *P. aeruginosa* exotoxin A increased the ABR threshold over the whole frequency range by 5–25 dB, especially in the high tones. All threshold shifts were of combined conductive and cochlear type and reversible. Deterioration began at 24–48 hours, and recovery occurred at 2–4 weeks. Serous fluid effusion occurred at 24 or 48 hours, causing conductive hearing loss. Latency–intensity curves showed a cochlear component along with conductive hearing loss. On morphologic assessment by scanning electron microscopy, slight and inconsistent derangement of OHCs was observed (Fig 2).

*Conclusions.*—Reversible changes in function occur after exposure of the rat cochlea to exotoxin. The electrophysiologic changes were mild, most marked at 48 hours after exposure, expressed mostly in the high-frequency region tonotopically adjacent to the round window membrane, and both conductive and cochlear in nature. Interindividual susceptibility

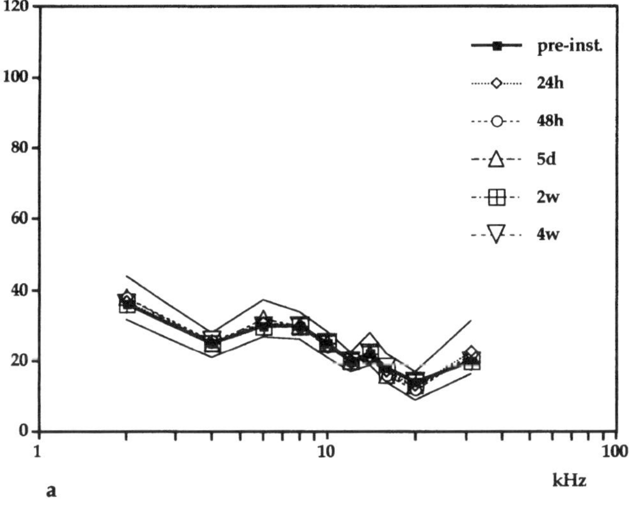


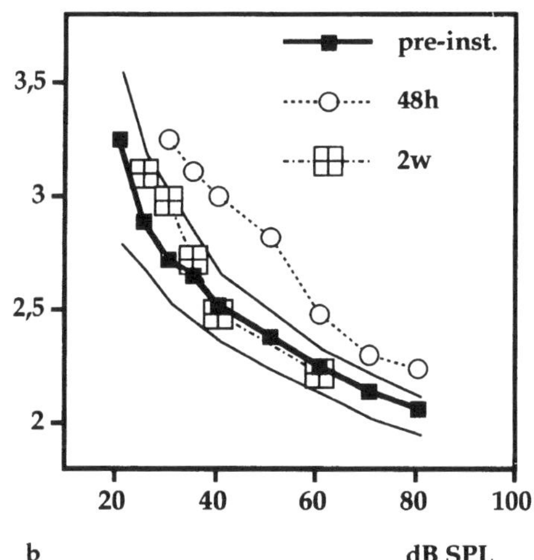


FIGURE 2.—**A,** auditory brainstem response threshold mean values for saline-instilled control rats ($n$ = 6) before and at 24 and 48 hours, 5 days, and 1 and 2 weeks after exposure, superimposed on grey zone of means ±2 SD for normal Sprague-Dawley rats at our laboratory. No noticeable changes in threshold means occurred during the 2-week period. **B,** means of latency–intensity values of PaExoA-instilled rats ($n$ = 10) before instillation and at 48 hours and 2 weeks, superimposed on grey zone of means ±2 SD of interindividual variability. The 48-hour curve is both shifted upward in parallel (conductive component) and has a steeper slope out of the 2 SD zone (cochlear damage). (Courtesy of Stenqvist M, Anniko M, Pettersson Å: Effect of *Pseudomonas aeruginosa* exotoxin A on inner ear function. *Acta Otolaryngol* 117:73–79, 1997.)

to toxins varied substantially. In the human cochlea, the basal turn represents the highest frequencies, which are rarely measured, possibly explaining why inner ear damage is rarely found in clinical practice.

▶ This animal study clearly demonstrates cochlear lesions with great involvement of the high frequencies localized to the basal turn. What is interesting is that not only the conductive but the cochlear type of hearing loss was reversible, which suggests toxic or serous labyrinthitis. This could be followed by suppurative labyrinthitis, which would destroy the cochlea and might, in fact, lead to meningitis and other problems, if this were an individual instead of an animal. It is interesting that studies of this type invariably show involvement of the cochlea with greater involvement of the high frequencies. *P. aeruginosa* is known to be a virulent bacterium in chronic ear infections; thus, it is relevant to hear of its possible toxic effect on cochlear function.

**M.M. Paparella, M.D.**

## Extended High Frequency Hearing and History of Acute Otitis Media in 14-year-old Children in Finland

Laitila P, Karma P, Sipilä M, et al (Helsinki Univ)
*Acta Otolaryngol* Suppl 529:27–29, 1997                                    3–3

*Background.*—The effects of acute otitis media (AOM), a very common disease, on hearing have not been adequately explored. In the past, hearing loss has been reported at high frequencies after AOM, although others have found AOM attacks in children to have almost negligible effects on hearing. Large unselected groups of children 14 years of age or younger were examined in a population-based study.

*Methods.*—Five hundred seventy-three white boys and girls were examined at an outpatient clinic where they had been treated regularly from birth up to 2 years. The definition used for AOM after middle-ear effusion was otologic symptoms, a fever, tugging or rubbing the ear, irritability, vomiting, and diarrhea or a respiratory infection in conjunction with the aforementioned features. A history of ear morbidity was carefully considered in research subjects, and otoscopy, otomicroscopy, and typanometry were performed. The number of AOM attacks was considered in each research subject.

*Results.*—Children were divided into groups: (1) no history of AOM (97), (2) 1–2 attacks (118), (3) 3–7 attacks (153), and (4) 8 or more attacks (205). Middle ear pathologic conditions of varying degrees were found in 46 research subjects. There was no significant variance between results gathered from right and left ears.

*Conclusion.*—Extended high frequency hearing may be effected negatively by many AOM attacks early in life. However, the clinical impact of this loss appears fairly slight. The mechanism for this loss of hearing warrants further study.

▶ This study is important in that it assesses 14-year-olds, who are sufficiently old to have had some longevity after severe bouts of otitis media, to see whether toxins and enzymes have spread through the round window so as to damage the basal turn. It should be remembered that the average adult cochlea is approximately 31 mm long and that the basal turn is generally silent and not measured with routine audiometry. Only high-frequency audiometry, as well as possibly other electrophysiologic methods, can assess the basal turn. These authors found a statistically significant frequency of basal turn hearing loss in these children. We need further studies because, from all our animal studies and human studies to date, we have found that infection frequently contaminates the basal turn. Certainly, as these children grow older, this could be a part of what might later in life be called adult deafness, including presbycusis.

**M.M. Paparella, M.D.**

## Experimental Sensorineural Hearing Loss Following Drill-induced Ossicular Chain Injury

Gjuric M, Schneider W, Buhr W, et al. (Univ of Erlangen-Nuremberg, Germany)

*Acta Otolaryngol (Stockh)* 117:497–500, 1997                     3–4

*Introduction.*—Inadvertent injury to the ossicular chain during drilling in the epitympanum or in the middle ear cavity, a potential cause of acute sensorineural hearing loss in the course of surgery on the middle ear, has not been widely examined in the literature. A guinea pig model was used

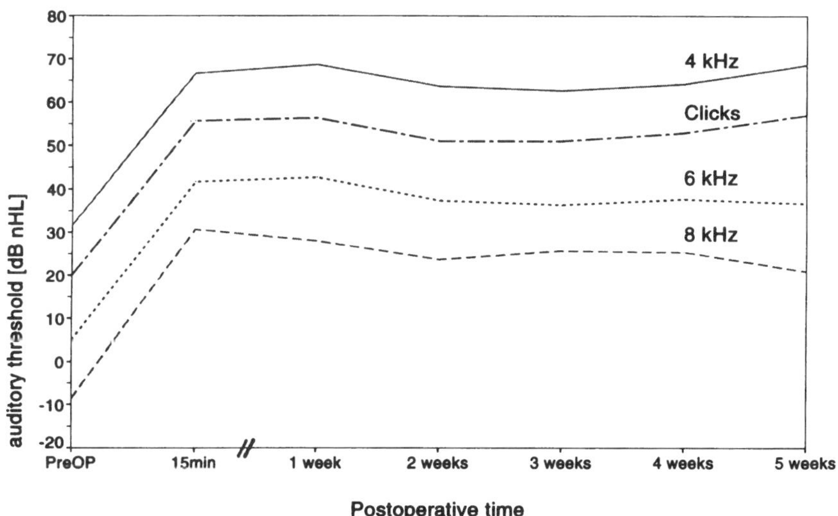


FIGURE 1.—Mean values of the auditory threshold shifts for clicks and bursts in 15 guinea pigs after drilling on the incus. (Courtesy of Gjuric M, Schneider W, Buhr W, et al: Experimental sensorineural hearing loss following drill-induced ossicular chain injury. *Acta Otolaryngol* 117:497–500, 1997.)

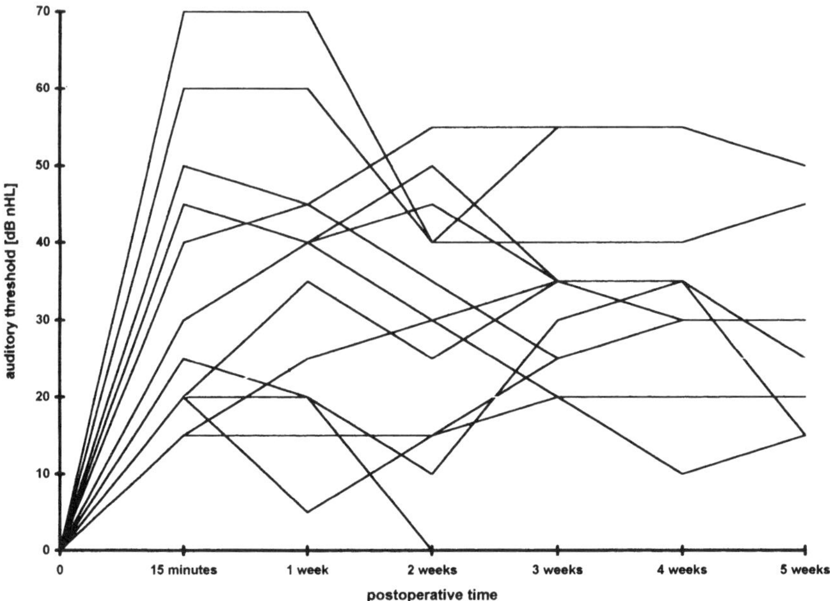

FIGURE 2.—Time course of air-conduction, click-evoked CAP thresholds after drilling in 15 guinea pigs. (Courtesy of Gjuric M, Schneider W, Buhr W, et al: Experimental sensorineural hearing loss following drill-induced ossicular chain injury. *Acta Otolaryngol* 117:497–500, 1997.)

to characterize the effects on hearing of a drill-induced injury to the body of the incus.

*Methods.*—Twenty-three white Dunktin-Hartley guinea pigs with normal otoscopic findings and normal Preyer reflex thresholds were used. Acoustically evoked compound action potentials (CAP) were recorded in anesthetized animals before drilling, a minute after drilling, after closure of the wound, and weekly for 5 weeks after surgery. Three control guinea pigs had the bulla opened but no further manipulations.

*Results.*—Auditory thresholds for clicks and tone-bursts remained stable (within 10 dB nHL) in control animals during the 5-week observation period. Drilling in the experimental group resulted in a threshold shift within seconds, and the shift remained stable during the 5 weeks of follow-up. Fifteen minutes after drilling, the threshold shift averaged 35.7 dB for clicks, 35 dB nHL for 4 kHz bursts, 36.7 dB nHL for 6 kHz bursts, and 39 dB nHL for 8 kHz bursts (Fig 1). Responses in individual animals showed considerable variation, with minimum deterioration in threshold (15 dB) and maximum deterioration for clicks (70 dB nHL) (Fig 2). A disarticulation of the incudostapedial joint, performed in 5 animals before drilling, did not reduce the threshold shift.

*Conclusion.*—In this guinea pig model, drilling on the ossicular chain with a 1.4 mm diamond bur for 10 seconds resulted in significant andirreversible hearing loss. Responses to the procedures varied according to the individual susceptibility of the cochlea to mechanical trauma. Drilling around an intact ossicular chain must be done with great care to avoid permanent sensorineural hearing loss.

▶ In this day of modern otology, the surgeon needs to continue to be careful that rotating burs, particularly bone-cutting burs, do not bump into the ossicular chain, because they will indeed cause acoustic trauma, as this study so eloquently describes. Caution is mandatory when drilling around an intact ossicular chain, particularly when drilling in the aditus using a transmastoid approach to surgery on the endolymphatic sac, tympanomastoidectomy, and so forth.

**M.M. Paparella, M.D.**

**Intratympanic Gentamicin for Treatment of Intractable Ménière's Disease: A Preliminary Report**
Rauch SD, Oas JG (Harvard Med School, Boston)
*Laryngoscope* 107:49–55, 1997                                             3–5

*Background.*—Approximately 5% of patients with Ménière's disease fail to respond to conservative medical treatment. Alternative management in such cases has consisted of either drainage operations, such as cochleosacculotomy, or destructive operations, such as labyrinthectomy. "Chemical" labyrinthectomy can be achieved with intratympanic gentamicin (ITG), but hearing loss occurs in some patients. Two protocols using ITG were compared for their effects on vertigo and on hearing.

*Methods.*—Participants in the study were 15 women and 6 men with intractable classic Ménière's disease. The treatment protocol was designed to balance the risk of hearing loss from an overdose of gentamicin to the patients' desire for a short duration of therapy. Patients initially received a 30 mg/mL dilution in injectable saline given in 2 consecutive doses 24 hours apart and repeated weekly. The dose was later increased to 40 mg/mL. Of the 9 patients in this treatment group, 1 lost hearing 4 days after the fourth injection. The second protocol consisted of 40 mg/mL gentamicin administered at 8 AM and 5 PM for 2–4 consecutive days. This schedule was reduced to a maximum of 4 injections in the first week when 2 of the first 4 patients experienced profound sensorineural hearing loss.

*Results.*—Follow-up ranged from 3 to 31 months. Of 21 patients, 20 responded initially to ITG with complete control of episodic vertigo. Six responders experienced relapsing symptoms within 12 months, but retreatment was successful in 75%. Hearing was preserved or improved in 62% of patients and worsened in 24%. Results of tests of hearing were not available for 14% of patients. We were able to reduce hearing loss when the cumulative dose of ITG was 4 or fewer injections in the first week.

*Conclusion.*—In this small series of patients, intratympanic gentamicin therapy succeeded in controlling or significantly improving vertiginous attacks of Ménière's disease in 95% of patients and preserving or improving hearing in 81%. Compared with surgical treatment, ITG offers lower cost, lower medical risk, and substantially less posttreatment discomfort.

▶ This study is of interest. There seems to be a newly awakened interest in the use of intratympanic gentamicin for treatment of intractable Ménière's disease. Subscribers to the YEAR BOOK might be interested to know that the ototoxic treatment of Ménière's disease is not new; in fact it goes back to the late 1940s, when Dr. Hansen in Minneapolis and Dr. Fowler at Columbia University in New York first used these methods to treat patients with intractable Ménière's disease. This method was then popularized by Schuknecht during the 1950s and 1960s. Streptomycin was the ototoxic agent used then, and gentamicin was used subsequently by many.

This technique involves instillation of an ototoxic drug in the middle ear, hopefully to locate it generally in the region of the round window niche. It is then absorbed by the round window and passes through the cochlea until it creates its ototoxic damage to specific vestibular sensory cells in the vestibular labyrinth. For this reason, it should not be surprising that, as this article indicates, patients (in this study, 24%) demonstrated worsening of hearing. Other studies have indicated that a third or more of such patients may develop worsening of hearing. This study also shows that relapse or recurrence of vertigo can take place subsequently. These studies should be done longitudinally, as long-term studies.

**M.M. Paprella, M.D.**

---

**Low-Dose Intratympanic Gentamicin and the Treatment of Ménière's Disease: Preliminary Results**
Driscoll CLW, Kasperbauer JL, Facer GW, et al (Mayo Clinic, Rochester, Minn)
*Laryngoscope* 107:83–89, 1997                                                    3–6

---

*Introduction.*—Vertigo is often the most disabling symptom of unilateral Ménière's disease, but treatment by means of labyrinthectomy sacrifices residual hearing. The ideal therapy would control vertigo while preserving cochlear function. Patients reported here were treated with a single injection of gentamicin. In most cases, this low-dose regimen controlled vertigo without significantly altering pure tone averages or speech discrimination scores.

*Methods.*—The prospective study enrolled 23 patients with severe, limiting vertigo that was unresponsive to at least 6 months of medical management. All underwent a preprocedure evaluation, which included an audiogram, CT or MRI, and electronystagmography. A single dose of gentamicin (10–80 mg) was injected into the middle ear space with a 3½-inch, 25-gauge needle. The patient remained recumbent for 40 minutes, turning the head to maximize retention of gentamicin and coverage of the round window membrane. Repeated audiologic and vestibular testing was performed 2–4 weeks later.

*Results.*—Patients had a mean age of 58 years and an average follow-up time of 13.3 months. Of 19 patients who were evaluated for frequency of vertigo, 16 had no episodes during the last 6 months of follow-up. The remaining 3 patients reported that their episodes were less frequent and less intense, and none required a surgical labyrinthectomy. Both mean pure tone averages and mean speech discrimination scores were unchanged. All but 1 experienced worsening of hearing in the high frequencies. Caloric function was reduced in 93% of cases. There was no relationship between higher doses of gentamicin and higher risk of hearing loss.

*Conclusion.*—Low-dose intratympanic gentamicin is a simple treatment, which safely and effectively controls vertigo in most patients with unilateral Ménière's disease. There is little risk to hearing, and even low concentrations (10 ng/mL) of gentamicin may prove adequate to prevent vertigo.

▶ The key point to be made in this article is from the title itself—preliminary results. This was a very short-term study; thus we have not had a sufficiently long period to find out whether this method is indeed efficacious. As mentioned in my comments in the preceding article, Abstract 3–5, the concept of using ototoxic medication topically as well as systemically is not new; it has been used during the past 50 years. My assumption all along has been that one needs to eliminate function in the vestibular cells, which clearly low-dose gentamicin would not do. Thus, a long-term study is needed, with controls, to have any thought about whether these preliminary studies will hold up over time. It should be remembered, by readers and subscribers of the YEAR BOOK, however, that any time one uses gentamicin, one is destroying the inner ear. I think there are other methods, medical and conservative surgical methods, which have as their objective the preservation and possible restoration of cells and not their destruction. It is a simple truism that whether one uses labyrinthectomy or destroys the vestibular nerve through sectioning or uses ototoxic drugs, once a structure is destroyed it no longer can be replaced or improved.

**M.M. Paparella, M.D.**

---

## A New Adhesive Bonding Material for the Cementation of Implantable Devices in Otologic Surgery

Maniglia AJ, Nakabayashi N, Paparella MM, et al (Case Western Reserve Univ, Cleveland, Ohio; Tokyo Med and Dental Univ; Univ of Minnesota, Minneapolis)
*Am J Otol* 18:322–327, 1997                                    3–7

---

*Introduction.*—The need for adhesives that permanently cement metalloprostheses to bone is important in otologic surgery now that cochlear implantation and implantable hearing devices are available. There are no U.S. Food and Drug Administration(FDA)-approved adhesive bone cements available at this time for use in otologic surgery. A new cement, 5%

4-methacryoyloxyethyl trimellitate anhydride in methyl methacrylate with polymethylmethacrylate powder initiated by tri-*n*-butyl borane, designated as 4-META/MMA-TBB opaque resin, has been cleared by the FDA as a dental adhesive. Experimental findings demonstrate the long-term clinical efficacy and biocompatibility of this product as an adhesive agent for use in otologic surgery.

*Methods.*—An electromagnetic, semi-implantable hearing device was implanted into the middle ears of 6 cats. The 4-META/MMA-TBB resin was used to cement a titanium-encased magnet to the incus. The animals were killed at a mean of 9.6 months to analyze the temporal bones, specifically the magnet–incus complex.

*Results.*—In all cats, the titanium-encapsulated magnet was firmly adherent to all incudes. There were no failures of the cement–bone interface. Histopathologic examination of the implanted temporal bones indicated an absence of inflammation in the middle ear. A unique "hybrid layer" in the bone-side subsurface of the bone–cement interface was observed by using transmission electron microscopy. These findings indicate that the resin–bone interface was completely sealed without any formation of a capsule.

*Conclusion.*—The efficacy and biocompatibility of 4-META/MMA-TBB for the cementation of implantable prostheses is demonstrated with these experimental findings. This adhesive system is not yet available for clinical otologic use because FDA approval is pending.

▶ These authors describe a new cement that holds promise for cementing prosthetic alloplastic materials in the middle ear. This new cement, 4-META/MMA-TBB opaque resin, has shown good adhesive properties but has also appeared to be quite innocuous in studies of temporal bones to date. The material seems to be biocompatible and may find clinical application during otologic surgery, especially when prostheses are used in the middle ear.

**M.M. Paparella, M.D.**

---

**Use of an Implantable Hearing Device**
Yellin W, Roland PS, Culbertson M, et al (Univ of Texas, Dallas)
*Am J Otolaryngol* 18:33–37, 1997                                    3–8

---

*Objective.*—The XOMED Audiant Bone Conductor has proved to be a safe implantable amplification device for some patients with conductive hearing loss but intact cochlear function. The device consists of a magnetic screw in a titanium-aluminum-vanadium cup that is subcutaneously implanted in the temporal bone, and an electromagnetically coupled external induction coil. Vibrations are sent to the cochlea by the internal magnet in response to stimulation from acoustic energy picked up by the microphone. The efficacy of the XOMED device was evaluated in 24 patients.

*Patients.*—The XOMED device was implanted in 24 patients aged 10 months to 24 years. In addition to meeting audiologic criteria, all patients were dissatisfied with bone-conduction hearing aids, could not obtain adequate amplification from air-conducted hearing aids because of surgical distortion, or had chronic ear infection. Twenty-three patients were interviewed by telephone about their use of the device and the benefit obtained. The interviews were performed an average of 34 months after surgery.

*Findings.*—Eleven of the patients were still using their XOMED device. All patients in this group were completely dependent on the device for amplification. The other 12 patients were not using the device, either because they were not getting enough amplification from the device or because of problems with magnet strength.

*Conclusions.*—Some patients achieve good results with the XOMED Audiant Bone Conductor whereas others do not. The findings of this study have led the authors to change their criteria for XOMED implantation. With stricter criteria, the device should be a viable amplification alternative for patients who do not benefit from more conventional devices.

▶ We have had a few patients in which this device was implanted and have had somewhat similar but perhaps less optimistic results than these authors indicate. These authors did a very nice comparative study of patients, and find that 11 patients continued to use the implantable hearing device whereas 12 patients are not using their device. We have found that most of our patients have preferred not to use the device even after the implantation, but our numbers are smaller compared with these authors'. It is hoped that an improved device and stricter patient criteria, as the authors indicate, will lead to a viable amplification alternative for patients who are candidates and who are not candidates for other surgical corrective methods of therapy.

**M.M. Paparella, M.D.**

---

**Temporal Bone Pathology of a Patient With Cochlear Implant**
Nakai Y, Sakashita T, Kubo T, et al (Univ Med School, Osaka, Japan; Otsu Red Cross Hosp, Shiga, Japan)
*ORL J Otorhinolaryngol Relat Spec* 59:230–234, 1997          3–9

---

*Introduction.*—Cochlear implants are now a widely used treatment for patients with profound total hearing loss. Implantation is known to cause a foreign body reaction, but there have been few opportunities for histologic examination of the temporal bone from a human recipient. The patient reported on here died 2½ years after cochlear implantation, and his temporal bone was harvested for histologic and electron-microscopic evaluation.

*Case Report.*—The man, 66, had used a hearing aid since age 7 when a head injury led to bilateral hearing loss. Ten years after total deafness developed, the patient had a Nucleus 22-channel cochlear implant inserted. Hearing was restored, and the patient

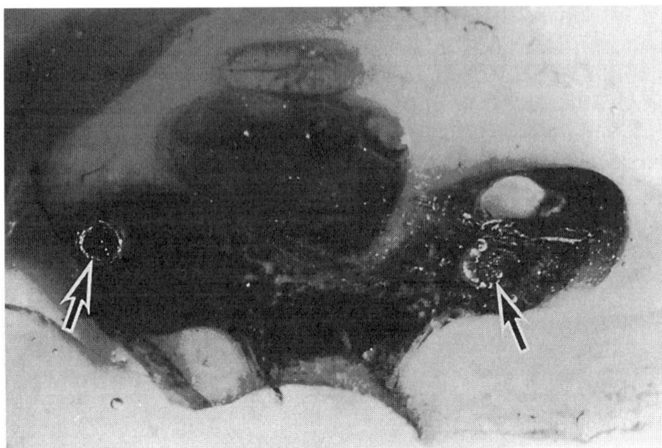

FIGURE 4.—The electrode is inserted in the scala tympani *(arrows)*. (Courtesy of Nakai Y, Sakashita T, Kubo T, et al: Temporal bone pathology of a patient with cochlear implant. *ORL J Otorhinolaryngol Relat Spec* 59:230–234, 1997. Reproduced with permission of Karger, AG, Basel.)

was quite satisfied with results of the implant. When he died of lung cancer 27 months after surgery, an autopsy was performed, and the temporal bone was harvested. The cochlea was then embedded in epoxy resin and sectioned for light and electron microscopy.

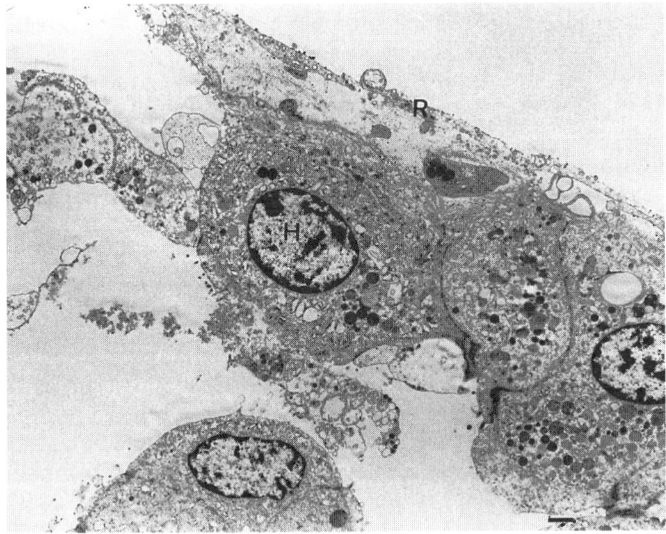

FIGURE 9.—Electron micrograph showing degenerated hair cell *(H)* in the organ of Corti. *R*, Reissner's membrane. (Courtesy of Nakai Y, Sakashita T, Kubo T, et al: Temporal bone pathology of a patient with cochlear implant. *ORL J Otorhinolaryngol Relat Spec* 59:230–234, 1997. Reproduced with permission of Karger, AG, Basel.)

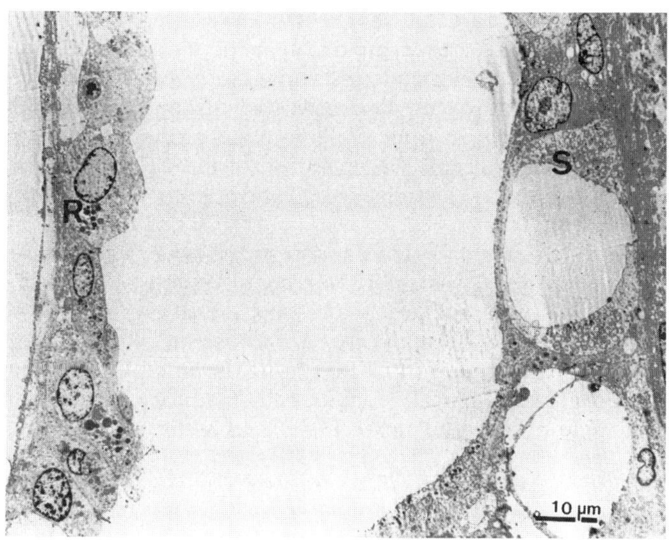

FIGURE 8.—Electron micrograph showing degenerated stria vascularis (*S*) and Reissner's membrane (*R*). (Courtesy of Nakai Y, Sakashita T, Kubo T, et al: Temporal bone pathology of a patient with cochlear implant. *ORL J Otorhinolaryngol Relat Spec* 59:230–234, 1997. Reproduced with permission of Karger, AG, Basel.)

*Results.*—No inflammation was observed at the site, and the receiver-stimulator was firmly embedded in new bone. The mastoid cavity was preserved and had a thin mucosal lining. Dacron mesh tie used for fixing the electrodes had been almost entirely absorbed, remnants were surrounded by fibrous tissue. The tympanic cavity appeared normal, with little foreign body reaction in the round window. Examination of the cut

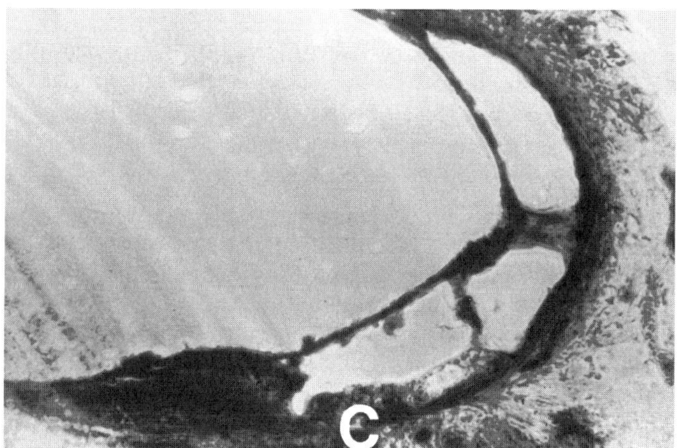

FIGURE 7.—Cross section of the cochlea. The scala media has collapsed as a result of atrophy of stria vascularis. The organ of Corti *(C)* has degenerated, and no tectorial membrane is observed. (Courtesy of Nakai Y, Sakashita T, Kubo T, et al: Temporal bone pathology of a patient with cochlear implant. *ORL J Otorhinolaryngol Relat Spec* 59:230–234, 1997. Reproduced with permission of Karger, AG, Basel.)

surface of the cochlea revealed the electrodes inserted 17 mm above the basal turn (Fig 4) in the scala tympani, near the modiolus. Fibrous tissue was present at the site of electrode-insertion. Nerve fibers were detected in the osseous spiral lamina, but hair cells had disappeared (Fig 9) in the organ of Corti. Fewer than normal nerve fibers and spiral ganglion cells were present in the modiolus. Degeneration of the stria vascularis (Fig 8) had caused collapse of the scala media, and the cochlear duct had collapsed (Fig 7).

*Discussion.*—Threshold (T) level and dynamic range (DR) are related to function of the inner ear and ability to recognize sounds of speech. In this patient, the T level of some electrodes was increased, and DR was decreased, 1 year after surgery, perhaps because of slight foreign body reaction or senile degeneration of nerves in the inner ear. Despite a decrease in the number of spiral ganglion cells, auditory stimulation of the remaining ganglion cells and nerve fibers had achieved a reasonable response.

▶ Cochlear implants have been established and certainly are very helpful for those who have deafness, particularly postlingual deafness. The jury is still out concerning whether the cochlear implant causes damage to the inner ear and to what extent. There can be no doubt that some damage is caused in all patients, and, of course, I would suspect that the amount of damage caused by the cochlear implant as direct trauma and/or reaction to a possible foreign body in the inner ear will depend on the individual pathologic status of the cochlea in each person. This article very nicely demonstrates a number of changes that took place in the inner ear, including changes in the stria vascularis and cochlear duct, which can be attributable to the presence of the implant.

**M.M. Paparella, M.D.**

---

**Cochlear Implant in the Child Under Two Years of Age: Skull Growth, Otitis Media, and Selection**
Hoffman RA (New York Univ)
*Otolaryngol Head Neck Surg* 117:217–219, 1997                    3–10

---

*Background.*—Performing cochlear implantation in young children can provide adequate hearing for the development of receptive and expressive language. Under current Food and Drug Administration (FDA) guidelines, the lower age limit for cochlear implantation is 2 years. However, earlier implantation could have important advantages in terms of speech and language acquisition. Important considerations in performing cochlear implantation in children younger than 2 years are discussed.

*Cochlear Implants Before Age 2.*—From an anatomic standpoint, cochlear implant surgery appears to be feasible in children younger than 2 years. The labyrinth is fully formed at birth, and the middle ear is of near-normal size. Skin thickness is a consideration, but problems can be overcome simply by seating the electronics in a deep well. Furthermore, the anatomy can be assessed preoperatively by CT. The temporal bone continues to grow through adolescence. However, surgical techniques are available to prevent the receiver-stimulator from extruding and the electrode from migrating. Studies suggest that electrode migration is no more common in children than adults, and that device migration is less common in children. There has been concern that cochlear implantation could be associated with an increased risk of otitis media in children. However, experimental studies suggest that a fibrous tissue sheath forms around the electrode during the first few weeks, sealing off the cochleostomy and serving as a barrier to the spread of infection.

The need for accurate diagnosis can be met by frequency-specific evoked-response audiometry, along with behavioral testing. There is a need for a more objective approach to measuring and documenting the speech and language progress in the under-2 age group, however. The Nucleus 22-channel device and the Clarion 16-electrode bipolar array are currently being tested for use in children. Because of its greater thickness, the Clarion device may necessitate a larger well to avoid device migration or flap complications. It has not been studied for use in children younger than 2 years. The Nucleus device has been placed in 78 children younger than 2 years, including 69 aged 18 to 23 months. No surgical complications have been reported. Data on hearing and on speech and language acquisition are still to come.

*Discussion.*—From a technical standpoint, it should be feasible to perform cochlear implantation in children younger than 2 years old. Most of the concerns raised about this procedure have been satisfactorily answered. The major remaining issue is to establish that the child is a candidate for the procedure.

▶ Dr. Hoffman makes a good point in this study, that there are some examples when the child younger than 2 years of age would be better served by having an implantation instead of waiting for too long a period before, for example, ossification fills the inner ear as a result of labyrinthitis ossificans. At the same time, the success of implantation below the age of 2 will clearly depend on the etiologic basis, the pathogenesis, and the pathologic condition that led to deafness in that child. Thus, congenital genetic deafness with dysplasia of sensorineural elements will have a less desirable result from implantation than will implantation in a child who is deaf before age 2 because of an acquired cause such as infection or trauma.

**M.M. Paparella, M.D.**

## Cochlear Implantation in the Presence of Chronic Suppurative Otitis Media

Axon PR, Mawman DJ, Upile T, et al (Manchester Royal Infirmary, England)
*J Laryngol Otol* 111:228–232, 1997                                      3–11

*Introduction.*—Cochlear implantation is most commonly performed in middle ears free of pathologic conditions. The procedure is typically an uncomplicated single-stage operation. Chronic suppurative otitis media (CSOM) may be the cause of profound deafness in some patients, or it may be an incidental finding; it presents a surgical challenge. Reported are 9 patients with CSOM who underwent cochlear implantation.

*Methods.*—Nine of 157 patients (5.7%) who underwent cochlear implants had CSOM. Four patients had a simple tympanic membrane perforation, 4 had pre-existing mastoid cavities, and 1 had a cholesteatoma in the ear chosen for implantation. Patients underwent high-definition axial CT scans of the petrous bones, and pure tone audiometry and speech audiometry, preoperatively. After implantation, free field audiometry, Bench Kowal Bamford sentence tests, consonant confusion tests, and environmental sound recognition were performed. Patients with simple perforations underwent a staged procedure with myringoplasty, then cochlear implantation 3 months later. Patients with a cholesteatoma or with a unstable mastoid cavity underwent staged procedures that included a mastoidectomy or revised mastoidectomy with obliteration of the middle ear and mastoid using a superiorly pedicled temporalis muscle flap and blind sac closure of the external meatal skin. Six months later, patients underwent a second-stage procedure to confirm healthy middle-ear cleft and insertion of the implant. Patients with stable mastoid cavities underwent a 1-staged procedure involving obliteration of the cavity and implantation of the electrode.

*Results.*—At 18-month follow-up examinations, there were no problems with breakdown of the graft, recurrent disease, or extrusion of the implant. The performance in audiometry and language testing was improved in all patients between 9 and 18 months postoperatively.

*Conclusion.*—Cochlear implantation in 9 patients with CSOM and profound deafness was successful, and all patients benefited from the procedure(s). It is important to individualize treatment approaches in these patients.

▶ These authors describe their method of cochlear implantation in the presence of CSOM. The title of the article, however, may be a slight misnomer in that these patients had their chronic otitis media treated, and the patient must have a dry ear before the implant is inserted as a secondary procedure. This is certainly logical, as one obviously would not wish to enter the inner ear in any way in the presence of an active infection. Various other methods could be used, but the principle here is that the disease needs to be brought under control—the patient requires a safe, dry ear—and then the cochlear implantation can be considered.

**M.M. Paparella, M.D.**

## Meningitis After Cochlear Implantation in Mondini Malformation
Page EL, Eby TL (Univ of Alabama, Birmingham)
*Otolaryngol Head Neck Surg* 116:104–106, 1997
3–12

*Background.*—The potential for CSF leakage and subsequent meningitis after cochlear implantation in patients with a malformed cochlea has been recognized, but no reports of this complication have been published to date. A patient with a Mondini malformation in whom delayed CSF otorhinorrhea developed with resulting meningitis after cochlear implantation was described.

*Case Report.*—Boy, 5, was hospitalized because of recurrent bacterial meningitis. He had bilateral Mondini malformations, resulting in profound sensorineural hearing loss. Two years earlier, he had had a posterior fossa craniotomy for fenestration of a cerebropontine angle arachnoid cyst, followed by cochlear implantation several months later. He did well after these procedures. About 1 year later, the boy fell and bumped his head. He did not lose consciousness or show rhinorrhea, but 2 weeks later he required hospitalization for a febrile illness. Sinusitis was diagnosed, and a 6-day course of IV antibiotics was delivered. Three months later, severe bacterial meningitis developed, resulting in quadriparesis. Endotracheal intubation was required. A CT scan of the temporal bones showed opacification of the left middle ear and mastoid. The cochlear implant was in an appropriate place. The meningitis resolved after 10 days of IV antibiotics. However, prolonged ventilation was needed because of his profound weakness. He was discharged at 5 weeks, after gradually regaining strength in all his extremities. Rhinorrhea recurred after discharge, and 3 months later he was hospitalized again with meningitis. A CT scan showed opacification again, with the electrode of the cochlear implant encroaching on the floor of the middle cranial fossa. A CSF leak was confirmed by a radionuclide cisternogram. The boy was treated with IV antibiotics for 1 week, then underwent middle ear exploration. Extensive scar tissue was noted around the wire for the electrode array. The opening into the mastoid was enlarged with a diamond burr, and clear fluid was observed. On inspection of the cochleostomy site, the fluid was found to be leaking out around the electrode insertion site. Temporalis fascia was packed around the electrode array and into the vestibule to stop the leakage, and temporalis muscle was placed in the middle ear space on top of the fascia. After wound closure, the neurosurgery service inserted a lumbar drain. The boy did well after the operation, with no further rhinorrhea or meningitis. The 2-month follow-up CT scan showed a well-pneumatized mastoid cavity.

*Conclusions.*—Although this complication appears to be rare, the cochleostomy must be sealed carefully at the initial operation in children with inner ear malformations. Any episode of meningitis after surgery must be explored thoroughly to exclude CSF leakage from the labyrinth.

▶ *Mondini malformation* refers to a bony as well as a membranous dysgenesis of the inner ear. There can be an enlarged cochlear aqueduct as well as an enlarged vestibular aqueduct. As this case demonstrates, a delayed CSF otorhinorrhea can result and, as in this case, not only develop but also lead to meningitis after cochlear implantation in a child with Mondini malformation. Thus, in the future, it would behoove those who are considering cochlear implantation in cases of Mondini malformation to try to compensate for this feature by various techniques (e.g., perhaps by causing less trauma in the cochlea and perhaps by grafting the middle ear–inner ear interactive barrier, including the round window niche).

**M.M. Paparella, M.D.**

# 4  Otosclerosis

**Genetics of Otosclerosis**
Sabitha R, Ramalingam R, Ramalingam KK, et al (KKR ENT Hosp and Research Inst, Kilpauk, Madras, India)
*J Laryngol Otol* 111:109–112, 1997                                    4–1

*Background.*—Otosclerosis is a genetic disorder that affects ear bone remodeling in early to middle adulthood. The current study explored the genetics of otosclerosis in Indian populations.

*Patients and Findings.*—One hundred fifty-one families with otosclerosis with 153 probands were included. The mean ages of the male and female probands at disease onset were 24.1 years and 25.7 years, respectively. Very low expression rates were found among the offspring (5% to 6%), siblings (about 22%), and parents (about 30%) of the probands. In second-degree relatives, the expression rate was about 70%. The expression rate among siblings was 22.4% and rose to more than 50% when matings between 2 individuals with normal hearing (N) with proband alone affected were excluded. This increased to about 61% when siblings younger than 15 years were excluded. When only parents of affected A × N, A × A, and N × N − OR matings (excluding N × N matings) were considered, the expression rate among parents was 71% and 37% in siblings. However, the rate remained low at 10% to 12% in offspring, regardless of whether children younger than 15 years were included.

*Conclusions.*—Otosclerosis appears to be a heterogenous disease. The role of nongenetic factors is probably much more important than is appreciated. Further research with a larger sample is needed to better define the role of genetic and nongenetic factors in the manifestation of otosclerosis.

▶ The question raised in this study of the genetics of otosclerosis is not only valid but also important. When we see patients with otosclorosis, it is amazing to me, if this is supposed to be an autosomal dominant disease, how many patients really do not have a family history of otosclerosis in their identifiable relatives. Thus, other factors, including heterogeneity, need to be searched for. It is quite likely that these patients may have had relatives with otosclerosis generations ago but have no knowledge of a linkage. It is still my impression and belief that otosclerosis is a genetically induced disease. There are many other diseases, congenital or acquired, that can cause stapedial fixation that are not otosclerosis because they do not have otospongiosis as a correlatable pathologic lesion.

**M.M. Paparella, M.D.**

---

**Dehiscences of the Horizontal Segment of the Facial Canal in Otosclerosis**
Tange RA, de Bruijn AJG (Academic Med Centre, Amsterdam)
*ORL J Otorhinolaryngol Relat Spec* 59:277–279, 1997                    4–2

---

*Introduction.*—Dehiscences of the facial canal are common, occurring in more than 50% of the temporal bones, and are seen most often in the region of the oval window. Reports of the incidence of natural dehiscences of the horizontal segment of the facial canal are based primarily on cadaver studies, and findings vary. The present study is based on operative observations of the facial canal in 427 cases of middle ear surgery for otosclerosis.

*Methods.*—All information on middle ear surgery at the study institution has been stored in a database from 1982. Since then, 427 consecutive stapes operations for otosclerosis have been performed by the same surgeon. The facial canal was carefully inspected and palpated under microscopic view in all cases. Four grades of stapes fixation were identified intraoperatively: grade I, stapes fixation without otosclerotic change of the footplate; grade II, fixation with a single otosclerotic focus; grade III, stapes fixation with more than 1 otosclerotic focus; and grade IV, total obliteration of the oval niche by otosclerosis. Patients received systemic and oral antibiotic prophylaxis; no postoperative infections or dead ears occurred.

*Results.*—The patient group included 268 women and 169 men with an average age of 40.4 years. A dehiscence of the facial canal was observed in 14 (3.27%), 7 men and 7 women. The location of the dehiscence was just above the oval window niche in all cases; defect size ranged from 2 mm to 5 mm. Gradations of stapes fixation for the entire group of 427 operations were: grade I, 97 cases; grade II, 154 cases; grade III, 144 cases; and grade IV, 32 cases. Distribution of grades in patients with a dehiscence of the facial canal were, respectively, 1, 3, 8, and 2 cases. All cases of dehiscence of the facial canal exhibited a normally shaped stapes suprastructure. In 1 patient with a dehiscence, the facial nerve was exposed and herniated into the oval window after removal of the stapes suprastructure.

*Discussion.*—The incidence of dehiscence in this study, 3.27%, is lower than that of previous reports. Histologic cadaver studies have yielded rates as high as 74%, perhaps because very small dehiscences can be detected by histology. Dehiscences in the bony facial canal should be considered anomalies, and their occurrence in otosclerosis is sporadic.

▶ These authors find a low incidence of dehiscence of the Fallopian canal in cases of otosclerosis during surgery for otosclerosis. It is very possible that studies of temporal bones might reveal dehiscences that might not be identified during exploratory tympanotomy and through the microscope. Nevertheless, the incidence is far lower than that found in temporal bones in general, in which dehiscences may be 50% to 60% or greater. If indeed the incidence is lower in patients with otosclerosis, one wonders if there is any rationale for this having to do with the genealogy and development of the disease process itself.

**M.M. Paparella, M.D.**

## Stapedectomy in Combat Pilots

Katzav J, Lippy WH, Shamiss A, et al (Israel Air Force Aeromedical Ctr, Tel Hashomer; Warren Otologic Group, Ohio)
*Am J Otol* 17:847–849, 1996

4–3

*Background.*—Although stapedectomy is now a safe, effective procedure for improving conductive hearing loss from otosclerosis, several complications may occur. An oval window fistula, which can be manifested by sudden incapacitating vertigo, is most feared by pilots and air crew. Fear of this complication and its implications for continued flying can cause pilots, crew members, and their otologists to delay treatment of otosclerosis for as long as possible. The outcomes of stapedectomies in a group of Israeli Air Force fighter pilots were reported.

*Patients and Outcomes.*—Nine stapedectomies were performed in 6 high-performance pilots with otosclerosis between 1977 and 1995. The Robinson-vein graft technique was performed, which has been found to have a low rate of fistula formation compared with wire-Gelfoam stapedectomies. In all patients, postoperative pure tone average (PTA) air conduction thresholds were within 10 dB of their preoperative PTA bone conduction thresholds. Thus, the outcomes were considered successful in all patients. The pilots were able to return to full active duty free from vestibular symptoms.

*Conclusions.*—These findings suggest that high-performance pilots may safely return to full flight status after stapedectomy. Full flight status may be resumed as soon as 3 months after surgery without endangering flight safety.

▶ This study and topic are somewhat similar to those in the last article, Abstract 4–2, in that combat pilots certainly endure alterations in barometric pressure as well as rapid accelerating motion during flight. It is reassuring to know that after a successful stapedectomy, combat pilots can return to full duty. Thus it would seem that patients who have had successful stapedial surgery can return to duty in almost all aspects of life. If the patient, however, has a complicated problem and does not do well postoperatively, certainly clinical judgments against full return to duty may be made in exceptional cases.

**M.M. Paparella, M.D.**

## Barotrauma After Stapes Surgery: A Survey of Recommended Restrictions and Clinical Experiences

Harrill WC, Jenkins HA, Coker NJ (Baylor College of Medicine, Houston)
*Am J Otol* 17:835–846, 1996                                    4–4

*Background.*—Although many reports of barotrauma after stapes surgery have been published, there are no generally accepted restrictions on activities likely to produce rapid barometric pressure changes after such surgery. A consensus on the postoperative barorestrictions after stapes surgery was sought, and the clinical barotrauma experience of patients undergoing such surgery was assessed.

*Methods.*—A 34-item survey was mailed to 419 active members of the American Otological Society and the American Neurotology Society. The physicians were queried about the necessity of postoperative restrictions on air travel, snorkeling, and scuba diving after stapes surgery. Recommendations for the use of ventilation tubes and hyperbaric oxygen treatment were also elicited. Two hundred eighty-four surveys were returned, for a response rate of 67.8%. Fifty-three of these surveys were not complete and excluded from the final analysis.

*Findings.*—No consensus was reached on restrictions from activities such as air travel, snorkeling, or scuba diving. However, there were no significant differences in the prevalence of barotrauma reported by patients in the responding physicians' practices based on their individual recommendations for restrictions.

*Conclusions.*—This lack of consensus among otologists on activity restriction after stapes surgery is surprising. The survey respondents had conflicting opinions about the postoperative management of otosclerotic patients. However, complications from the surveyed activities can result in permanent postoperative hearing loss, and therefore further study is needed.

▶ These authors surveyed 419 members of the American Otological Society and found a wide variety of advice provided to patients regarding alterations in barometric pressure after stapedial surgery. As they indicate, no consensus was demonstrated, but it seems reasonable that patients should not fly for at least 2 weeks, and should not do anything resembling scuba diving during that time. Some physicians advise patients never to snorkel or scuba dive. We have had patients do this successfully, but I would recommend against scuba diving for a month or so after surgery, whereas flying can usually take place safely about 2 weeks after successful stapedectomy.

**M.M. Paparella, M.D.**

## Stapedectomy vs Stapedotomy: Do You Really Need a Laser?

Sedwick JD, Louden CL, Shelton C (Univ of Utah, Salt Lake City)
*Arch Otolaryngol Head Neck Surg* 123:177–180, 1997                    4–5

*Background.*—Many different techniques are currently used to perform stapedectomy, including lasers. The efficacies of different methods in improving hearing in patients with a conductive hearing loss from otosclerosis were compared.

*Methods.*—The records of 875 patients undergoing primary stapedectomies at 1 center were reviewed. The 550 patients with otosclerosis and adequate postoperative bone conduction threshold data were included. Large and small fenestra techniques were compared, as well as the use of drills vs. lasers.

*Findings.*—The rates of closure of the air-bone gap were similar for small fenestra stapedotomy and large fenestra techniques. Small fenestra stapedotomy had a slightly lower rate of postoperative sensorineural hearing loss, particularly at higher frequencies. In patients undergoing the small fenestra technique, no significant differences were found in postoperative air-bone gap closure or postoperative sensorineural hearing loss, regardless of whether the fenestra was produced by laser or microdrill.

*Conclusions.*—Although there was a statistically significant difference between the large and small fenestra methods in postoperative sensorineural hearing loss at higher frequency, this difference is probably not significant clinically. Thus, similar good results can be obtained by an experienced surgeon using the large or small fenestra method. The laser and microdrill also appear to be equally safe and effective in the creation of the fenestra.

▶ A small percentage of ear surgeons feel that the laser is essential for stapedectomy and/or stapedotomy. My personal findings are congruent with these authors', who find that the experience of the surgeon is more important than what tools are used. They find that, whether a microdrill or a laser is used, equally good results can be obtained. I do not use the laser during stapedectomy and find that my results have been better in recent years than they were in former years. The fewer pieces of equipment I have to cope with, the easier it is to concentrate on the pathologic findings and the technique, all of which benefits the patient.

**M.M. Paparella, M.D.**

## Stapedectomy in Patients With Small Air-Bone Gaps

Lippy WH, Burkey JM, Schuring AG, et al (Warren Otologic Group, Ohio)
*Laryngoscope* 107:919–922, 1997                    4–6

*Introduction.*—Success rates have been high (up to 97%) in patients treated with stapedectomy to eliminate a conductive hearing loss or a conductive component in a mixed hearing loss resulting from otosclerosis.

The minimum air-bone gap proposed as an indicator for stapedectomy has ranged from less than 25 dB to 40 dB. In some cases, however, the primary author has performed stapedectomies in patients with very small air-bone gaps. The results for such patients were examined to provide criteria for outcome.

*Methods.*—Clinical records were reviewed to identify patients who had a stapedectomy to correct an air-bone gap of 10 dB or less. In most cases, surgery was undertaken to prevent the need for a hearing aid or to restore symmetrical hearing. Air-bone gap was confirmed preoperatively by audiologists. Only patients with word recognition scores (WRSs) of 80% or better were selected for surgery. The ear was explored, but stapedectomy was performed only if otosclerosis was found. Results of baseline audiograms were compared with tests performed 6 months postoperatively.

*Results.*—The 154 patients who underwent surgery represented 1.1% of the total number of stapedectomies, stapedial mobilizations, and explorations performed over a 35-year period. The mean patient age was 52.6 years, and 68.2% were women. Stapedectomy was performed in 136, a stapedial mobilization in 1, and exploration in only 17. Average hearing thresholds after stapedectomy improved through the speech frequencies of 500, 1,000, and 2,000 Hz, but they were essentially unchanged at 4,000 Hz. Surgery had no effect on mean WRSs. The mean pure-tone average (PTA) hearing improvement was 16.7 dB, and 80.5% of patients had a PTA hearing improvement greater than the largest preoperative air-bone gap (10 dB). A PTA closure down to 0 dB was achieved in 89.7% of patients receiving stapedectomies.

*Conclusion.*—Stapedectomy was effective in treating selected patients with a small air-bone gap ($\leq$10 dB) caused by otosclerosis. Surgery was performed only when patients' history and otologic examination, and the results of audiometric, impedance, and tuning fork tests were consistent with otosclerosis.

▶ Carhart's notch, or the measurement of prestapedectomy thresholds for bone conduction, is notoriously difficult. This may be another reason why these patients with small air-bone gaps have such good results. I find that in my patients, similarly, half or more have closure of the preoperative air-bone gap. Thus, an apparently small air-bone gap might have a better result postoperatively than otherwise might be anticipated. These patients also should always have testing done with a tuning fork, Weber testing, and particularly Rinne testing. This will afford a way of assessing the accuracy of the air-bone gap as measured by audiometry. A general rule I follow is that if patients do not have a definitely negative Rinne at both 500 and 1,000 cps, I do not generally consider them adequate candidates for stapedectomy. This rule could apply to these patients with small air-bone gaps as well, and often is more revealing than audiological measurement because of the Carhart's notch phenomenon.

**M.M. Paparella, M.D.**

**Revision Stapedectomy: Intraoperative Findings, Results, and Review of the Literature**

Han WW, Incesulu A, McKenna MJ, et al (Harvard Med School, Boston; Massachusetts Eye and Ear Infirmary, Boston; Brigham and Women's Hosp, Boston)

*Laryngoscope* 107:1185–1192, 1997                                    4–7

*Introduction.*—Postoperative hearing results have not been as good in revision stapedectomies as in primary cases. A retrospective review of 74 revision procedures was conducted to evaluate the surgical techniques employed, assess postrevision hearing outcomes, and determine the mechanisms of primary stapedectomy failure and predictors of surgical results.

*Methods.*—The 74 consecutive revision stapedectomies were performed in 64 patients from 1986 to 1995. Three surgeons performed all the operations using the same techniques. Indications for revision surgery were recurrent or persistent conductive hearing loss or vertigo. Postoperative audiologic evaluations were conducted at 6 weeks and at 1-year intervals. The threshold at 4,000 Hz was used instead of at 3,000 Hz to calculate pure-tone average (PTA).

*Results.*—The 74 cases included 56 first revisions, 16 second revisions, and 2 third revisions. Most patients (82.4%) underwent revision because of recurrent conductive hearing loss. The mean interval between primary and revision surgeries was 81.9 months; mean follow-up after revision was 18.2 months. Common intraoperative findings were incus erosion (particularly in multiple revisions), prosthesis displacement, and oval window closure. The success rate of postoperative air-bone gap closure to within 10 dB after revision surgery was 51.6% when calculated by postoperative air minus preoperative bone. The rate was slightly lower (45.6%) when American Academy of Otolaryngology—Head and Neck Surgery guidelines (postoperative air minus postoperative bone) were used. Hearing results after revision were worse in patients who had persistent conductive hearing loss after the initial procedure. There were 4 cases of sensorineural hearing loss. Postoperative results were not affected by use of the argon laser versus a handheld drill or by the ossicle to which the prosthesis was attached.

*Discussion.*—There is agreement that revision stapedectomy surgery is more technically challenging than a primary procedure, and patients are less likely to have optimal hearing results. Outcome was better in patients who showed improvement at primary stapedectomy and subsequently experienced recurrent conductive hearing loss or vertigo than among those whose initial results were unsatisfactory.

▶ Revision stapedectomy can be a very difficult procedure, and it is helpful if the surgeon has experience in dealing with cases of revision, since myriad observations can be identified, as are identified in this study. This study also points out the pitfalls and problems of the various pathologic conditions that can occur after stapedectomy, and the problems encountered in attempts to resolve those difficulties. As always in revisional stapedectomy, the results certainly will not be as desirable as in primary stapedectomy, a fact indicated by long-term follow-up of these cases of revision.

**M.M. Paparella, M.D.**

### Revision Stapes Surgery

Somers T, Govaerts P, de Varebeke SJ, et al (Univ of Antwerp, Belgium)
*J Laryngol Otol* 111:233–239, 1997                                                4–8

*Background.*—The relative frequency of revision stapes operations is increasing. The prognosis of such surgery was investigated in a retrospective analysis of 1 series.

*Methods.*—Data on 332 otosclerosis revision operations were analyzed. The type of procedure done primarily, the alleged cause of failure, and the technical solution applied were noted.

*Findings.*—Revision surgery was required in 3.4% of patients undergoing primary total stapedectomy, 2.2% undergoing partial stapedectomy, and 2% undergoing stapedotomy. The reason for revision surgery varied according to the initial procedure. A migrated piston, too short piston, and a lateralized graft occurred almost exclusively after total stapedectomies. The median hearing gain after revision of stapedotomy and partial stapedectomy was greater than after revision surgery for total stapedectomy but significantly lower than that after primary surgery. The outcomes of revision surgery were better after primary interventions with the use of a piston or piston–wire than after primary interventions with a wire-type prosthesis. The risk for sensorineural loss associated with revision surgery was 1%, which was no higher than that after primary surgery (Figs 1 and 2).

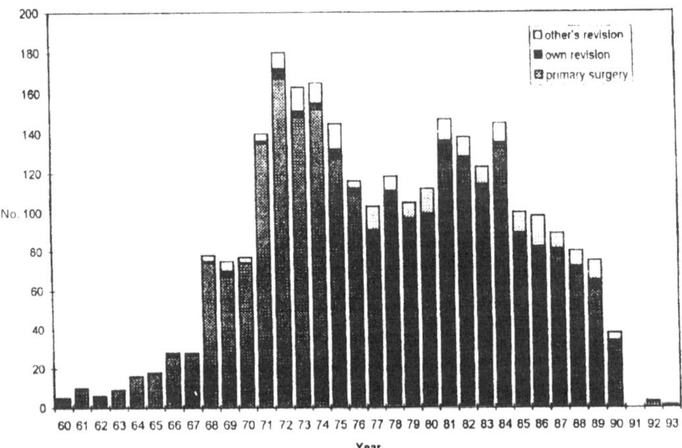


FIGURE 1.—Number of otosclerosis operations performed yearly by J. Marquet during his career, with emphasis on incidence of revision surgery in comparison with primary surgery. (Courtesy of Somers T, Govaerts P, de Varebeke SJ, et al: Revision stapes surgery. *J Laryngol Otol* 111:233–239, 1997.)

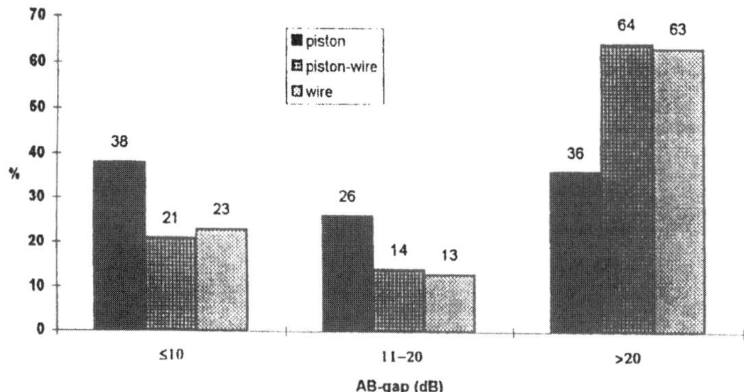


FIGURE 2.—Air-bone (AB) gap closure 6 months after revision according to the prosthetic material used during primary surgery. (Courtesy of Somers T, Govaerts P, de Varebeke SJ, et al: Revision stapes surgery. *J Laryngol Otol* 111:233–239, 1997.)

*Conclusions.*—The risk for sensorineural loss is apparently no greater after revision surgery than after primary surgery, as long as fibrosis in the oval window is managed with extreme care. The stapedotomy method is the preferred primary method, as the need for revision surgery is reduced after this procedure and the hearing outcomes after stapedotomy revisions are better than after stapedectomy revision surgery.

▶ These authors describe their findings and results in 332 patients with otosclerosis requiring revisional procedures. They identify the pathologic conditions found in such cases and conclude that the need for revisional surgery was higher after primary total stapedectomy (3.4%) than after partial stapedectomy (2.2%) or stapedotomy (2%). I wonder if this difference is statistically significant. Nevertheless, these observations are of interest and should be compared with other series and the experience of others who perform revisional procedures on the stapes.

**M.M. Paparella, M.D.**

# 5 Facial Nerve and Tumors

**Prognostic Factors in Carcinoma of the External Auditory Canal**
Testa JRG, Fukuda Y, Kowalski LP (Universidade Federal de São Paulo, Brazil; AC Camargo Hosp, São Paulo, Brazil)
*Arch Otolaryngol Head Neck Surg* 123:720–724, 1997                5–1

*Introduction.*—Less than 1% of malignant tumors of the head and neck are carcinomas of the external auditory canal. Radiography shows the size of the tumor and the adjacent structures involved. Treatment is by complete resection of the tumor, preferably en bloc. A 42-year carcinoma experience with external auditory canal (EAC) at a single medical center was reviewed to determine the prognostic factors associated with this tumor.

*Patients.*—The experience included 79 patients: 56 men and 23 women; mean age was 62 years. The tumors were squamous cell carcinomas in 56% of patients and basal cell carcinomas in 43%. Thirty-four patients had stage T1 to T2 tumors, 43 had stage T3 to T4 tumors, and 2 had stage TX tumors. Nodal staging was N0 in 68 patients and N1 in 11. Fifty-nine patients were initially treated by surgery, consisting of meatal resection in 47%, partial resection of the temporal bone in 19%, subtotal resection of the temporal bone in 8%, and total resection in 1%. Nine patients were initially treated by radiotherapy, and 11 received only supportive therapy. Patients' outcomes and prognostic factors were analyzed.

*Results.*—Twenty-nine patients had local recurrences and 2 had metastasis to the neck. Patients treated by surgery had a 5-year survival rate of 65%, compared with 29% for those treated by radiotherapy and 63% for those treated by a combination of surgery and radiotherapy. Survival was significantly better for the patients with basal cell carcinoma and for patients with disease in lower stages, but it was unaffected by the type of surgery performed. On univariate analysis, survival was significantly related to type of tumor, involvement of bone, and stage of the tumor.

*Conclusion.*—For patients with squamous cell carcinoma of the EAC, early diagnosis and radical surgery are the keys to survival. Type of tumor, involvement of bone, and stage of the tumor are significant prognostic factors. The staging system used for surgically treated squamous cell carcinoma of the ear is validated by these findings.

▶ These authors clearly describe how diseases of the EAC suspected of being carcinomas or tumors should be watched and treated aggressively. As the authors state, every effort must be undertaken to make an early diagnosis and perform appropriate, but radical, surgical resection of squamous cell carcinomas in the EAC before invasion and serious problems can develop. We are in total agreement with this thesis. It is important for the practicing otolaryngologist to consider tumors that can develop in the EAC and to be suspicious of any lesion that does not heal or that continues to suggest a form of squamous cell carcinoma or another type of tumor, benign or malignant.

**M.M. Paparella, M.D.**

---

**Anomalously Coursing Facial Nerves Above and Below the Oval Window: Three Case Reports**
Huang T-S (Chang Gung Mem Hosp, Taiwan, Republic of China)
*Otolaryngol Head Neck Surg* 116:438–441, 1997                5–2

---

*Introduction.*—Instances of an anomalously coursing, dehiscent facial nerve either covering the oval window or running inferior to it along the bony promontory are extremely rare. Described are 3 patients with facial nerves coursing over and below the oval window.

*Case 1.*—A man, 41, was given a diagnosis of otosclerosis on follow-up evaluation of hearing impairment in the right ear since early childhood. During a middle-ear exploration, the facial nerve was found to be dehiscent and running inferiorly to the oval window along the promontory wall (Fig 2). A small-fenestra stapedotomy was performed. The patient experienced no facial paralysis after surgery and regained some hearing.

*Case 2.*—A woman, 38, was seen for impaired hearing in her left ear of 10 years' duration. The left middle ear was explored for a tentative diagnosis of congenital conductive deafness. An exposed, prolapsing facial nerve was seen coursing over and obscuring the entire oval window. The stapedial superstructure was missing, and the stapedial tendon was connected to the long process of the incus. An ossicular reconstruction was attempted; the cleft was too narrow to permit unambiguous identification, so contact with a footplate may or may not have been achieved. At follow-up, hearing was neither improved or worsened.

*Case 3.*—A woman, 23, was examined for bilateral hearing loss since childhood. A surgical exploration of the right ear was performed for a diagnosis of bilateral otosclerosis. A dehiscent facial nerve was observed to overlay and occlude the oval window; the

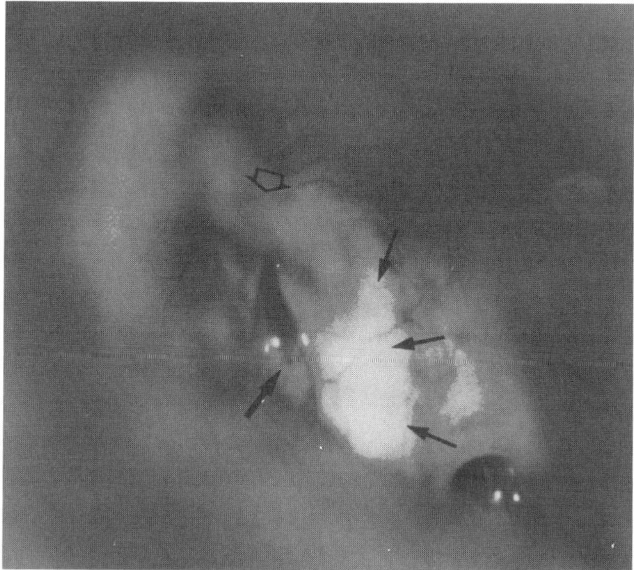

**FIGURE 2.**—Abnormal coursing of dehiscent facial nerve (*short arrows*) below oval window, ill-defined footplate of stapes (*long arrow*), and deformed and shortened incus (*blank arrow*) in case 1. (Courtesy of Huang T-S: Anomalously coursing facial nerves above and below the oval window: Three case reports. *Otolaryngol Head Neck Surg* 116:438–441, 1997.)

anterior and posterior crura of the stapes were not connected to the footplate and were resting on the facial nerve (Fig 4), and the tympanic sulcus was circumferentially contracted relative to the external ear canal. The operation was aborted because of fear of damaging the facial nerve. Surgery on the left ear was not at-

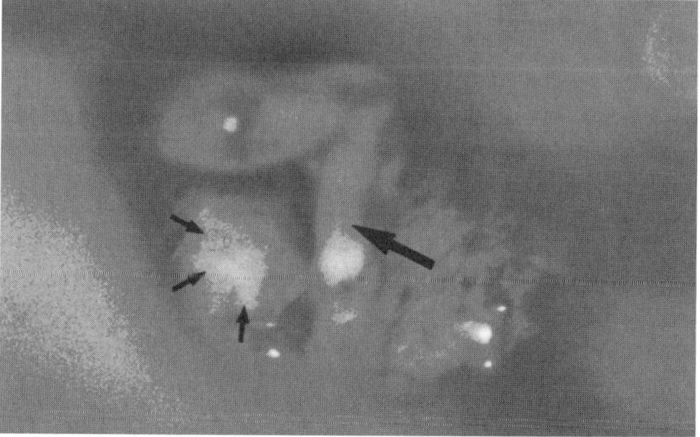

**FIGURE 4.**—Abnormal coursing of dehiscent facial nerve (*short arrows*) over oval window and remnant of crura (*long arrow*) resting on facial nerve in case 3. (Courtesy of Huang T-S: Anomalously coursing facial nerves above and below the oval window: Three case reports. *Otolaryngol Head Neck Surg* 116:438–441, 1997.)

tempted because symptoms and test results for both ears were similar and hearing improvement was not expected.

*Conclusion.*—Reported are 3 patients with rare anomalously coursing facial nerves and 1 coincidence of an abnormally contracted tympanic ring. These findings should alert surgeons to risk of surgical damage.

▶ I have observed findings in other patients during the past several decades similar to the ones that this author indicates in these 3 patients. It is rare, but the facial nerve may be seen as either a bifurcated nerve or a single nerve below the oval window. This should be looked for, especially during reconstruction and when dealing with congenital otologic problems.

**M.M. Paparella, M.D.**

---

**Acute Otitis Media and Facial Paralysis in Children**
Elliott CA, Zalzal GH, Gottlieb WR (George Washington Univ, Washington, DC)
*Ann Otol Rhinol Laryngol* 105:58–62, 1996                    5–3

---

*Background.*—Acute otitis media can be associated with incomplete facial paralysis, which resolves after myringotomy and adequate antibiotic treatment. However, such paralysis may progress to complete paralysis, despite seemingly adequate treatment. The outcomes of facial paralysis associated with acute otitis media in patients treated without facial nerve decompression were investigated.

*Methods and Findings.*—Ten children with facial paralysis after the onset of acute otitis media were included. Eight had incomplete paralysis, and 2, complete paralysis. In the first group, 7 patients had a rapid return of function after myringotomy and IV antibiotics. The remaining patient in this group had a delayed recovery, with return of complete function taking 9 months. In the 2 children with complete paralysis, mastoidectomy was needed to control otorrhea and fever after initial myringotomy and antibiotic therapy. Recovery was prolonged in both of these patients, requiring 3 and 7 months, respectively.

*Conclusions.*—Wide myringotomy and antibiotic treatment result in rapid improvement in most patients with incomplete paralysis associated with acute otitis media. Patients with complete paralysis have a more protracted recovery. However, excellent return of function can be expected with mastoidectomy without facial nerve decompression.

▶ These authors describe very nicely how acute otitis media can result in incomplete or complete facial paralysis. A myringotomy will allow pus to exit the middle ear. If, after myringotomy and appropriate antibiotics, paralysis continues, the patient may be a candidate for a simple mastoidectomy, as the authors indicate. We find that assessing these patients for neurapraxia vs. axonotmesis is valid, just as we would assess patients who have Bell's palsy. If the paralysis persists, however, simple mastoidectomy and decompression can be considered. When these kinds of patients are decompressed, however, we do not open the sheath but simply remove diseased bone from over the Fallopian canal.

**M.M. Paparella, M.D.**

**Facial Nerve Palsy in Mastoid Surgery**
Nilssen ELK, Wormald PJ (Groote Schuur Hosp, Cape Town, Republic of South Africa)
*J Laryngol Otol* 111:113–116, 1997                                  5–4

*Background.*—With the introduction of the microscope and otologic drill, the risk of facial nerve injury during mastoid surgery has declined markedly. However, the facial nerve continues to be at risk during mastoid surgery. There are no recent publications that accurately quantify the incidence of this severe complication or that discuss its management.

*Methods and Findings.*—A total of 1,024 consecutive mastoidectomies done between 1985 and 1994 were reviewed. Seventeen palsies occurred. Seven were complete, and 10 were incomplete. Four patients with complete palsies had decompression only and recovered to House Brackmann grade 2 or better. The remaining 3 had decompression and grafting, of whom 2 (available for follow-up) recovered to House Brackmann grade 4 only. All patients with partial palsies (except for 1 lost to follow-up) treated conservatively with pack removal, toilet, and topical therapy recovered to House Brackmann grade 2 or better.

*Conclusions.*—Although many patients with facial nerve palsy after mastoid surgery can have acceptable outcomes with proper treatment, residual dysfunction is likely to occur in patients with severe injuries. These patients may experience many months of disability and cosmetic disfigurement. Otologic surgeons must be careful to avoid this complication.

▶ These authors describe a problem important to all otologic surgeons: the problem of facial nerve palsy resulting from mastoid surgery. They identified 17 palsies in their series; 7 were complete and 10 were incomplete. They describe a useful protocol to follow in management of these patients. They discuss techniques that may allow the surgeon to avoid trauma to the facial nerve. The experience and skill of the surgeon play a role, but the ability to identify and deal with pathologic and anatomical–developmental anomalies will also aid in avoiding facial nerve palsy. An interesting survey that appeared in the literature recently indicates that experienced surgeons tend not to require monitoring of the facial nerve during mastoid surgery, although younger surgeons find that this is helpful to them. Certainly, they should use whatever helps them to enhance safety while at the same time treating the disease process.

**M.M. Paparella, M.D.**

### Treatment of Ramsay Hunt Syndrome With Acyclovir-Prednisone: Significance of Early Diagnosis and Treatment

Murakami S, Hato N, Horiuchi J, et al (Ehime Univ, Japan)
*Ann Neurol* 41:353–357, 1997                                              5–5

*Background.*—Ramsay Hunt syndrome is characterized by paralysis of the facial nerve and vestibulocochlear dysfunction associated with the eruption of varicella-zoster virus (VZV) on the pinna. It is the second most common cause of acute facial paralysis. The antiviral agent acyclovir is used to treat this syndrome, but its effectiveness has not been well established. A retrospective analysis was performed of the effects of combined therapy using acyclovir and prednisone on the facial nerve and on recovery of hearing of 80 patients with Ramsay Hunt syndrome.

*Study Design.*—The study group consisted of 41 men and 39 women between the ages of 15 and 75 years with facial paralysis attributable to Ramsay Hunt syndrome, seen from 1989 to 1995. Twenty-two of these patients also had hearing loss. Treatment was initiated as patients were seen from 1–10 days after onset. Evaluation of voluntary facial movement and nerve excitability testing (NET) were performed to analyze the effect of treatment on function in the facial nerve. Patients were divided into 3 groups: group A, treatment initiated within 3 days of the onset of facial paralysis; group B, between 4 and 7 days after onset; and group C, between 8 and 10 days after onset. The effect of IV vs. oral administration was also examined.

*Results.*—Among the 28 patients who initiated treatment within 3 days of the onset of facial paralysis, complete recovery occurred in 75%. Among the 23 patients who initiated treatment more than 7 days after the onset of facial paralysis, recovery was complete in only 30%. The difference between these 2 groups was significant. Nerve excitability testing demonstrated that early treatment with acyclovir-prednisone reduced degeneration of nerve. Hearing recovery was also improved among patients who received early treatment. There was no significant difference in outcome between IV and oral treatment.

*Conclusions.*—This retrospective, observational study indicated that early treatment with acyclovir-prednisone has a beneficial effect on the outcome for patients with Ramsay Hunt syndrome. A reliable test to detect this syndrome should be developed and disseminated, to permit treatment to be initiated as early as possible.

▶ These authors have a fairly large series of patients who have Ramsay Hunt syndrome. The study emphasizes the use of acyclovir-prednisone as treatment in 80 patients with Ramsay Hunt. The only way to do a double-blind study, of course, is to assess patients with and without the use of these drugs, individually and/or together. Nevertheless, this study suggests that the combination of drugs utilized may be beneficial for patients, particularly when used as early as possible.

**M.M. Paparella, M.D.**

**Uncommon Lesions Presenting as Tumors of the Internal Auditory Canal and Cerebellopontine Angle**
Kohan D, Downey LL, Lim J, et al (New York Univ; Beth Israel Med Ctr, New York)
*Am J Otol* 18:386–392, 1997                                              5–6

*Introduction.*—Distinguishing among intracranial lesions has important therapeutic and prognostic implications. Almost 10% of all intracranial tumors are located at the cerebellopontine angle (CPA) and internal auditory canal (IAC). A retrospective review of charts identified cases of surgically managed IAC and CPA tumors and analyzed these lesions for distinguishing characteristics.

*Methods.*—Of 426 surgical cases identified during the period from January 1985 to April 1996, 24 involved lesions at the CPA and IAC. The remaining patients had acoustic neuromas (90.1%) or meningiomas (4.2%). Patients with CPA or IAC were 17 women with a mean age of 40.6 years and 7 men with a mean age of 41.9 years. Imaging studies included contrast-enhanced MRI (94% of patients) and contrast-enhanced CT (16%); 1 patient had a CT cisternogram. Data on these cases were analyzed for clinical presentation, diagnostic–radiologic workup, surgical management, histologic diagnosis, and therapeutic outcome.

*Results.*—The most frequently identified tumors among CPA and IAC lesions were epidermoid cysts and lipomas (4 cases of each). Patients with epidermoids experienced slow-onset hearing loss and aural fullness, and 1 with a large tumor had seizures. Patients with lipomas had slowly progressive cochleovestibular symptoms; 1 had a mild facial palsy. Two patients with slowly progressive profound sensorineural hearing loss were found to have facial nerve neuromas. Arachnoid cysts were detected in 2 patients with slowly progressive cochleovestibular complaints. Choroid plexus papillomas were diagnosed in 2 patients, 1 with mild weakness in a lower extremity, headaches, and aural fullness, and another with disequilibrium. Contrast-enhanced MRI demonstrated metastatic adenocarcinomas (Fig 2) in 2 patients and an invasive malignant lymphoma in 1 patient (Fig 3). Other lesions were represented by 1 case each: metastatic neuroblastoma, ependymoma, cholesterol cyst, angioleiomyoma, venous hemangioma, cavernous angioma, and pontine glioma.

*Conclusion.*—Tumor differentiation among lesions of the CPA and IAC is challenging, but a comprehensive picture of the pathology may be achieved by integrating clinical history, physical findings, audiovestibular test results, and imaging studies, especially MRI. Although the variety of lesions in these areas is considerable, their clinical manifestations are often similar.

▶ This article is helpful in reminding us that not all lesions in the cerebellopontine angle tumor are vestibular schwannomas (or acoustic tumors). One can have cholesteatomas, as this article indicates. These tumors include a variety of types including primary and sometimes secondary, or

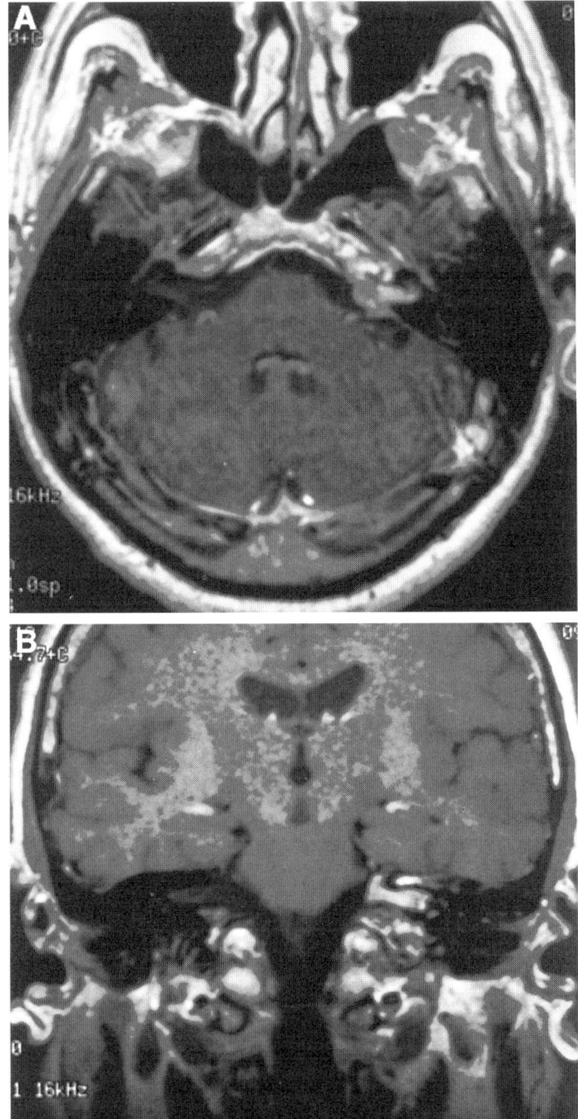

FIGURE 2.—Left IAC metastatic pulmonary adenocarcinoma. MR T1-weighted image with contrast axial (A) and coronal (B) views demonstrate heterogeneous lesions filling IAC. C, black and white micrograph of hematoxylin-eosin stain demonstrates adenocarcinoma. (Courtesy of Kohan D, Downey LL, Lim J, et al: Uncommon lesions presenting as tumors of the internal auditory canal and cerebello-pontine angle. *Am J Otol* 18:386–392, 1997.)

(*Continued*)

FIGURE 2 (cont.)

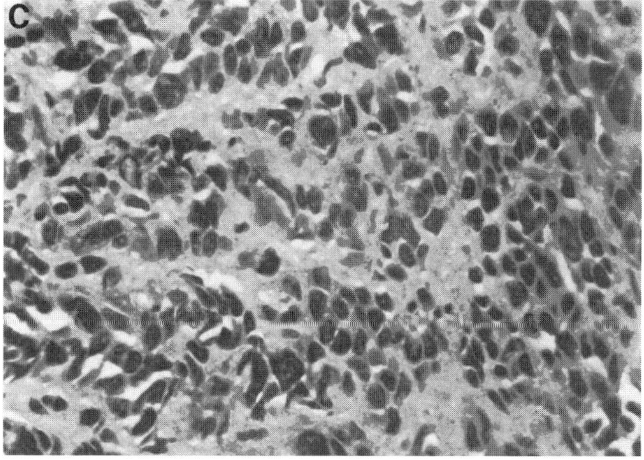

metastatic, lesions. This article presents the helpful fact that sometimes preoperative imaging and surgical findings show distinguishing characteristics of some of these unusual types of tumors in the cerebellopontine angle and in the internal auditory canal.

**M.M. Paparella, M.D.**

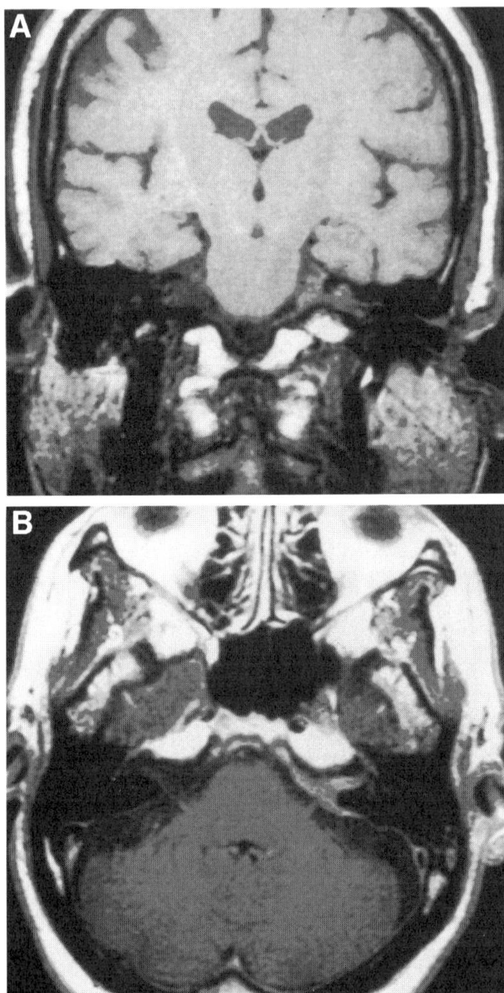

FIGURE 3.—Left IAC and cerebellopontine angle malignant lymphoma. **A,** coronal MR T1-weighted noncontrast scan shows lesion. MR T1-weighted images with contrast axial (**B**) and coronal (**C**) views demonstrate tumor enhancement and dural tail. (Courtesy of Kohan D, Downey LL, Lim J, et al: Uncommon lesions presenting as tumors of the internal auditory canal and cerebellopontine angle. *Am J Otol* 18:386–392, 1997.)

(Continued)

FIGURE 3 (cont.)

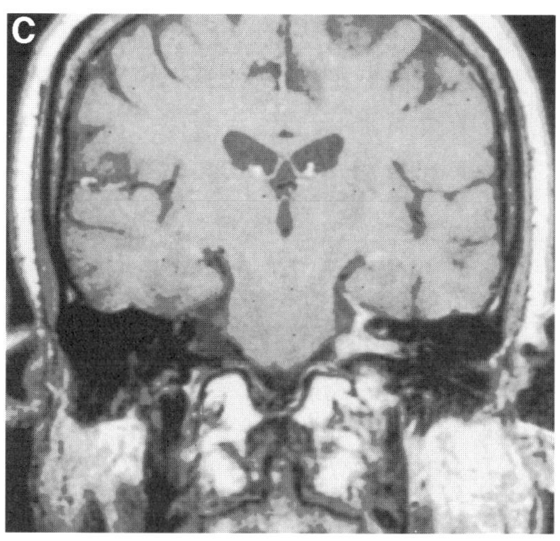


## Management of 1,000 Vestibular Schwannomas (Acoustic Neuromas): Clinical Presentation

Matthies C, Samii M (Nordstadt Hosp, Hannover, Germany)
*Neurosurgery* 40:1–10, 1997                                            5–7

*Purpose.*—During the last few decades, continued advances have occurred in the management of vestibular schwannomas (VS), also called acoustic neuromas. The symptoms of VS and their impact on the surgical results have been well studied. However, there are still few data on how the clinical characteristics of the patient correlate with the size or extension of the tumor or the cranial nerve damage that has occurred. The clinical presentation of 1,000 cases of VS was analyzed.

*Methods.*—One of the authors operated on 1,000 VS during a 15-year period. A total of 962 patients were operated on, consisting of 522 females and 440 males, with a mean age of 48 and 45 years, respectively. The incidence of subjective complaints was analyzed in terms of the objective morbidity. The sequence and duration of symptoms were examined, and the relationship between symptoms and tumor size and extension was assessed.

*Results.*—The symptoms were related to the acoustic nerve in 95% of cases, the vestibular nerve in 61%, the trigeminal nerve in 9%, and the facial nerve in 6%. Hearing loss had been present for a mean of 3.7 years, facial paresis for 1.9 years, and trigeminal disturbances for 1.3 years. There was no direct correlation between the incidence and duration of symptoms and the size of the tumor. The diagnosis was often made as a result of symptoms related to tumor extension—for example, trigeminal disturbances in patients with large tumors compressing the brain stem, or tinnitus in patients with small neuromas. The duration of symptoms was shorter in patients with symptoms related to the trigeminal or facial nerve. The patients subjectively perceived only one third to two thirds of the nerve disturbances demonstrated.

Twenty-three percent of patients had chronic deafness before surgery, whereas 3% had sudden deafness. Sudden deafness sometimes occurred in a patient with a long-standing but moderate hearing deficit. Tinnitus was more likely in hearing patients, but 46% of patients with preoperative deafness still had tinnitus. Vestibular disturbances tended to manifest as unsteadiness while walking or as vertigo. The vestibular symptoms were usually fluctuating rather than constant.

*Conclusions.*—The clinical findings in patients with VS may not reflect underlying differences in tumor biology. Small intrameatal tumors may have a duration of symptoms suggestive of larger tumors, and commonly cause vestibular symptoms and tinnitus. In contrast, patients with larger tumors compressing the brain stem may be younger and have a shorter duration of symptoms. Both of these characteristics suggest fast tumor growth. The analysis may lend new insight into the dynamics of tumor growth and the affected neural tissues.

▶ It is unusual to see such a large number of tumors reviewed in terms of clinical presentation. I think that this summary is helpful for general otolaryngologists/otologists, so that they can better identify these lesions in patients seen in their offices.

**M.M. Paparella, M.D.**

---

**Management of 1,000 Vestibular Schwannomas (Acoustic Neuromas): The Facial Nerve—Preservation and Restitution of Function**
Samii M, Matthies C (Nordstadt Hosp, Hannover, Germany)
*Neurosurgery* 40:684–695, 1997                                    5–8

---

*Background.*—Facial nerve paresis or paralysis continues to be a common sequela of surgery for vestibular schwannomas. Criteria for the indication, timing, and type of treatment for patients with palsies despite anatomical nerve continuity and for patients with loss of anatomical continuity were defined.

*Methods.*—Between 1978 and 1993, 1,000 vestibular schwannomas were treated surgically at the Nordstadt Hospital. Complete removal was possible in 979 patients. In 21, removal was deliberately partial. The facial nerve was preserved anatomically in 93% and was anatomically severed in 6%. In the 42 patients with nerve discontinuity, immediate nerve reconstruction was performed in the same surgical setting using 1 of the following procedures: within the cerbellopontine angle, intracranial–in-

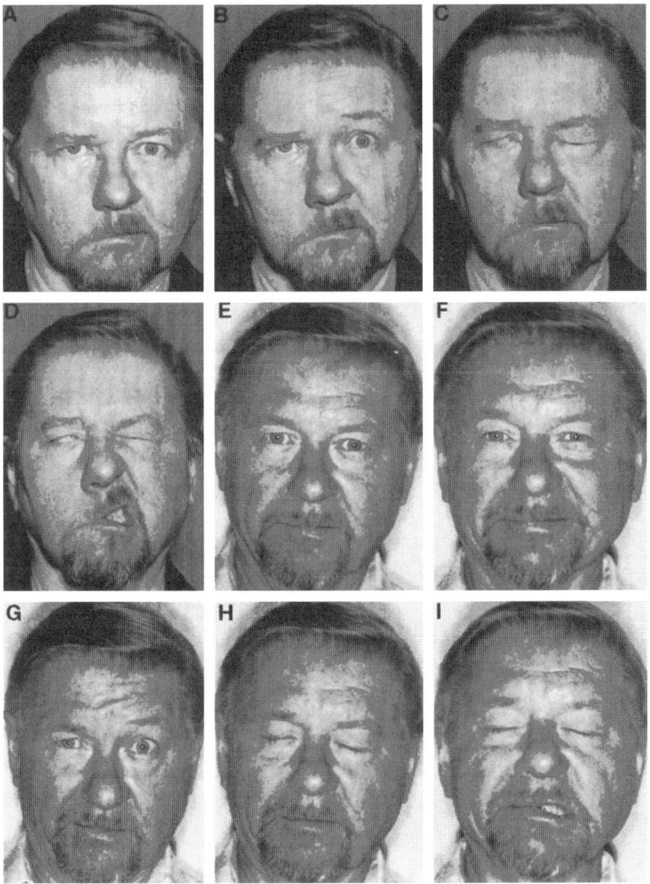

FIGURE 1.—At resection of a vestibular schwannoma, facial nerve discontinuity was bridged by a 20-mm sural transplant for an intracranial reconstruction in this 56-year-old man. His initial paralysis with facial asymmetry (**A**), lack of frowning (**B**), lagophthalmus (**C**), and lack of any mouth control on the right (**D**) started to improve after 5 months, and a satisfactory result was documented after 2 years (**E–I**). There is good facial symmetry at rest (**E**), during movement with good emotional expressivity (**F**), some recovery of frowning (**G**), complete eye closure (**H**), and some mouth angle control and some residual autoparalytic syndrome (**I**). (Courtesy of Samii M, Matthies C: Management of 1,000 vestibular schwannomas (acoustic neuromas): The facial nerve—preservation and restitution of function. *Neurosurgery* 40:684–695, 1997.)

tratemporal, or intracranial–extracranial. Early reanimation by combination with the hypoglossal nerve was achieved in most patients with loss of the proximal facial nerve stump at the brainstem within weeks after surgery. A hypoglossal–facial combination was applied in a few patients with anatomical nerve continuity but absence of reinnervation for 10–12 months. Patients with partial or complete palsies were treated in a special follow-up program of regular controls and modulation of physiotherapeutic treatment every 3–6 months.

*Findings.*—Sixty-one percent to 70% of patients undergoing intracranial nerve reconstruction at the cerebellopontine angle regained complete eye closure, and the overall result was comparable to House-Brackmann grade 3. In 79% of patients undergoing hypoglossal–facial reanimation, outcomes were comparable to grade 3. The interval between paralysis onset and the reconstructive procedure was important to the quality of outcome (Fig 1).

*Conclusions.*—Intraoperative monitoring aids in the preservation of facial nerve continuity and function. Early nerve reconstruction is indicated when continuity is lost. A scheduled follow-up program for all patients with incomplete or complete palsies is important.

▶ This article was selected because it is of interest from 2 points of view: (1) it involves an extremely large collection of cases (1,000 vestibular schwannomas) and (2) it was published in a neurosurgical journal by Drs. Samii and Matthies. The facial nerve was preserved in 93% of their cases and was anatomically severed in 60 cases or 6%. It is interesting to compare results of preservation with results indicated in publications by neurotologists in collaborative association with neurosurgery. Up to 70% of the patients regained complete eye closure after intracranial nerve reconstruction, which, to me at least, was a surprisingly good result. This article will be interesting when neurotologists compare their results to large series such as described here by neurosurgeons.

**M.M. Paparella, M.D.**

---

**Management of Acoustic Neuroma in the Elderly Population**
Glasscock ME III, Pappas DG Jr, Manolidis S, et al (Otology Group, Nashville, Tenn; Pappas Ear Clinic, Birmingham, Ala)
*Am J Otol* 18:236–242, 1997                                                      5–9

---

*Introduction.*—Acoustic neuromas (AN) are being detected earlier because of advances in audiologic and imaging techniques. Age-related factors make removal of small, asymptomatic ANs in elderly patients controversial. Nonoperative and operative experience in patients 70 years and older are described.

*Methods.*—Tumor size was observed by serial imaging for a mean of 28.5 months in 34 elderly patients. Of these, 8 subsequently underwent surgery for significant growth of the tumor. Twelve patients were managed surgically at the time of diagnosis. The mean follow-up time was 49.3 months.

*Results.*—The overall mean tumor size at the initial visit was 1.3 cm (Fig 1). The mean annual rate of growth of the tumor for patients in the watched group was 0.29 cm per year (Fig 2). Fifteen patients had no growth of the tumor, or regression in its size, during follow-up. Eight patients experienced accelerated tumor growth. Of these, 4 patients described symptoms of renewed onset. The mean rate of growth in tumors in

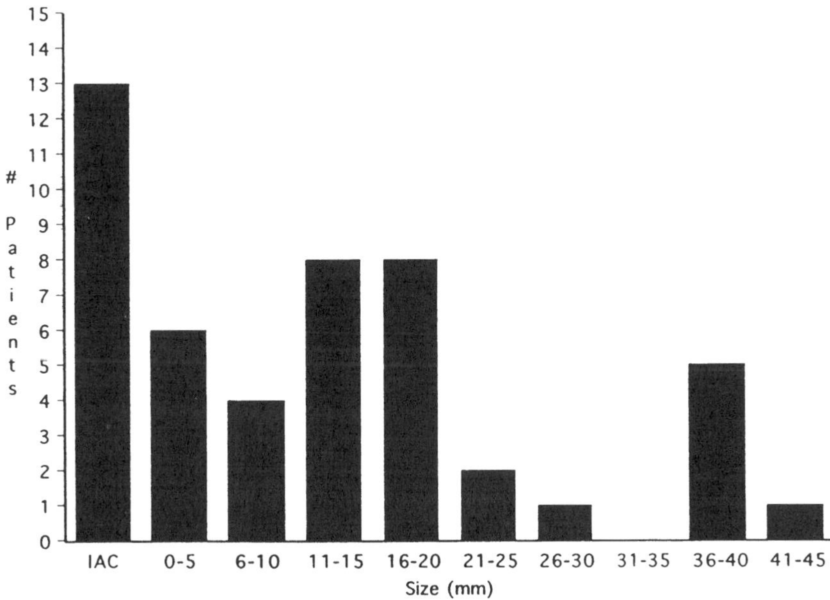


**FIGURE 1.**—Distribution of size of tumors. (Courtesy of Glasscock ME III, Pappas DG Jr, Manolidis S, et al: Management of acoustic neuroma in the elderly population. *Am J Otol* 18:236–242, 1997.)

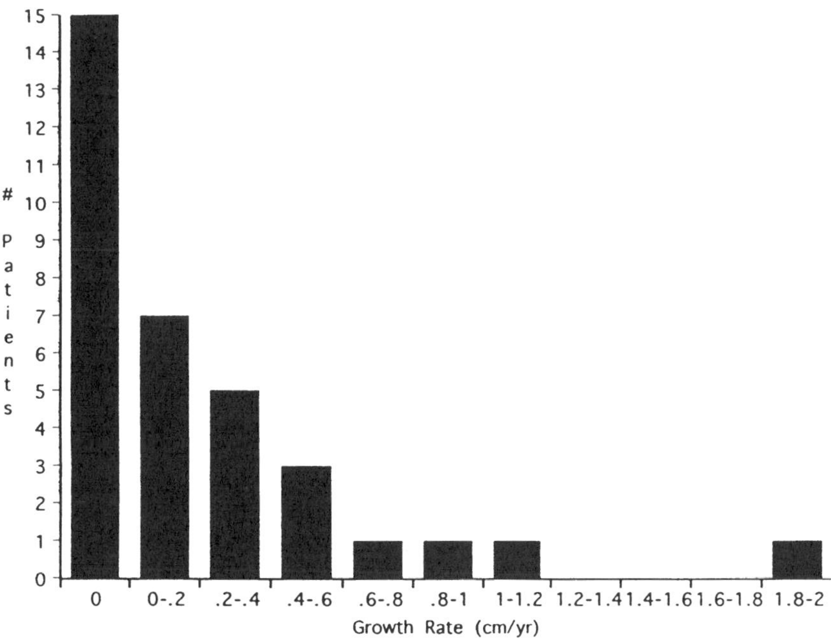


**FIGURE 2.**—Distribution of growth rate of tumors. (Courtesy of Glasscock ME III, Pappas DG Jr, Manolidis S, et al: Management of acoustic neuroma in the elderly population. *Am J Otol* 18:236–242, 1997.)

this cohort was 0.82 cm per year. Excluding the 8 patients whose nonoperative management failed, the rate of growth of the tumors in the remaining 26 patients was 0.13 cm per year. At final followup, 30 patients were alive (23 with disease and 7 disease-free). Three patients died of unrelated causes. The mean size of tumors at the time of resection in the group undergoing surgery was 2.8 cm. Resection was reported as complete in 17 patients and near total in 3 patients. Twelve patients had postoperative complications, and 1 patient died perioperatively of a myocardial infarction after resection of the tumor.

*Conclusion.*—A trial of conservative, nonoperative management is recommended for elderly patients with small ANs. Early surgical intervention is required in patients with significant growth or size of tumors, or neurologic deterioration, to avoid the problems associated with removal of larger tumors.

▶ By assessing growth-rate factors of ANs in elderly patients, these authors have arrived at a practical and applicable solution: when elderly patients are seen with small ANs, they can be observed, but when the tumors' growth, size, or neurologic deterioration is demonstrated, surgical intervention, along with assessment of the general health status of the patient, is required to avoid complications experienced with the removal of larger tumors.

**M.M. Paparella, M.D.**

---

**Radiation-induced Tumors of the Temporal Bone**
Lustig LR, Jackler RK, Lanser MJ (Univ of California, San Francisco)
*Am J Otol* 18:230–235, 1997                                             5–10

---

*Introduction.*—Not much is known about the long-term, adverse sequellae of radiation on the temporal bone. The most serious complication of radiotherapy is probably the radiation-induced tumor. These neoplasms are rare in the temporal bone but are inclined to be aggressive and are often lethal. Five patients with radiation-induced malignant tumors of the temporal bone are described.

> *Case 1.*—A man, 42, was seen 17 years after being treated with radiotherapy and after 4 attempts at removal of an acoustic neuroma. Squamous cell carcinoma of the external auditory canal was discovered. After resection and 2 series of radiotherapy, he was disease-free at 3 years.
>
> *Case 2.*—A woman, 19, was given a diagnosis of a grade II astrocytoma and underwent a craniotomy and radiotherapy. She was seen 8 years later for progressive right-sided hearing loss. An MRI scan showed a 15- × 20- × 25-mm intensely enhanced mass involving the right petrous bone (Fig 1). A biopsy showed an osteogenic sarcoma. She received chemotherapy but died 14 months after diagnosis of the osteogenic sarcoma.

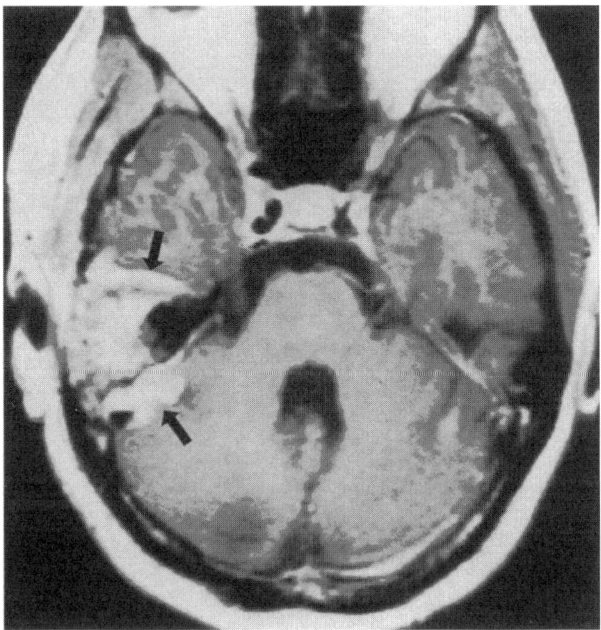

**FIGURE 1.**—Axial T1 MRI with gadolinium enhancement of case 2. The lesion is a 15- × 20- × 25-mm intensely enhancing mass involving the right petrous bone with extension into both the posterior and middle cranial fossae (*arrows*). (Courtesy of Lustig LR, Jackler RK, Lanser MJ: Radiation-induced tumors of the temporal bone. *Am J Otol* 18:230–235, 1997.)

*Case 3.*—A man, 40, was treated surgically and with radiation twice within a 14-month period for a malignant meningioma. Seven years later, he had a recurrence for which he underwent a third craniotomy and radiotherapy. Four years later, he was seen for a postauricular pain and swelling over the right mastoid process. An MRI showed an erosive lesion in the right temporal bone (Fig 2). He was surgically treated for fibrosarcoma, then underwent 5 cycles of chemotherapy. He died 1 year later.

*Case 4.*—A woman, 43, was seen for asymptomatic swelling of the left supra-auricular region 17 years after removal of a grade III astrocytoma and radiotherapy. A biopsy of the lesion revealed an osteosarcoma. She was treated with chemotherapy. An MRI scan 10 months later showed recurrence of the tumor (Fig 3). The patient died 2 months later.

*Case 5.*—A man, 30, was treated with surgery and radiotherapy for glomus jugulare. At age 46 years, he underwent aggressive resection for a low-grade fibrosarcoma arising within and displacing the old glomus tumor. He did not respond to chemotherapy and died 7 months later.

*Conclusion.*—Early results of radiosurgery are promising in some patients, but the adverse sequelae of radiotherapy are not evident for several

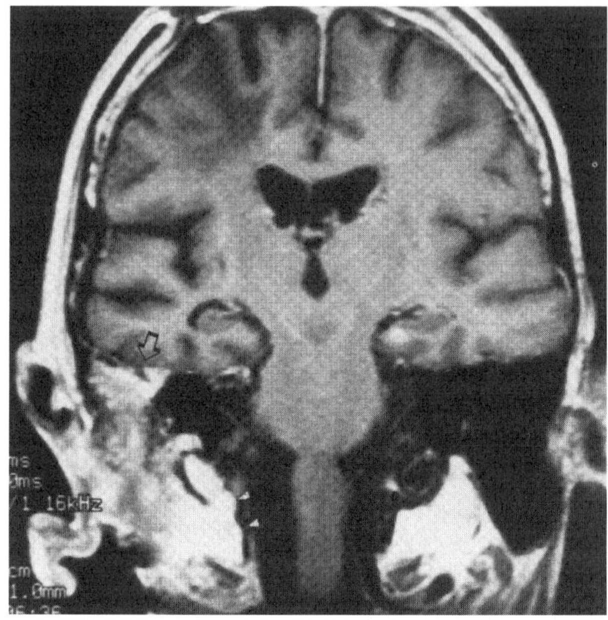

FIGURE 2.—Coronal T1 MRI with gadolinium enhancement of case 3. The radiation-induced tumor (*arrow*) involves the right temporal bone with extension of the tumor mass around the ipsilateral parotid gland and extension into the upper neck. (Courtesy of Lustig LR, Jackler RK, Lanser MJ: Radiation-induced tumors of the temporal bone. *Am J Otol* 18:230–235, 1997.)

years. Radiation-associated malignancies are highly lethal and have a latency of several years. This must be considered in young and otherwise healthy patients.

▶ Radiation administered to the temporal bone, as is well established, can cause osteoradionecrosis. It is interesting to consider the possibility that radiation may also help induce tumors in the temporal bone. Of course, one always wonders whether such tumors might have arisen in the absence of radionecrosis, that is, whether the radionecrosis may be coincidental. Nevertheless, these authors describe a compelling relationship between radiotherapy and the causes of 2 osteosarcomas, 2 fibrosarcomas, and 1 squamous cell carcinoma. The conclusion seems quite logical: if a benign tumor is present, one should eradicate it and avoid radiotherapy, whenever possible. We have had occasion to irradiate many temporal bones over the years, for a variety of reasons, and have yet to identify a radiation-induced tumor. From this study, of course, we will be on the lookout for such possible occurrences in the future.

**M.M. Paparella, M.D.**

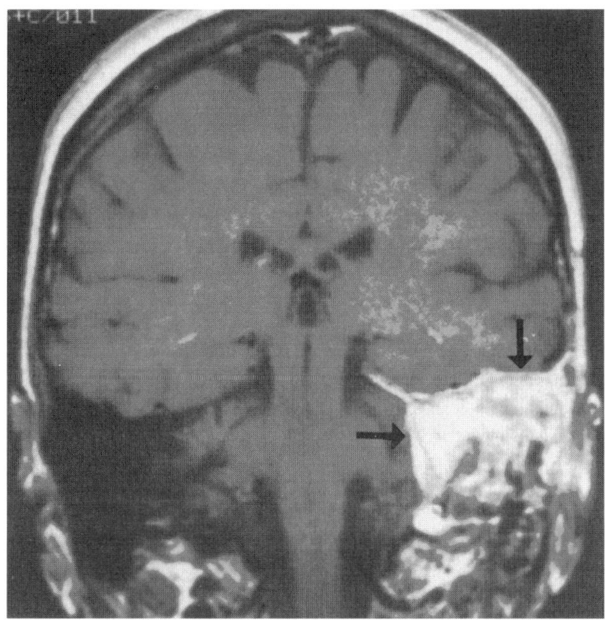

FIGURE 3.—Coronal T1 MRI with gadolinium enhancement of case 4. The scan demonstrates a large left petrous apex lesion (*arrows*) extending to the skin surface, involving the external auditory canal, and invading the cerebellum inferiorly. (Courtesy of Lustig LR, Jackler RK, Lanser MJ: Radiation-induced tumors of the temporal bone. *Am J Otol* 18:230–235, 1997.)

## Endolymphatic Sac Tumor: A Case Report and Review of the Literature

Reijneveld J, Hanlo P, Groenewoud G, et al (Univ Hosp Utrecht, The Netherlands; Univ Hosp Nijmegen, The Netherlands)
*Surg Neurol* 48:368–373, 1997

5–11

*Introduction.*—Papillary tumors of the temporal bone are rare tumors with an aggressive behavior pattern. These neoplasms were once thought to arise from the middle ear, but it has recently been shown that they actually originate from the endolymphatic sac. A case history and literature review of endolymphatic sac tumor (ELST) are presented. The first case is described below.

 *Case.*—A 63-year-old woman had a mass lesion of the temporal bone, which had been growing progressively for more than 35 years. The result was unilateral palsy involving the fifth to eleventh cranial nerves, progressive ataxia, and a pyramidal and pseudobulbar syndrome. Imaging studies revealed tumor invasion of the pars squamosa and petrosa of the temporal bone, with extension into the middle and posterior fossa. The tumor was hypervascular on angiographic evaluation. Nonradical surgery, including brain stem decompression, was performed to remove the tumor. The tumor proved to be a papillary ELST on pathologic examination. The patient recovered gradually and continues to be in neurologically stable condition. At follow-up, the intracranial tumor mass had increased only slightly. Further, cosmetic surgery was needed to deal with extensive extracranial expansion.

*Literature Review.*—Including the authors' case, 37 patients with ELST have been reported in the literature. There were 23 women and 14 men, average age 41 years. Major clinical manifestations were unilateral hearing loss, facial weakness, otitis, tinnitus, and vertigo. Imaging studies showed the tumors were centered between the sigmoid sinus and the internal auditory canal along the posterior petrosal plate. There was sometimes bone erosion toward the vestibule of the labyrinth. The vascular or hypervascular nature of the mass was demonstrated by angiography. Although intracranial extension was almost always present, there was just 1 case of brain invasion and none of distant metastasis. Preoperative diagnosis was difficult; the lesion was often mistaken for paraganglioma. Complete removal of all tumor was difficult to achieve. At an average follow-up of 58 months in 33 patients, 76% were without evidence of tumor growth, 12% were alive with recurrences, and 12% were dead.

*Discussion.*—Endolymphatic sac tumor is a rare but aggressive entity. It is essential to differentiate this tumor from more benign middle ear adenomas, because the treatment and prognosis are different. Radical resection is the treatment of choice, but complete resection is usually impossible. There is continued debate as to the role of radiation therapy. Patients should receive annual imaging follow-up for more than 10 years.

▶ These authors describe a very rare tumor in the region of the endolymphatic sac: a papillary tumor. These tumors can involve not only the region of the sac but can also extend intracranially. They are correct in that the treatment of choice would be radical resection, and as the authors mention, such resection can be difficult because of the location of the tumor.

**M.M. Paparella, M.D.**

---

**Value of Fat Suppression Magnetic Resonance Imaging in the Diagnosis of Lipomas of the Internal Auditory Canal**
Hara A, Takahashi K, Ito Z, et al (Univ of Tsukuba, Japan)
*Ann Otol Rhinol Laryngol* 106:343–347, 1997                5–12

---

*Background.*—Fat suppression methods in MRI have been found to suppress strong signals from fatty tissues that interfere with signals from adjacent areas. Two current case reports were presented to illustrate the value of fat suppression techniques in MRI to confirm the diagnosis of

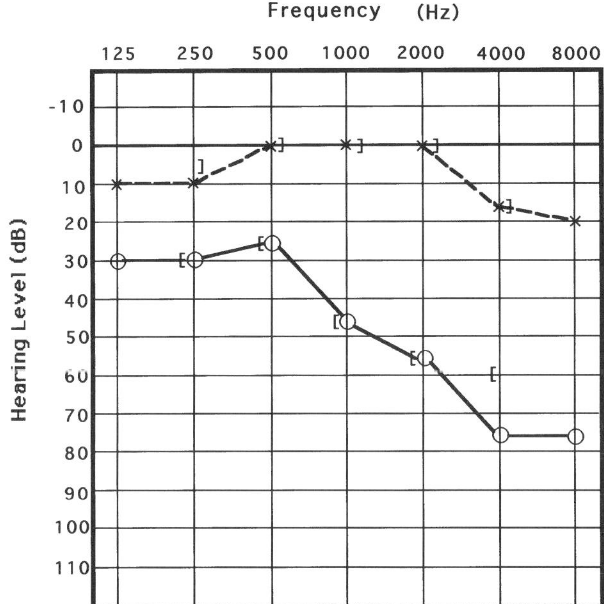


FIGURE 1.—(Case 1). Audiogram performed Nov. 8, 1993, showing sensorineural hearing loss at high frequencies with pure tone average of 42.5 dB on right. (Courtesy of Hara A, Takahashi K, Ito Z, et al: Value of fat suppression magnetic resonance imaging in the diagnosis of lipomas of the internal auditory canal. *Ann Otol Rhinol Laryngol* 106:343–347, 1997.)

cerebellopontine angle (CPA) and internal auditory canal (IAC) lipomas. The first case is described below.

> *Case Report.*—Man, 51, reported right hearing impairment of 10 years' duration and right-sided tinnitus. He had no vertigo, otalgia, or facial weakness. Audiography demonstrated a right high-frequency sensorineural hearing loss with a pure tone average of 42.5 dB (Fig 1) and a 50% speech discrimination. Axial T1-weighted MRI showed a 5 × 10 mm hyperintense tumor in the right IAC, and T2-weighted images showed a decreased signal intensity. In T1-weighted images, fat suppression markedly affected the signal from the hyperintense tumor in the right IAC. A homogeneous enhancement of the IAC lesion appeared on gadolinium-enhanced, fat-suppressed T1-weighted images (Fig 2). For 1.5 years, MR images obtained every 6 months showed no change in tumor size.

*Conclusions.*—This is the first report of MRI findings using a fat suppression technique in patients with CPA lipomas. With fat-suppression methods, MRI can confirm the diagnosis of CPA lipoma and even help avoid postoperative morbidity in patients without severe or progressive symptoms.

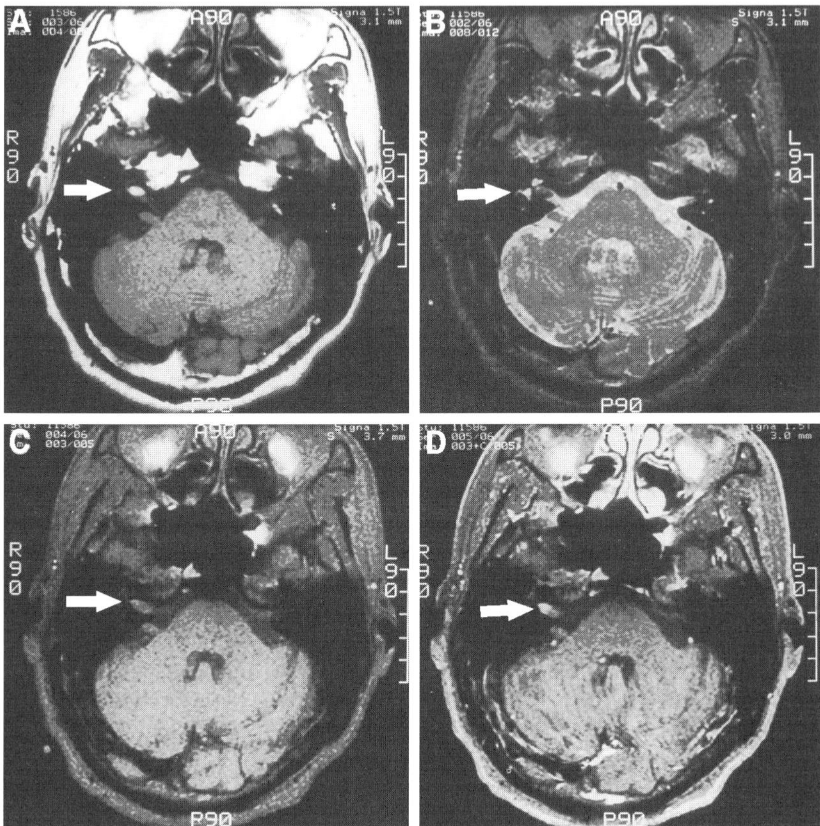

FIGURE 2.—(Case 1). Magnetic resonance imaging findings. *Arrows*—tumor. **A,** T1-weighted images revealed hyperintense tumor 5 × 10 mm in diameter in right internal auditory canal (IAC). **B,** signal from tumor in right IAC was hypointense on T2-weighted MRI. **C,** T1-weighted images with fat suppression. Hyperintense signal was markedly suppressed. **D,** gadolinium enhancement was clearly demonstrated in fat-suppressed, T1-weighted MRI. (Courtesy of Hara A, Takahashi K, Ito Z, et al: Value of fat suppression magnetic resonance imaging in the diagnosis of lipomas of the internal auditory canal. *Ann Otol Rhinol Laryngol* 106:343–347, 1997.)

▶ Lipomas in the CPA or in the IAC or both are extremely rare; there were apparently only 33 cases reported in the literature. Thus, these 2 cases are of interest because differential diagnosis in this region can sometimes be more than difficult. These authors describe their methods and technique, which will be helpful to neurotologists in the process of making a differential diagnosis of lesions in this region. The usefulness of the fat suppression techniques in MRI is described also, which helps confirm a diagnosis in this area.

**M.M. Paparella, M.D.**

# 6 External Ear, Middle Ear, and Mastoid

---

**Necrotizing External Otitis in Patients With AIDS**
Ress BD, Luntz M, Telischi FF, et al (Univ of Miami, Fla)
*Laryngoscope* 107:456–460, 1997
6–1

---

*Introduction.*—Necrotizing external otitis (NEO) is a severe, invasive external otitis that primarily affects elderly patients with diabetes and is usually caused by *Pseudomonas aeruginosa*. There are several documented reports of patients with NEO but without diabetes who have some other underlying disease resulting in neutropenia or immunosuppression. Re-

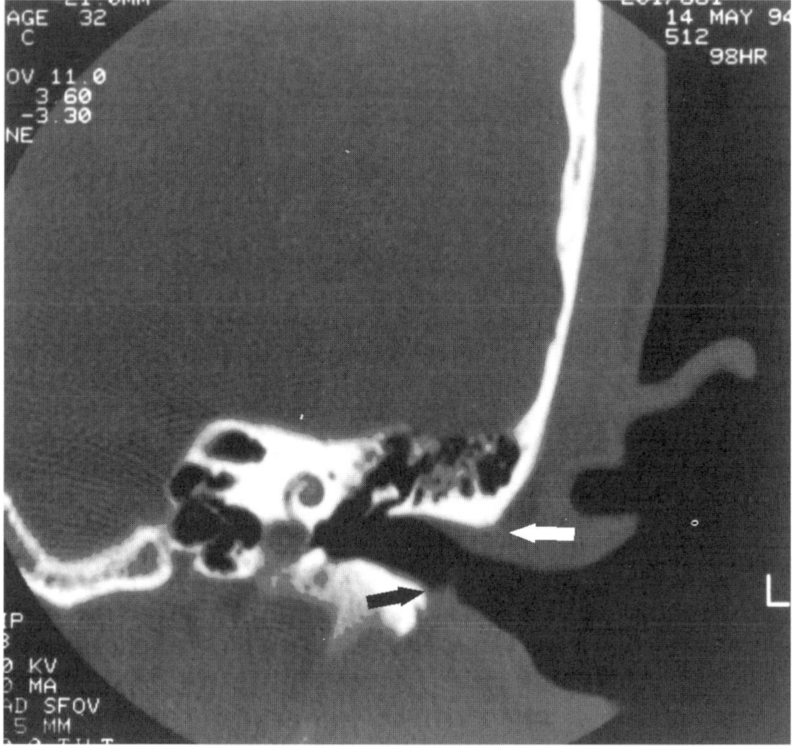

**FIGURE 1.**—Coronal high-resolution CT scan of patient with stage I necrotizing external otitis demonstrating soft-tissue changes in the external auditory canal. Edema is noted along the superior aspect of the bony external auditory canal (*arrow*), and debris can be seen in the floor of the external auditory canal (*arrowhead*). (Courtesy of Ress BD, Luntz M, Telischi FF, et al: Necrotizing external otitis in patients with AIDS. *Laryngoscope* 107:456–460, 1997. Copyright Triological Society.)

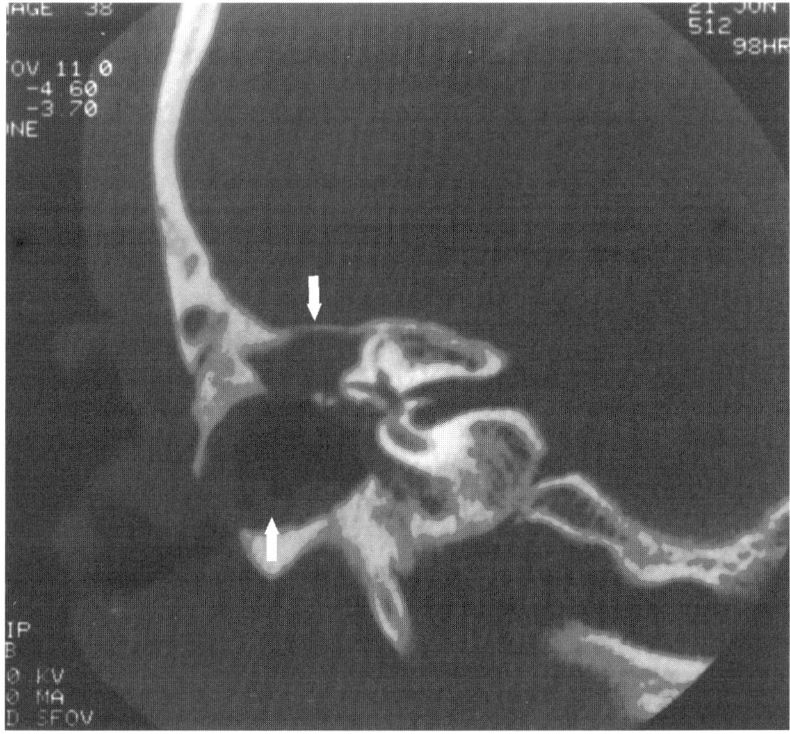

FIGURE 2.—Coronal high-resolution CT scan of patient with stage II necrotizing external otitis demonstrating both soft-tissue and bony involvement of the temporal bone. There is bony destruction in the posterior and inferior external auditory canal (*arrowhead*). A large necrotizing cavity containing soft-tissue debris and bony fragmentation is confined to the temporal bone superiorly by an intact tegmen tympani (*arrow*). (Courtesy of Ress BD, Luntz M, Telischi FF, et al: Necrotizing external otitis in patients with AIDS. *Laryngoscope* 107:456–460, 1997. Copyright Triological Society.)

ported is a retrospective review of the largest known series of patients with NEO and AIDS.

*Methods.*—Medical records of 7 patients with NEO and AIDS were reviewed. High-resolution CT (HRCT) studies for all 7 patients were reviewed by a single neuroradiologist. Findings were compared with those of patients with NEO and no AIDS.

*Results.*—Associated opportunistic diseases were present in all patients. None of the patients had diabetes. Two patients had organized granulation tissue in the external auditory canal (EAC). The EAC and masticator space were involved, in all patients. Patients with stage I disease had involvement of the middle ear and mastoid, parapharyngeal space, or infratemporal area (Fig 1). In stage II disease, the eustachian tube and nasopharynx were involved, and there was erosion of the temporal bone (Fig 2). In stage III disease, there was bony erosion of the skull base extending beyond the confines of the temporal bone, or intracranial extension with involvement of the contralateral side. *P. aeruginosa* was not the main pathologic organism. The outcome of NEO was significantly worse in patients with NEO and AIDS than for those with NEO but no AIDS.

*Conclusion.*—Patients with NEO and AIDS are more likely than patients with classically described NEO to be younger, not have granulation tissue in the EAC, have organisms other than *P. aeruginosa* in EAC cultures, and have worse outcomes. Reliable anatomical and prognostic information may be gained from HRCT.

▶ These authors bring to the attention of the practicing otolaryngologist the fact that malignant external otitis can appear to be similar in patients with AIDS but may have a differing foundation from what has previously been described for this disease. These patients were much younger and did not have diabetes, and *P. aeruginosa* was not necessarily the dominant pathologic organism. As the authors indicate, we should be watchful for this terrible disease so that these patients with AIDS can be managed when they are seen with malignant external otitis.

**M.M. Paparella, M.D.**

## Total Ear Replantation

Kind GM, Buncke GM, Placik OJ, et al (Davies Med Ctr, San Francisco)
*Plast Reconstr Surg* 99:1858–1867, 1997                                    6–2

*Introduction.*—Since the first report of successful microsurgical replantation of the ear in 1980, only 12 successful ear replantations have appeared in reports in English. Reported are 4 patients successfully treated with microvascular ear replantation.

*Case 1.*—A man, 21, was involved in a motor vehicle accident in which his right ear was completely amputated; he also sustained a compression fracture of his cervical spine. The ear was anastomosed and seemed well perfused immediately. He was treated with heparin and intermittent leech therapy for ear congestion. The ear was completely viable at 1 week, except for the necrotic inferior half of the lobe, which was excised and revised during spinal fusion 1 week later.

*Case 2.*—A man, 26, was seen after part of his left external ear was bitten off during an altercation. The ear was anastomosed, and perfusion was good until 14 hours postoperatively when the replanted part showed signs of venous congestion for which he received heparin and intermittent leech therapy. At 6 weeks, he underwent excision of demarcated areas, and a Z-plasty closure was used.

*Case 3.*—A man, 51, sustained a shear-force injury and amputation of the right ear when he fell against a door. The ear was reattached and revascularized. He was treated with heparin and intermittent leech therapy for congestion. On postoperative day 3, he had arterial thrombosis for which the artery was opened and cleared of a clot. Further heparin, then coumadin, therapy was successful.

*Case 4.*—A man, 28, was involved in an altercation in which the entire right auricle was completely avulsed. The ear was anastomosed after being forcibly extracted from the assailant's mouth. He was treated with heparin postoperatively. A small area of skin loss was detected at the inferior helical rim, but the patient refused further treatment and was lost to follow-up.

*Conclusion.*—Successful revascularization and superior aesthetic results were achieved in 4 patients with amputated ears using different techniques: vein grafts, primary vascular repair, and repair by means of pedicled superficial temporal vessels. All patients required blood transfusions after medicinal leech therapy.

▶ We have had occasion in the past to see pinnae or portions of auricles removed during bites and were able to sterilize the removed portion of the pinna and suture it with a good result and a good take. This study indicates that restoring an amputated ear with microsurgical techniques can result in even greater incidences of success. This article is of interest especially in light of the recent Holyfield–Tyson fight in which Holyfield lost a portion of his ear; in that case, the pinna was allowed to granulate and heal without any attempt at reimplantation.

**M.M. Paparella, M.D.**

---

## Epithelial Migration in Keratosis Obturans

Corbridge RJ, Michaels L, Wright T (Royal Natl Throat Nose and Ear Hosp, London; Univ College, London)
*Am J Otolaryngol* 17:411–414, 1996                                              6–3

---

*Introduction.*—Patients with keratosis obturans have a cholesteatoma-like mass within the deep external auditory meatus. A problem with migration of the auditory epithelium has been suggested in this condition but has never been proved. Abnormal pathways of tympanic membrane epithelium were demonstrated in 2 patients with keratosis.

*Methods.*—Two patients with keratosis obturans—a 37-year-old woman and a 50-year-old man—were studied. The eardrums were marked with dye, and then follow-up photographs were obtained to compare the pathways and speed of migration of the markings.

*Results.*—In 1 patient, migration was significantly delayed only in the affected ear. The migratory pattern was abnormal as well, with the epithelium moving in an anterior direction across the entire eardrum. The second patient also showed delayed migration. The pattern in this case was downward toward the par tensa, and from there inferiorly across the entire tympanic membrane.

*Discussion.*—Defective migration of the tympanic membrane epithelium may be the basis of keratosis obturans. Migration is delayed and has an abnormal pattern in the affected ear only. Damage to the basal epithelial layer of the tympanic membrane is a possible causative factor.

▶ Keratosis obturans can be a difficult problem that sometimes requires periodic, frequent, and difficult cleansing in the physician's office, only to find the keratomatous and desquamated epithelial material to recur so rapidly. These authors have done a nice little study in a few patients, in which they argue that keratosis obturans develops as a result of abnormal epithelial migration across the tympanic membrane to the ear canal. I certainly think this is most likely true. Nevertheless, this does not describe the entire etiology or pathogenesis of this disease—genetic and other factors most likely also play a role.

**M.M. Paparella, M.D.**

---

**Otitis Media in 2253 Pittsburgh-area Infants: Prevalence and Risk Factors During the First Two Years of Life**
Paradise JL, Rockette HE, Colborn DK, et al (Univ of Pittsburgh, Pa; Children's Hosp of Pittsburgh, Pa)
*Pediatrics* 99:318–333, 1997                                              6–4

---

*Introduction.*—The peak incidence and prevalence of otitis media occurs in the first 2 years of life. Reported are prospective epidemiologic findings regarding the relationships between early-life otitis media and later developmental impairment in 2,253 Pittsburgh-area children who represent a broad sociodemographic spectrum.

*Methods.*—Healthy infants seen for primary care by age 2 months in diverse public and private institutions and physicians' practices were intensely monitored for middle-ear status throughout their first 2 years of life by pneumatic otoscopy and tympanometry.

*Results.*—The incidence for having 1 or more episodes of middle-ear effusion (MEE) was 47.8% for children between the ages of 61 days and 6 months, 78.9% for children between the ages of 61 days and 12 months, and 91.1% for children between the ages of 61 days and 24 months. The mean cumulative proportion of days with MEE was 20.4% for the first year of life and 16.6% for the second year of life. The incidence of MEE was highest in urban infants and lowest in suburban infants, especially in the early months of life. The mean cumulative proportions of days with MEE were higher among boys than girls, higher among black than white children, and higher among children with Medicaid than among those with private health insurance. The cumulative proportions of days with MEE varied according to the number of smokers in the household and the number of other children to whom the child was exposed. Significant risk factors related to the cumulative proportion of days with MEE in the first year of life were grouping by study-site, sex, the socioeconomic index, breastfeeding for 4 or more months, the number of smokers in the household, and the child exposure index. In the second year, these factors were sex, the socioeconomic index, and the child exposure index.

*Conclusion.*—The prevalence of otitis media in the first 2 years of life in black infants with lower socioeconomic status seems to be as high as or higher than among white infants with lower socioeconomic status and is definitely higher than among middle-class white infants. The most significant risk factors for otitis media seem to be low socioeconomic status and repeated exposure to large numbers of other children.

▶ These authors report their findings from a comprehensive long-term study. The findings are of interest to all physicians, especially otologists. The emphasis was on the first 2 years of life, and the authors find that the incidence of otitis media in minorities such as black infants appears to be as high as in white infants. They find that environmental factors, such as low socio economic status and repeated exposure to large numbers of other children, particularly those with similar infections, whether at home or in daycare centers, predisposed to otitis media with effusion. This study is of interest but would have even more merit if we knew what happened to these children after the age of 2 years, during later childhood, or even during adulthood, in terms of those who had a continuation of difficulties. In addition, It is my observation that black patients tend to have a lesser incidence of otitis media; this study would suggest that the opposite might be true.

**M.M. Paparella, M.D.**

---

**Patterns of Persistent Otitis Media in the First Year of Life in Aboriginal and Non-Aboriginal Infants**
Boswell JB, Nienhuys TG (Menzies School of Health Research, Darwin, Australia)
*Ann Otol Rhinol Laryngol* 105:893–900, 1996                                        6–5

---

*Objective.*—Otitis media (OM) is extremely common among Australian Aboriginal children. For school-age children of this group, the prevalence of chronic OM and conductive hearing loss may be as high as 80%. However, relatively little is known about the onset and natural history of this disease in infancy and early childhood. In other racial groups, early-onset OM has been linked to an increased risk of chronic and persistent ear disease in later childhood. The course of OM during the first year of life was studied in Aboriginal and non-Aboriginal Australian infants.

*Methods.*—The study included 41 Aboriginal and 17 non-Aboriginal infants. All infants underwent repeated otoscopy and tympanometry, starting soon after birth. Patterns of OM disease during the first year of life were compared for the 2 groups. In addition, conditional probabilities were calculated for changes in the condition of the ears at consecutive examinations. The data were used to develop a model of the course of OM in Aboriginal infants.

*Results.*—None of the Aboriginal infants studied had normal ear health throughout the entire study period. Thirty-five percent had persistent perforations, and 19% had intermittent perforations that closed by the next examination. The non-Aboriginal infants were found to have occasional cases of OM with effusion or acute OM, which resolved within 1 month. In contrast, the Aboriginal infants had persistent disease that rarely or never normalized. After a normal examination, the Aboriginal infants were 3 times more likely to develop OM with effusion (OME) and 4 times more likely to develop acute OM (AOM) than their non-Aboriginal peers. The data suggested a model of ear disease in Aboriginal children progressing from OME to AOM to tympanic membrane perforation and chronic suppurative OM (CSOM).

*Conclusions.*—The binaural pattern of chronic OM detected in Aboriginal school-age children is probably already established in the first year of life. The data may be helpful in the early detection and management of Aboriginal infants with OM. Children with a binaural pattern suggesting long-term tympanic membrane perforation have the most to gain from early detection and treatment.

▶ Many of us were recently at the World Congress meeting in Sydney, Australia, where one of the leading politicians of the country did speak about OM in Aboriginal children. Most of us were astonished to hear what a high incidence this group of patients has, in terms of not only OME but chronic OM. The gentleman indicated that approximately half of Aboriginal children in school have perforated eardrums and chronic OM. Thus, this study is of interest, not only because it alerts us to a population who have an extremely high prevalence of OM but also because, by studying such populations, we will gain insight into the natural history as well as racial, genetic, and environmental factors as they impact on the problem of OM.

**M.M. Paparella, M.D.**

## How Common Is Recurrent Acute Otitis Media?

Alho O-P (Univ of Oulu, Finland)
*Acta Otolaryngol (Stockh)* Suppl 529:8–10, 1997                    6–6

*Background.*—Criteria for recurrent acute otitis media (RAOM) are defined, and those children who need prophylaxis and special surveillance, taking the resources available into consideration, are identified in this population-based study.

*Methods.*—Two thousand four hundred and eleven randomly sampled research subjects had their ears and hearing checked at 3, 6, 12, 18, and 24 months. Examinations included pneumatic otoscopy, and myringotomy was used to relieve symptoms. The definition of AOM was acute symptoms in combination with inflammation of the tympanic membrane as gauged by pneumo-otoscopic signs. Chronic otitis media effusion was diagnosed with middle ear effusion behind the tympanic membrane and also with otomicroscopic findings. Pneumatic otoscopy and myringotomy (90% of cases) were used in cases of middle ear effusion.

*Results.*—Four thousand one hundred and seventy AOM cases were recorded in 1,503 children. One hundred and eighteen children had more than 4 episodes in 6 months, 375 had 3, and 825 had 2. In the subsequent 6-month period, 5% of these 1,503 children experienced chronic otitis media with effusion. Of the group with more than 4 episodes, 10% had further occurrences in the second 6-month period; 12% of the children with 3 episodes and 7% of the children with 2 episodes had recurrences.

*Conclusion.*—In past population studies, the percentage of children with RAOM varied from 2% to 41%. However, RAOM has commonly been defined as 3 recurrences in 6 months. Using this definition, 15% of children studied exhibited RAOM. This figure is reasonable with regard to resources, if all these children were to be given preventive medicine. However, the diagnosis of RAOM was not a good predictor that future otitis episodes would occur. Spontaneous recovery often occurred with age without administering prophylaxis.

▶ I found this article interesting in that it really indicates a very high incidence of recurrent otitis media in this population: 34% of children had 2 episodes within 6 months, 15% had 3 episodes, and 5% had 4 episodes within 6 months. These figures are somewhat higher than I might have anticipated. Also, high numbers of children had continued episodes during the subsequent 6 months, and some went on to have chronic disease. Recurrent AOM, which can occur over an ear constantly filled with fluid, can indeed lead to recurrent problems; in fact, it can lead to long-term problems characterized by intractably pathologic tissue along a continuum, as has been demonstrated in many animals and humans to date.

**M.M. Paparella, M.D.**

## Bacteriological Findings and Persistence of Middle Ear Effusion in Otitis Media With Effusion

Jero J, Karma P (Helsinki Univ)
*Acta Otolaryngol (Stockh)* Suppl 529:22–26, 1997

6–7

*Objective.*—There is continuing debate over the cause and pathogenesis of otitis media with effusion (OME). The authors believe that OME can occur along a continuum with acute otitis media (AOM). After bacterial AOM, inflammation could continue in the middle ear mucosa, with little involvement of viable bacteria. If this hypothesis is correct, then the findings of viable bacteria might vary in differing phases of otitis media and OME. The bacteriologic findings of middle ear effusion (MEE) in children with asymptomatic OME were studied.

*Methods.*—The study included 165 children, from infancy to age 12 years, with asymptomatic OME. Samples of MEE were obtained at tympanostomy, with the patients under general anesthesia, in 1993–1994. The culture findings of MEE were analyzed and correlated with the persistence of MEE.

*Results.*—The mean duration of persistent MEE was 3.5 months. The culture results showed major otitis pathogens—*Streptococcus pneumoniae, Haemophilus influenzae, Branhamella catarrhalis*, and *Streptococcus pyogenes*—in 41% of patients younger than 2 years old vs. 17% of older children. The younger children also had a higher rate of respiratory infections and episodes of AOM during the preceding 6 months. Patients with MEE persisting for less than 2 months had higher rates of *S. pneumoniae* and *H. influenzae*—25% and 38%, respectively—than patients with longer durations of MEE—8% and 3%, respectively. No such relationship was observed for other bacteria. Past the 2-month point, there was little change in the occurrence of different bacteria until the 6-month point. Beyond that, no bacteria were cultured. Eight percent of children with previous adenotomy had major otitis pathogens cultured from MEE, compared with 32% of children who had not undergone adenotomy. None of the children who had undergone adenotomy had *S. pneumoniae, B. catarrhalis*, or *S. pyogenes* cultured from MEE, compared with 25% of children who had not had adenotomy.

*Conclusions.*—In children with OME, bacterial pathogens are more likely to be cultured from MEE if the effusion has persisted for less than 2 months, compared with longer durations of perfusion. This bacteriologic pattern is similar to that of AOM, suggesting that the 2-month interval represents a transitory phase between AOM and established OME. Beyond 2 months, positive culture findings from MEE become rare. The true role of bacteria in established OME remains to be determined.

▶ This study is somewhat comparable with other studies that again show a high incidence of bacterial involvement in noninfected ears; these are children who have OME or middle ear effusion without any evidence of infection, thus not requiring any antibiotics from a clinical point of view. Nevertheless, these authors identify positive culture results in 41% of the children younger than 2 years of age and 17% of the older children. Major pathogens included *S. pneumoniae, H. influenzae, B. catarrhalis*, and *S. pyogenes*. This study is in agreement with other studies suggesting that dormant pathogens along with other factors such as eustachian tubal dysfunction, obstructive sites, and so forth, can in some instances lead to continuing infectious problems including chronic infectious problems in the middle ear cleft.

**M.M. Paparella, M.D.**

### Modulation of Middle Ear Epithelial Function by Steroids: Clinical Relevance

Tan C-T, Escoubet B, van den Abbeele T, et al (Université Paris VII; Natl Taiwan Univ, Taipei)
*Acta Otolaryngol (Stockh)* 117:284–288, 1997                                     6–8

*Introduction.*—Active sodium transport has been found in the middle ear epithelium. For the efficiency of the mucociliary clearance, removing solutes from apical fluid is important. In the treatment of otitis media in children, the efficacy of steroid therapy is still controversial. To evaluate changes in ion transport induced by glucocorticoids, a short-circuit current technique was used.

*Methods.*—A short-circuit technique was used with the MESV cell line. Biolectric measurements were taken, as was a measurement of the ouabain-sensitive $^{86}$Rb uptake. Other tests included an RNase protection assay and cRNAs probes, and a statistical analysis was conducted.

*Results.*—A dose- and time-dependent increase in short-circuit current was produced by MESV cells by dexamethasone. Specific glucocorticoid antagonist RU-38486 inhibited this effect, which was related to a sodium transport. This was proved because the dexamethasone-induced increase in short-circuit current was prevented or abolished by apical addition of the specific sodium channel inhibitor benzamil or by a substitution of sodium with N-methylglucamine in the incubation medium. The expression of the α subunit sodium channel mRNA was increased by dexamethasone, according to the results of the RNase protection assay. Through an increase in the transcription of sodium channels, steroids directly modulate sodium transport across the middle ear epithelium.

*Conclusion.*—A direct effect of steroids on the middle ear epithelium was seen in these experiments, which support the use of steroids in treating chronic otitis. Corticosteroid-induced improvement in fluid clearance from the middle ear may be a component of the beneficial effect of steroid therapy in treating otitis media. In the course of chronic otitis, this process might allow dry out of the middle ear cavities and enhance the healing process.

▶ As these authors appropriately indicate, the usefulness of steroid therapy for treating otitis media in children is controversial; in fact, I think most studies indicate that there is no definite positive effect. Nevertheless, these authors, while using cell cultures and bio electric measuring techniques, find a beneficial effect for steroid therapy under the conditions of these experiments. In humans, however, it may well be a different story, because humans may have different anatomical development in the temporal bone, may have obstructive sites throughout the middle ear cleft, and may have inspissated and intractably pathologic tissue, and indeed those factors will mitigate against improvement with steroids. So these other considerations in treating pathogenesis in humans need to be considered.

**M.M. Paparella, M.D.**

## Acute Mastoiditis in Children: A 12-Year Retrospective Study

Harley EH, Sdralis T, Berkowitz RG (Royal Children's Hosp, Melbourne, Australia)

*Otolaryngol Head Neck Surg* 116:26–30, 1997                                    6–9

*Introduction.*—A retrospective study was performed of 12 years of experience with acute mastoiditis in an Australian pediatric population.

*Study Design.*—The charts of all children admitted to The Royal Children's Hospital from 1982 to 1993 with a diagnosis of acute mastoiditis were reviewed. The complete records of 57 children who had 58 episodes of acute mastoiditis formed the basis for this report. Gender, age, clinical history, and radiographic and laboratory data were collected for all patients in the group studied.

*Findings.*—Children in the group studied were aged 3 months to 15 years. In 54% of patients, acute mastoiditis was the first evidence of otitis media. Pain and fever lasting for more than 4 days were the most common symptoms. The most common organism recovered was *Streptococcus pneumoniae*. All children were given intravenous antibiotics, and 41 underwent an adjunctive drainage procedure. There were no significant differences in cure-rates for children treated surgically with myringotomies with or without tubes and those managed aggressively with mastoidectomies.

*Conclusions.*—Acute mastoiditis occurred mainly in infants and young children, and could be the first symptom of otitis media. Persistent pain and fever were the most common symptoms. Conservative treatment with intravenous antibiotics coupled with myringotomy or myringotomy plus tube-insertion is appropriate for children without signs of intratemporal or intracranial complications of acute mastoiditis such as sigmoid sinus thrombosis or abscess in the central nervous system. Posttreatment follow-up is necessary because the first sign of cholesteatoma may be acute mastoiditis.

▶ These days in the United States, we do not often see patients who have acute mastoiditis, particularly children. This 12-year retrospective study from Melbourne, Australia, therefore affords us an opportunity to reexamine this question, which indeed occurs but certainly not so commonly as it did in earlier decades and particularly in the preantibiotic era. These authors conclude that, from their study, acute mastoiditis occurs mostly in young children and may be the first evidence of ear disease. This is certainly a clinical nugget that we can maintain in memory for diagnosis of future, similar problems in young patients. Intravenous antibiotics combined with myringotomy, with or without tubal insertion, are appropriate, thus reserving mastoidectomy for obstinate problems.

**M.M. Paparella, M.D.**

### The Role of Surgery in Tuberculous Mastoiditis: Appropriate Chemotherapy is not Always Enough

Weiner GM, O'Connell JE, Pahor AL (City Hosp NHS Trust, Birmingham, England)
*J Laryngol Otol* 111:752–753, 1997                6–10

*Background.*—Although rare, tuberculosis of the middle ear can cause serious morbidity. It is generally believed that surgery is not necessary for the treatment of middle-ear tuberculosis. This article reports on a baby who required surgery for the management of tuberculous otitis media.

*Case.*—Boy, 19 months, was evaluated for left-sided otalgia and hearing loss that did not improve with antibiotics. Acute otitis media was diagnosed after myringotomy, but bacteriologic examination of the pus was negative and there was still no response to antibiotics. Radiographs showed ectopic calcification in the middle ear and lung opacity at the right hilum. On CT scanning, granulation tissue was found in the middle ear and mastoid with destruction of the bony septae in the mastoid cavity. Tuberculosis was diagnosed after biopsy of the postnasal space, and treatment with isoniazid and rifampicin was started.

Three weeks later, the patient was seen for right facial paralysis. Mastoid surgery revealed granulation tissue surrounding the ossicles, with dehiscence of the horizontal segment of the facial canal. The facial palsy resolved within 3 weeks after surgery. By 6 months, after completing chemotherapy, the patient had a dry and stable ear.

*Discussion.*—Despite appropriate chemotherapy, surgery may sometimes be needed for tuberculosis of the middle ear. The granulation tissue in the middle ear may be slow to resolve, posing an ongoing threat to nerve integrity.

▶ It would be rare in the United States, and perhaps somewhat more common in developing countries, that tuberculous chronic otitis media and chronic mastoiditis can still be a problem. The authors indicate that it has not been described previously that surgery might be necessary for these patients after chemotherapy. I cannot cite specific articles, but it is generally fairly well understood that, indeed, these patients may require surgery even after appropriate chemotherapy. I have personally treated several such patients, and the only way to remove intractably pathologic tissue, particularly in the middle ear cleft including the mastoid, is through surgery after chemotherapy is used in patients who have tuberculosis as a cause of their chronic otitis media and chronic mastoiditis.

**M.M. Paparella, M.D.**

## Secretory Otitis Media in Adults: II. The Role of Mastoid Pneumatization as a Prognostic Factor

Sadé J, Fuchs C (Tel Aviv Univ, Israel)
*Ann Otol Rhinol Laryngol* 106:37–40, 1997

6–11

*Background.*—In a previous study, the authors reported that adult ears with poor mastoid pneumatization are at high risk for secretory otitis media (SOM). In this study, the correlation between the size of adult mastoid pneumatization and the probability that an adult ear with SOM will develop into chronic SOM or retraction of the tympanic membrane was investigated.

*Methods and Findings.*—Seventy-two adults with SOM were followed up for a mean of 33 months. Secretory otitis media became chronic, and tympanic membrane retraction appeared to be a function of the pneumatization of the mastoid. Chronic SOM developed in 52.2% of ears with pneumatization of less than 6 cm², compared with 20% of ears with pneumatization of 6 cm² and greater. Atelectasis developed in 37.3% of the poorly pneumatized ears compared with only 5.7% of well-pneumatized ears.

*Conclusions.*—These data support previous studies that view the mastoid pneumatic system as an organ, as a middle ear pressure buffer. The sequelae observed may be linked pathogenetically to the extent of pneumatization, because both the SOM and sequelae appeared many years after formation and maturation of the pneumatic system. Negative pressure and chronic sequelae rarely occur in well-pneumatized ears. Ears with poorly pneumatized mastoids do not have the physiologic function of such a pressure buffer. Thus, ears that tend to develop a negative gas balance will develop a negative pressure more readily when their pneumatic system is underdeveloped and, consequently, will be more prone to chronic sequelae.

▶ Dr. Sadé is well known as an expert in studying the pathogenesis of otitis media. Thus, his findings are of interest and certainly quite valid. As always, however, the question is what comes first, the chicken or the egg? It may well be that the same pathogenetic mechanisms that lead to otitis media with effusion or secretory otitis media (the term used by Europeans) may also lead to hypoventilation, as well as hypopneumatization of the middle ear cleft, including the mastoid air-cell system. Nevertheless, Sadé and Fuchs' discussion regarding gaseous exchanges is relevant to understanding this all-too-common disease.

**M.M. Paparella, M.D.**

**Development of Tympanosclerosis: Can Predicting Factors Be Identified?**
Forséni M, Eriksson A, Bagger-Sjöbäck D, et al (Karolinska Inst, Stockholm)
*Am J Otol* 18:298–303, 1997                                    6–12

*Objective.*—Tympanosclerosis occurs because of calcification of the connective tissue in the middle ear. Some cases of tympanosclerosis occur after mild inflammatory otitis media, while some more aggressive infections heal without tympanosclerosis, perhaps because of individual variations in inflammatory response. There may be factors triggering an immunologic chain reaction that leads to formation of tympanosclerosis. If these factors could be identified, the information might be useful in predicting which patients are at risk of tympanosclerosis, or in preventing or treating the disease. A technique for immunohistochemical staining of the delicate tympanic membrane (TM) and its bony frame was developed.

*Methods.*—Healthy male Sprague-Dawley rats underwent inoculation into the middle ear of a *Streptococcus pneumoniae*, type 3, in suspension; this caused acute otitis media. One week to 6 months later, the animals were killed for evaluation of the TM and its bony frame. Immunohistochemical processing was performed by a new "free-floating technique" in which the entire specimen was briefly prefixed, incubated en bloc with primary antibodies, and decalcified in edetic acid. Immunohistochemical staining was performed with primary antibodies against macrophages.

*Results.*—By 1 month after induction of the infection, myringosclerosis was confirmed in 30% of rats. The disease appeared as white chalky patches in the TM, most commonly located close to the bony frame or the handle of the malleus. In the free-floating technique, antibodies against macrophages were precipitated in the TM itself and were more concentrated in the periphery, in the same area in which (under light microscopy and hematoxylin and eosin staining) macrophages were seen to be localized.

*Conclusions.*—This model demonstrates the successful induction of acute otitis media in rats, and of myringosclerosis in a subset of these. The new free-floating technique shows precipitation of antimacrophage antibodies close to the insertion of the TM in its bony frame, and to a lesser extent in the TM itself. This technique is valuable because it preserves antigenicity and offers good morphological presentation. The localization of macrophages in this experiment suggests that triggered inflammatory cells from the periphery might invade the TM, where they exert their effects.

▶ These authors have developed an interesting and nice new method in which immunohistochemical staining was accomplished in specimens that were stained en bloc before decalcification and sectioning. The pathologic correlate for tympanosclerosis is hyalinized collagen; there may or may not be calcification in such tissues, and, in fact, under the microscope in our laboratory, we may see many examples in which tympanosclerosis has not yet developed calcification. Nevertheless, these studies will be helpful in allowing us better to understand the genesis of tympanosclerosis, particularly in patients who have otitis media. We so often see extensive tympanosclerosis in the TM, and the patient may have normal hearing, or we may see a very small amount of tympanosclerosis in the TM, and the patient has considerable conductive hearing loss as a result of ossicular fixation to extensive tympanosclerotic plaques in the middle ear.

**M.M. Paparella, M.D.**

## Tensor Fold and Anterior Epitympanum
Palva T, Ramsay H, Böhling T (Univ of Helsinki)
*Am J Otol* 18:307–316, 1997

6–13

*Introduction.*—The anatomical and pathologic features of the epitympanic compartments have recently been updated from original data presented by Prussak in the 19th century. Now the anatomical and pathologic features of the anterior epitympanum and their role in surgery for chronic ear problems are described.

*Methods.*—Fifty-one fresh temporal bones were deeply frozen until dissection. After thawing, the bones were dissected, and anatomical details were photographed. There were 42 normal bones and 9 infected bones. Seven bones, 5 normal and 2 infected, were serially sectioned and evaluated histologically.

*Results.*—The distance between the roof of the tegme and the superior surface of the head of the malleus was short, and the interspace was usually sealed by a small fold. In all normal bones, the medial attic was open to the anterior epitympanum between the tensor tympani tendon and the attic roof; the central portion of the tensor fold could usually be seen through this opening. The transverse crest was seen in all dissected bones anterior to the head of the malleus. In 78% of specimens, the tensor fold was 40–80 degrees and was seldom horizontal, and as the fold of the angle increased so did the size of the supratubal recess. A membranous defect connecting the 2 spaces was observed in 14 ears (27%). When the tensor fold was intact, blockage of the tympanic isthmus produced inflammatory obliteration of the anterior epitympanum.

*Conclusion.*—About one fourth of the ears dissected showed membrane defects. Membranous defects in the tensor fold allow an additional direct route for aeration to the epitympanum. In ears with epitympanal pathologic features, transposition of the incus should be combined with resection of the thin portion of the tensor fold to preserve permanent attic aeration.

▶ These authors describe interesting anatomical details relating to the anterior epitympanum, and special attention is paid to the "tensor fold." They indicate that, in approximately one fourth of ears, this membrane may have a defect. That being the case, this might have some relationship to aeration of the epitympanum and, thus, to attic retraction.

**M.M. Paparella, M.D.**

---

**Correlation Between Retractions of the Pars Flaccida and the Pars Tensa**
Luntz M, Fuchs C, Sadé J (Univ of Tel Aviv, Israel)
*J Laryngol Otol* 111:322–324, 1997
6–14

---

*Background.*—Retraction of the pars flaccida (PF) and pars tensa (PT) can occur under negative intratympanic pressure. Atelectatic ears were studied to assess the relationship between PF and PT retractions and how the differences in their mechanical properties are reflected clinically.

*Methods.*—Retraction of the PT or the PF or both was found in 250 of 542 consecutively examined ears. The study excluded ears previously operated on and those with cholesteatoma or tympanic-membrane perforation. Both PT and PF retraction were graded according to the classifications of Sadé, and correlation between their degrees of retraction was assessed.

*Results.*—Eighty-seven percent of ears had PF retraction and 60% had PT retraction. Forty-seven percent of ears had both types of retraction and 53% had only 1 type. Of the ears with only 1 type of retraction, 75% had PF retraction and 25% had PT retraction. In ears with both types, the severity of retraction was positively correlated.

*Conclusions.*—Retraction of the PF is more common than retraction of the PT. The findings suggest that the flaccid portion of the tympanic membrane can retract under even mild negative intratympanic pressure. The mechanical properties of the tympanic membrane account for the positive correlation observed between the degrees of PF and PT retraction.

▶ These authors have done an interesting study, correlating the retraction characteristics of the PF or the PT, alone or together. This study is, as far as I know, the first time such a correlation has been drawn together. It is true that retractions in the PF often resemble more of a retraction-pocket, whereas retractions of the PT more often resemble atelectasis, with a somewhat different appearance and not necessarily a retraction-pocket per se. In any case, this study is of interest and has clinical relevance as well as relevance in terms of correlating pathology.

**M.M. Paparella, M.D.**

**Endoscopy and Otomicroscopy in the Estimation of Middle Ear Structures**

Karhuketo TS, Laippala PJ, Puhakka HJ, et al (Univ of Tampere, Finland)
*Acta Otolaryngol (Stockh)* 117:585–589, 1997                6–15

*Objective.*—In the anatomically normal ear, a straightforward-looking otomicroscope can visualize only certain structures. Thus, the condition of the middle ear may not be properly diagnosed if only an otomicroscope is used. With an endoscope, the surgeon can see around the corner, confirming the diagnosis and possibly avoiding the need for radical surgery. Endoscopy and otomicroscopy were compared for their ability to demonstrate structures in the middle ear.

*Methods.*—Studies were performed in blocks from 8 temporal bones from recently deceased patients. Each specimen of a middle ear was studied using a Zeiss OPMI-1 operating microscope and Olympus endoscopes. The examinations were performed 3 times each, in random order. A Gage design for repeatability and reproducibility was used to assess variation within and between the 2 techniques. Analysis of variance, with total variation divided into different components, was used for analysis of the data.

*Results.*—Endoscopy provided better visualization than otomicroscopy. In each specimen, the greater the angle of the endoscope, the more structures it could visualize. In every quadrant, any endoscope visualized more variables than the otomicroscope, and the 90-degree endoscope gave better visualization than the 30-degree endoscope. The exception was the posterosuperior quadrant, for which the 30-degree endoscope was superior. There was analogous variation between methods and trials.

*Conclusion.*—Endoscopy is superior to otomicroscopy for evaluation of the middle ear. The 90-degree endoscope is the best for visualizing anatomical structures and for getting a general view of the middle ear, although the 30-degree endoscope is better for the posterosuperior quadrant. Endoscopy appears to be an indispensable technique for diagnosis of pathologic conditions in the middle ear, raising the need for endoscopes and endoscopically assisted operative procedures.

▶ This study of temporal bones is of interest, but the problem is that it looks at normal temporal bones. When dealing with pathology, there can be a variety of abnormal anatomical, as well as pathological, findings that will preclude adequate endoscopy. I have seen many occasions in which, for example, there is blockage of the attic at the isthmus, or there can be adhesions or granulation tissues obstructing a variety of areas in the middle ear cleft—and of course anatomical obstructions can occur as well. Thus, we cannot simply rely on endoscopy to solve all these problems. It is helpful if there is a normal middle ear, but if there are pathologic conditions and anatomical obstruction, and if there is sufficient indication, the otolaryngologist should resort to exploratory tympanotomy when indicated, either transcanal or endaural, to adequately assess the pathologic conditions and to treat them.

**M.M. Paparella, M.D.**

---

**Efficacy of Ototopical Ciprofloxacin in Pediatric Patients With Otorrhea**
Wintermeyer SM, Hart MC, Nahata MC (Children's Hosp, Columbus, Ohio; Ohio State Univ. Columbus; The Wexner Inst for Pediatric Research, Columbus, Ohio )
*Otolaryngol Head Neck Surg* 116:450–453, 1997                                    6–16

---

*Introduction.*—Otorrhea occurs commonly among patients with tympanostomy tubes. The bacteriology of ear fluid in such cases varies according to the patient's age, and opportunistic pathogens increase with duration of the otorrhea. Ciprofloxacin, the only available oral antibiotic with antipseudomonal coverage, is not approved for pediatric use in its oral form. A study of 29 children with otorrhea and confirmed *Pseudomonas aeruginosa* in ear fluid evaluated the efficacy and safety of topical ciprofloxacin.

*Methods.*—The group of patients ranged in age from 1 to 14 years (mean 4.8 years). All had a history of placement of a tympanostomy tube. The mean duration of a history of ear disease was 3.3 years, and the mean duration of drainage from the ear for the current infection was 5 months. Excluded were patients with a documented hypersensitivity to quinolone antibiotics. Treatment consisted of 3 ciprofloxacin drops 3 times daily for 14 days in the affected ear or ears. Aural irrigation was performed twice daily before the drops were given. Effectiveness of the therapy was assessed on days 7 and 14. Patients with a complete cessation of drainage, a dry cavity, and no signs of infection were considered clinically cured.

*Results.*—After 14 days of treatment with ciprofloxacin drops, 18 of the 29 patients were cured; 8 showed improvement (a 50% reduction in days with drainage and/or minimal moisture in the cavity); 2 were cured after changing to an alternate therapy; and 1 showed no improvement. Two additional children were cured after 3 weeks of treatment. Of the cured patients, 6 had been only partially compliant with the treatment regimen. There were no adverse effects from ototopical ciprofloxacin, and the number of ear infections was significantly reduced in the year after the study.

*Conclusion.*—The use of topical ciprofloxacin in pediatric patients with otorrhea achieved a cure rate of nearly 70% and a cure improvement rate of 90%. Outcome was not significantly affected by age, gender, duration of acute drainage, use of aural irrigations, or the presence of multiple pathogens.

▶ *Pseudomonas aeruginosa* continues to be a problem in otology. It would be helpful if we did have a new type of eardrop that would be helpful in these patients. We have used tobramycin drops and now will use ciprofloxacin drops in such patients, in the event that this might be helpful in controlling particularly superficial *P. aeruginosa* infections. If, however, the infection emanates from the middle ear cleft, one might not find topical drops to be as helpful as the appropriate antibiotics directed against the *P. aeruginosa* organism.

**M.M. Paparella, M.D.**

---

**Continuous Twice Daily or Once Daily Amoxicillin Prophylaxis Compared With Placebo for Children With Recurrent Acute Otitis Media**
Roark R, Berman S (Univ of Colorado, Denver; Children's Hosp, Denver)
*Pediatr Infect Dis J* 16:376–381, 1997                                  6–17

---

*Purpose.*—Recurrent otitis media is a common and expensive problem in young children. Several studies have examined the ability of prophylactic antibiotics to prevent new episodes of acute otitis media (AOM), but none have compared the relative efficacy of once-daily vs. twice-daily dosing. This placebo-controlled study compared once-daily vs. twice-daily administration of amoxicillin for the prevention of recurrent AOM.

*Methods.*—The sample studied comprised 194 children (aged 3 months to 6 years) with recurrent AOM. All had had 3 confirmed episodes of AOM during the previous 6 months. Patients with ventilation tubes, anatomical defects, immunodeficiency disorders, or penicillin allergy were excluded. After exclusion of 36 noncompliant patients, the analysis included 158 evaluable subjects. The patients were randomized to receive amoxicillin, 20 mg/kg/day either once or twice daily. The patients were followed on a monthly basis and whenever symptoms of upper respiratory infection developed. Those with 2 new episodes of AOM were removed from the study. For all patients, incidence density (ID) figures were calculated, with stratification by age and season.

*Results.*—In a total of 7,243 patient-days at risk, the number of new episodes of AOM was 56, for an annual ID of 2.82. The ID figures were no different for patients receiving amoxicillin once a day vs. twice a day or at either dosage of amoxicillin vs. placebo. There were still no differences after stratification by age and season of enrollment. Sixty-three percent of patients receiving placebo remained free of AOM throughout the study, as did 64% of patients receiving amoxicillin once a day and 61% of those receiving the drug twice a day.

*Conclusion.*—In children with recurrent AOM, giving prophylactic amoxicillin—whether once or twice daily—is no more effective than placebo in preventing new episodes of AOM. The findings suggest that prophylactic amoxicillin should not be routinely prescribed for patients with recurrent AOM. Rather, individual episodes of AOM should be treated. Children with 5 or 6 episodes of AOM over a 1-year period may be considered for placement of tympanostomy tubes.

▶ We continue to see many young children who are receiving continuous maintenance-doses of antibiotics. We think this is a bad policy that drives the disease underground. We see much evidence of this in our otopathology laboratory. Here children and adults with chronic otitis media have had prolonged antibiotic treatments, and we see continuing disease in the middle ear cleft as well as the potential for making the bacteria more dormant and resistant, only to arise and reactivate at a later date. It is interesting, therefore, that this study suggests that there was no benefit of amoxicillin prophylaxis, compared with placebo, in preventing new episodes of AOM in the group studied. The use of amoxicillin prophylaxis should be discouraged.

We very much agree with these authors regarding the design of their study and also their conclusions, especially when one tries to assess the pathogenesis of these problems with or without treatment. In short, antibiotics should help eliminate bacterial infection and should not allow chronicity of the disease and its sequelae to take place.

**M.M. Paparella, M.D.**

---

**Myringotomy and Ventilation Tube Insertion: A Ten-Year Follow-up**
Riley DN, Herberger S, McBride G, et al (Tyrone County Hosp, Northern Ireland)
*J Laryngol Otol* 111:257–261, 1997                                      6–18

---

*Introduction.*—The most common surgical procedure for children in the United Kingdom is myringotomy and ventilation tube insertion, with a national average annual insertion rate of 5 children per 1,000. This surgery can lead to damage to the tympanic membrane, with other complications including long-term hearing loss, tympanosclerosis, atelectasis, tympanic membrane perforation, and cholesteatoma. An individual's social and intellectual development can be impaired by hearing loss. The prevalence of causes, level of hearing loss, and level of tympanic membrane perforation with associated morbidity was ascertained, as were the presence, extent, and site of tympanosclerosis.

*Methods.*—Eighty children who had myringotomy performed for otitis media with effusion were reviewed 10 years later. The children had surgery on a total of 158 ears, and hearing loss, tympanic membrane perforation, and tympanosclerosis were evaluated.

*Results.*—In 13 ears (8.2%), hearing losses were evident, with losses under 20 decibels in 7 ears. There were 6 ears with losses of more than 20 decibels (3.8%), with 5 children having bilateral losses of 30 decibels caused by a recurrence of effusions, a large dry posterior perforation, an infected anterior perforation, a cholesteatoma, a mastoidectomy, or ossiculoplasty. One ear had a type I tympanoplasty with a 50-decibel hearing loss. Myringotomy and ventilation tube insertion were directly associated in only 3 ears (1.9%). Seven children had perforations that persisted unilaterally, 3 of whom had tympanoplasties. In 39% of those who had a ventilation tube inserted (48 ears), tympanosclerosis was found.

*Conclusion.*—Hearing loss was not associated with tympanosclerosis. The site of myringotomy was not restricted to the site of tympanosclerosis.

Many patients had myringotomy in other areas of the tympanic membrane. Those ears which had more ventilation tube insertions seemed to have more extensive tympanosclerosis. A policy of "watchful waiting" is recommended because of the risk of perforation.

▶ It is interesting to assess the role of long-term follow-up after treatment for otitis media and/or otitis media with effusion. These authors look at a 10-year follow-up after myringotomy and insertion of ventilation tubes. They find a variety of lesions, such as perforations and tympanosclerosis, that could be expected in such a long-term study. My only point of disagreement with their observations is that tympanosclerosis was found only in those ears that had had ventilation tubes inserted.

Certainly, in our clinic and, on a routine basis, in other colleagues' clinics, we see tympanosclerosis in many patients, both children and adults, who have not had ventilation tubes inserted. In fact, most tympanosclerosis seen in the clinic is in such patients. Thus, one wonders about the control group for this particular long-term observation. The authors are correct in that usually tympanosclerosis is not associated with a hearing loss. The hearing loss will develop only if there is invasion of the middle ear such as encasement of the ossicles and fixation of the ossicles, including the stapes.

**M.M. Paparella, M.D.**

---

**Clinicopathological Consultation: Ear Cholesteatoma Versus Cholesterol Granuloma**
Ferlito A, Devaney KO, Rinaldo A, et al (Univ of Padua, Italy; Univ of Bari, Italy; Univ of Michigan, Ann Arbor; et al)
*Ann Otol Rhinol Laryngol* 106:79–85, 1997                    6–19

---

*Introduction.*—The differential diagnosis between cholesteatoma and cholesterol granuloma is very important in terms of treatment and clinical implications. These 2 conditions can occur simultaneously, however, and have often been confused in the literature. Each lesion is discussed separately in this study and a differential diagnosis based on distinct clinicopathologic features presented.

*Cholesteatoma.*—Cholesteatoma is an epidermoid cyst that often destroys adjacent tissue, particularly bone, and tends to recur even after radical surgery. Despite its name, cholesteatoma does not contain cholesterol crystals or fat and is not a neoplasm. The various terms by which this lesion has been known reflect a lack of agreement on its origin and nature. Several theories on the pathogenesis of cholesteatoma have been advanced, including congenital, immigration, metaplastic, and implantation. Macroscopically, the lesion is a whitish, friable mass of spongy consistency. Some are clinically undetectable, and others may grow to several centimeters in greatest dimension. The typical pattern of cholesteatoma consists of cystic content, the matrix, and the perimatrix. The acquired variety has a substantially thicker matrix than the congenital variety. Ultrastructural features are similar to those of normal epidermis. Complete surgical excision is the recommended treatment.

*Cholesterol Granuloma.*—This granulomatous lesion develops in the setting of hemorrhage, interference with clearance or drainage, and obstruction of air exchange or ventilation. The glistening, brownish or yellow lesion contains a large number of cholesterol crystals engulfed by multinucleated foreign body giant cells and embedded in fibrous granulation tissue. Cholesterol granulomas occur throughout the body as well as in the middle ear region. In the setting of middle ear disease, they may appear in association with cholesteatoma, chronic otitis media, middle ear adenomatous tumors, and endolymphatic sac tumors. Treatment consists of drainage and aeration or radical excision.

*Discussion.*—Cholesteatoma is a common epithelial lesion; cholesterol granuloma in an uncommon stromal lesion. The lesions often have a similar CT appearance, but MRI may distinguish between the two. Morphologically, cholesteatoma is an epidermoid cyst and cholesterol granuloma a reactive foreign body granuloma. Unlike cholesteatomas, cholesterol granulomas do not require aggressive management.

▶ In this article, the authors compare cholesteatoma with cholesterol granuloma. I agree with the authors in their thesis: namely, cholesteatoma would be a better term to apply to cholesterol granuloma, because a cholesteatoma is essentially a keratoma, whereas the granuloma does contain multiple cholesterin clefts. These are 2 different diseases; however, sometimes a cholesterol granuloma can be as serious as a cholesteatoma. I have 1 temporal bone in my collection, for example, that shows a cholesterol granuloma from otitis media destroying the petrous apex to present as a tumorous mass in the posterior cranial fossa. Thus, a cholesterol granuloma can destroy bone and cause complications, as does a cholesteatoma. Nevertheless, these are 2 different pathologic and distinct lesions, and management is predicated on an understanding of this difference.

**M.M. Paparella, M.D.**

---

**Repair of Chronic Tympanic Membrane Perforations With Fibroblast Growth Factor**

Kato M, Jackler RK (Univ of California, San Francisco)
*Otolaryngol Head Neck Surg* 115:538–547, 1996                    6–20

---

*Background.*—Several angiogenic growth factors accelerate wound healing. Previous animal experiments have shown that topical application of epidermal growth factor is effective in healing chronic tympanic membrane perforations. In theory, fibroblast growth factor may produce a better-healed membrane through preferential stimulation of the fibroblasts in the middle layer of the tympanic membrane. The effects of fibroblast growth factor exogenously applied to the chronically perforated tympanic membrane were assessed to test this hypothesis.

*Methods.*—Chinchillas were studied. A buffered solution of fibroblast growth factor was administered to a Gelfoam pledget placed over chronic tympanic membrane perforations. Gelfoam and the buffer solution only were applied to control ears.

*Findings.*—Complete closure of the tympanic membrane perforation occurred in 81% of the fibroblast growth factor–treated ears and in only 41% of the control ears. Healing required a mean of 4 weeks for the fibroblast growth factor–treated ears and 6.5 weeks for the control ears that healed. In a histologic analysis of the fibroblast growth factor–healed eardrums immediately after closure, hypertrophy of the squamous and fibrous layers of the tympanic membrane was observed. With time, the eardrum thinned to proportions comparable to those of a normal tympanic membrane. A substantial middle fibrous layer was observed. Screening ototoxicity assessment showed no structural damage to the organ of Corti after treatment with growth factor. In an assessment of possible systemic toxicity, 78% of the radioactivity was found to remain at the site of application.

*Conclusions.*—Favorable closure rates have been associated with fibroblast growth factor and epidermal growth factor in animal models of chronic tympanic membrane perforations. The available data on safety and efficacy in animal models warrant their use in human trials in the near future.

▶ These authors quite appropriately used a chinchilla model to test the efficacy and effects of using fibroblast growth factor. They find that there is no ototoxic effect on the inner ear, and that indeed healing histologic characteristics suggest a potential efficacy for humans. This is how studies should be done: first in animals and then carefully applied to humans. The authors are to be applauded for this approach, and it is hoped that this growth factor will find a useful role in tympanoplasty in patients.

**M.M. Paparella, M.D.**

## Clinical Importance of the Korner's Septum

Göksu N, Kemaloğlu YK, Köybaşioğlu A, et al (Gazi Univ, Ankara, Turkey)
*Am J Otol* 18:304–306, 1997                                    6–21

*Introduction.*—Korner's septum (KS) is described as a developmental variation that occurs at the junction point between the saccus anterior and saccus medius (middle or tympanic portion, cog) and between the saccus superior and saccus medius (dorsal or mastoid portion) (Fig 1). It has been suggested that the role of the cog and the supratubal recess is blockage of the attic, which increases the risk of attic retraction pockets and cholesteatoma. The prevalence of KS was evaluated in patients with chronic middle ear diseases and normal mastoids.

*Methods.*—Records of 688 patients who underwent mastoidectomies were reviewed retrospectively. The mean age of 389 males and 299 females

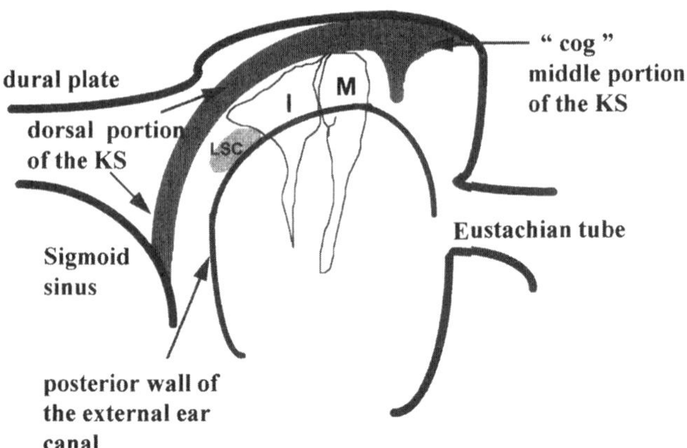



FIGURE 1.—Schematic drawing of Korner's septum (KS). The middle portion of KS (cog) facilitates narrowing and blockage of the passage between the protympanum, eustachian tube, and attic, while both dorsal and middle portions of KS contribute to block the passage between protympanum and antrum, as well as between mastoid cells and the antrum. *Abbreviations*: *I*, incus; *LSC*, lateral semicircular canal; *M*, malleus. (Courtesy of Göksu N, Kemaloğlu YK, Köybaşioğlu A et al: Clinical importance of the Korner's septum. *Am J Otol* 18:304–306, 1997.)

was 30.85 years (range, 8–67 years). The incidence of KS was correlated with the prevalence of retraction pockets (RPs) or retraction and/or adhesion of the whole tympanic membrane (R/A-TM).

*Results.*—Korner's septum was observed in 144 of 688 mastoidectomies (29.93%) and was found significantly more often in ears with chronic otitis media (COM) than in normal ears and mastoids (22.71% vs. 6.58%). Retraction pockets or R/A-TM were observed significantly more often in COM ears with KS compared with COM ears without KS (54.68% vs. 36.79%). Korner's syndrome was complete in 59.03% and incomplete in 33.33% of 144 patients. The anterior attic bony lamina (cog) was observed in 27 patients with KS.

*Conclusion.*—Findings indicate that KS is associated with COM; most patients with COM and KS also had RP or R/A-TM. Korner's septum is an important anatomical handicap that can make the patient susceptible to COM, especially when attic RPs, cholesteatoma, and adhesive otitis media are present, because KS contributes to attic blockage.

▶ These authors describe a high incidence of prominent KS associated with RPs in cholesteatomas. To me, the study requires further confirmation. We see many patients who have KSs that are extensive or slight, and we know that this abnormality may or may not be associated with an RP in the pars flaccida or in the posterior-superior quadrant. It is difficult to draw a direct relationship concerning this interaction and possible pathogenesis. This study is of interest and, as mentioned, should be confirmed by others before it is concluded this relationship is real. Nevertheless, this article does point out the importance of KS, and one needs to deal with this when doing tympanomastoid work or mastoid surgery for a variety of purposes.

**M.M. Paparella, M.D.**

## Revision Myringoplasty

Berger G, Ophir D, Berco E, et al (Tel Aviv Univ, Israel)
*J Laryngol Otol* 111:517–520, 1997

6–22

*Introduction.*—Although the success rate of myringoplasty is initially high, late reperforations develop in a considerable number of patients. Reported success rates for revision myringoplasty have ranged from only 60% to more than 80%. A retrospective study reviewed the short- and long-term results of 70 revision and 16 re-revision myringoplasty operations.

*Methods.*—The 86 revisions were performed in 78 patients between 1980 and 1995. Simple chronic otitis media was the reason for surgery in 90% of patients and traumatic perforation in 10%. Of 70 patients who underwent revision myringoplasty, 60 had had their first operation at the institution during this study; 48 operations were immediate failures, and 12 were late failures. Re-revision myringoplasty was performed in 16 patients after 2 successive failures of closure of the perforation. All ears were dry at revisioned surgery, with no evidence of active inflammation. The mean duration of postoperative follow-up was 22 months. Factors analyzed included cause of failure in the primary operation, location and size of perforation, patient's age, and seniority of the surgeon.

*Results.*—The most common causes of immediate failure of the primary myringoplasty had been infection and poor anterior adaptation, which accounted for 35% and 28.4%, respectively, of all failures in primary operations. Among late re-perforations, 7 had been attributed to atrophy of the graft without infection and 4 to infection. One patient required revision due to trauma. Most re-perforations were located anteriorly and involved less than half of the surface of the eardrum. The mean time between the primary operation and revision was 3 years. The overall success rate of revision was 52.8%. Twenty-seven failures of revision occurred immediately, and 6 developed later. The most common causes of failure in revision myringoplasty were complete no-take of the graft (39.4%) and necrosis of the graft associated with infection (27.3%). Re-revision was performed in 16 patients, with a success rate of 62.5%. Results of revision myringoplasty showed no relationship to patients' age, size or location of the perforation, or seniority of the surgeon.

*Conclusion.*—The success rate is lower in revision myringoplasty operations (54.7% overall) than it is in primary operations. Most failures of revisions occur immediately, and complete no-take of the graft is the leading cause. Reduced blood supply to the ears is the likely cause of no-take of a graft, whereas poor anterior adaptation of the graft can be considered a technical fault.

▶ These authors describe some aspects of myringoplasty, particularly revisional myringoplasty, that will be helpful to the practicing otologist. Certainly technique plays a role, but the ability of the patient to heal in the recipient site involved, and the surgeon's ability to take advantage of these recipient sites, also will dictate the success in myringoplasty. One should carefully define myringoplasty, compared with tympanoplasty. Certainly, tympanoplasty requiring greater recontruction of the tympanic membrane and underlying structures in the middle ear cleft is more formidable than a simple grafting or placement of a localized patch on the tympanic membrane. Nevertheless, these surgeons describe the problems involved in revision and some of the problems with technique and healing that can take place, and they offer suggestions concerning how to counteract those.

**M.M. Paparella, M.D.**

## A Comparison of the Biocompatibility of Three Absorbable Hemostatic Agents in the Rat Middle Ear

Liening DA, Lundy L, Silberberg B, et al (Brook Army Med Ctr, Houston; Michigan Ear Inst, Southfield; Providence Hosp; et al)
*Otolaryngol Head Neck Surg* 116:454–457, 1997                          6–23

*Introduction.*—In patients undergoing middle-ear surgery, Gelfoam absorbable gelatin sponge is a widely used hemostatic agent with few apparent side effects. However, in some patients fibrosis develops in the mesotympanum, and there is evidence to suggest that Gelfoam may be responsible for this. Gelfoam was compared with other absorbable hemostatic agents for its tendency to promote fibrosis in the middle ear of rats.

*Methods.*—The 3 materials tested were Gelfoam, Gelfilm absorbable gelatin sheet, and Instat absorbable collagen sheet. The materials were implanted into the middle ear of adult male Sprague-Dawley rats via a postauricular approach. Histologic changes in the temporal bone were assessed over time, using the other ear as a control.

*Results.*—The only animals to show any abnormal temporal bone findings were those implanted with Gelfoam. Three of 15 rats in this group had fibrosis, all severe. In the animals with fibrosis, the subepithelial layers were thickened and the ossicles were distorted. None of these abnormalities was present in any of the rats in the other groups.

*Conclusions.*—Studies in rats suggest that Gelfoam promotes fibrosis in the middle ear. No fibrosis is observed with Gelfilm or Instat. Gelfoam's ability to absorb blood and maintain its volume may permit it to serve as a scaffolding for fibroblast growth between the tympanic membrane and promontory, or between the promontory and ossicular mass. Further study of this phenomenon is warranted.

▶ This study is of interest and reflects some of our previous studies done in animals many years ago. Also, we have observed in surgery for chronic ear problems for some long time that when Gelfoam is implanted into the middle ear to serve as a support for a tympanoplastic graft, it can compromise aeration of the middle ear and lead to lack of air flow to the round window membrane. These authors demonstrate in an animal model what I think to be true, that Gelfoam in the middle ear serves as a framework that allows fibroblastic invasion, adhesions, and so forth to develop. For this reason and for many decades, whenever possible we try to avoid Gelfoam in the middle ear and will use other methods for reconstruction, including use of Gelfilm for certain patients who are having tympanoplasty, especially tympanoplasty for atelectasis.

**M.M. Paparella, M.D.**

---

## Acoustic Effect of Malleus Head Removal and Tensor Tympani Muscle Section on Middle Ear Reconstruction

Asai M, Roberson JB Jr, Goode RL (Stanford Univ, Calif; Palo Alto VA Med Ctr, Calif)
*Laryngoscope* 107:1217–1222, 1997

6–24

---

*Introduction.*—An incus replacement prosthesis (IRP) is often used to connect the malleus handle to the stapes head during reconstruction of middle ears with a damaged or missing incus. Some cases may also require resection of the malleus head and/or sectioning of the tensor tympani muscle (TTM) tendon. The acoustic effects of such procedures are difficult to evaluate because of the many other factors involved in postoperative hearing thresholds. A temporal bone model was used to evaluate the acoustic effect of malleus head removal and TTM section.

*Methods.*—Twenty temporal bones from individuals who ranged in age from 51 to 92 at the time of death were prepared for the experiments. All bones were obtained within 48 hours and all experiments performed within 6 days after death. Bones with abnormal tympanic membranes or middle ears were not used. Umbo and stapes displacement was measured before and after malleus head removal and TTM section plus incus replacement with an IRP.

*Results.*—Each of the 2 maneuvers resulted in improvement in the acoustic function of a cement IRP compared with the intact malleus and/or intact TTM situation, and combination of the 2 maneuvers appeared to have an additive effect. With both procedures, improvement was greatest (peak gain of 8 to 10 dB) at higher frequencies between 2 to 6 kHz. The effect of TTM section was less than that of malleus head removal.

*Conclusion.*—The removal of the malleus head results in an increase in umbo and stapes displacement at low and high frequencies. This effect is greatest with a cement IRP contacting the midmalleus. A similar, but lesser, effect occurs after section of the TTM tendon, and a combination of the 2 procedures can produce an additive effect. Findings suggest that postoperative hearing results can be improved by removal of the malleus head and/or section of the TTM when a malleus-to-stapes IRP is employed for middle ear reconstruction.

▶ These authors report an interesting study to assess the acoustical differences when the malleal head is removed and/or when the TTM tendon is sectioned in reconstruction of the middle ear. For many years and in many hundreds of patients, we have routinely sectioned the tensor tympani tendon in order to lateralize the malleus when placing either total or partial ossicular replacement prostheses. We have not found this, at least clinically, to have any deleterious acoustic effect. In fact, the contrary has been observed: that it helps not only to avoid extrusion of the prosthesis but helps to enhance reconstruction of the middle ear and enhance the overall hearing result. Nevertheless, in this study the experimenters looked at a model in temporal bone, and as always one will need to use living patients to assess the clinical efficacy of these maneuvers.

**M.M. Paparella, M.D.**

---

**Practical Use of Total and Partial Ossicular Replacement Prostheses in Ossiculoplasty**
Slater PW, Rizer FM, Schuring AG, et al (Warren Otologic Group, Ohio)
*Laryngoscope* 107:1193–1198, 1997                                         6–25

---

*Introduction.*—Over a 10-year period, more than 250 total and partial ossicular replacement prostheses (TORPs and PORPs) were performed by a single surgeon at the Warren (Ohio) Otologic Group. Outcome at both 6 months and 1 year was superior to that of previous reports. This retrospective review describes the technique used for ossicular reconstruction and compares hearing results in patients treated at the study center with those reported in the literature.

*Methods.*—After exclusion of patients who had TORPs for stapedectomies, 224 patients remained in the study group. All were implanted with either a porous polyethylene TORP or PORP, prostheses that do not require an intact malleus, are easily placed, and are suitable for an infected environment. Tragal cartilage was interposed between the drum and the prosthesis, and temporalis fascia was used for tympanic membrane reconstruction or support when required. Audiometric analysis was performed before surgery, at 6 months and 1 year, and annually thereafter. A PORP was used if the stapes' suprastructure was intact, and a TORP was employed when the suprastructure was absent or unsuitable.

*Results.*—Ninety-one patients had PORPs and 133 had TORPs; 29% of PORPs and 40% of TORPs were staged. Speech reception thresholds, which averaged 46 Db in the PORPs group and 56 dB in the TORPs group at baseline, improved to 30 dB and 38 dB, respectively, at 6 months. There were only 2 extrusions, 1 in each group. One patient in the TORP group had total sensory neural hearing loss. The air-bone gap was closed to within 20 dB in 67% of TORPs cases and in 81% of TORPs cases at 6 months. Relatively few patients were available for follow-up 1 to 2 years and beyond, but results remained good for closure of air-bone gap.

*Conclusion.*—The use of porous polyethylene TORPs and PORPs can yield excellent hearing results with low extrusion rates in patients undergoing ossicular reconstruction. Lysing the tensor tympani to lateralize the tympanic membrane is important, for this provides a more favorable platform for the cartilage prosthesis reconstruction to rest on.

▶ This study looks at a large series of TORPs and PORPs in reconstructive tympanoplasty while also comparing their results to results reported in the literature. Findings are similar to others published in that partial ossicular replacement prostheses (PORPs) provide better results in general than total replacement prostheses (TORPs). As always, it is not so much the prosthesis as the pathologic condition and the surgical procedure necessary to deal with the pathologic condition that will influence these factors, as well as eustachian tubal obstruction postoperatively. I would make a slit in my PORP in order to engage the stapedial tendon; these authors make a slit on both sides of the PORP so the prosthesis can act as a clothespin, attaching itself to the stapes. This also seems like a nice idea that I shall use in the future.

**M.M. Paparella, M.D.**

---

**Efficacy of Tympanomastoid Surgery for Control of Infection in Active Chronic Otitis Media**
Merchant SN, Wang P-C, Jang C-H, et al (Massachusetts Eye and Ear Infirmary, Boston; Harvard Med School, Boston)
*Laryngoscope* 107:872–877, 1997                                              6–26

---

*Introduction.*—A retrospective clinical study was conducted to assess the efficacy of tympanomastoid surgery in controlling infection in active chronic otitis media (COM) and to determine whether there were differences in outcome between active COM with cholesteatoma and active COM with granulation tissue but no cholesteatoma. Also investigated were factors that might influence outcome.

*Methods.*—Cases reviewed consisted of 170 procedures for active COM with cholesteatoma and 102 procedures for active COM with granulation tissue but no cholesteatoma. Excluded were patients with dry perforations of the tympanic membrane and patients with intermittently draining perforations. The majority of patients underwent a 1-stage mastoidectomy with tympanoplasty. Procedures were primary in 47% of cases and revisions in 53%. The mean follow-up time was 30 months, and all patients were monitored for at least 12 months. The following 4-point rating scale was developed to assess control of infection after surgery: 0 represents a totally dry, healed ear; 1 and 2 indicate adequate control of suppuration; and 3 indicates obvious failure to control infection.

*Results.*—Control of infection was scored as *adequate* in 248 (91%) cases. Persistent infection developed in the remaining 24 patients, but 10 were successfully treated with a combination of oral and topical antibiotics and/or delayed skin-grafting. The patients with COM with cholesteatoma did significantly better than those with COM with granulation tissue. Outcome was grade 0 in 59% of the group with cholesteatoma versus 47% of the group with granulation. Outcome was not influenced by extent of cholesteatoma or granulation tissue, primary versus revision surgery status, or canal–wall-up surgery versus canal–wall-down surgery.

*Conclusion.*—Tympanomastoid surgery effectively controlled infection in patients with active COM. Although the overall success rate was 95%, active COM with granulation tissue appears to be more difficult to control than COM with cholesteatoma.

▶ Of interest is that a large number of these patients did *not* have cholesteatoma. In fact, 102 were treated for chronic otitis media and chronic mastoiditis with granulation tissue alone. These authors institute a very clever 4-point rating system for assessing efficacy of results in these patients. Certainly achieving a dry, safe ear is of paramount importance, as these authors indicate, and hearing is a very important objective but only as a secondary consideration, as is also discussed and enunciated by these authors.

**M.M. Paparella, M.D.**

---

**Prognostic Factors in Complicated and Uncomplicated Chronic Otitis Media**
Panda NK, Sreedharan S, Mann SBS, et al (Postgraduate Inst of Med Education and Research, Chandigarh, India)
*Am J Otolaryngol* 17:391–396, 1996                                     6–27

---

*Background.*—Serious complications—aural, extracranial, and intracranial—can occur in patients with chronic suppurative otitis media. There is a need for some set of prognostic factors capable of identifying patients susceptible to otologic complications. These patients could then undergo early surgery. Factors associated with susceptibility to complications of chronic suppurative otitis media were determined prospectively.

*Methods.*—A total of 125 patients with complicated or uncomplicated chronic suppurative otitis media who were treated by mastoid surgery were studied. There were 45 patients with intracranial or extracranial complications of chronic suppurative otitis media (36%) and 30 patients with no complications but unsafe chronic suppurative otitis media. The 2 groups were compared for various factors, including age, sex, duration of ear discharge, otoscopic findings, presence of cholesteatoma or granulation, pneumatization, and aerobic and anaerobic culture results.

*Results.*—Fifty-five percent of patients with complications were younger than 15 years, compared with 28% of patients without complications. The duration of ear discharge was less than 5 years in 57% of patients with complications vs. 30% in those without. The otoscopic findings were similar between groups. At surgery, granulation tissue was found mainly in patients with complications. There was no significant difference between groups in the radiologic extent of mastoid pneumatization. However, patients in the group with complications who were older than 15 years were more likely to have lytic lesions. Anaerobic organisms were isolated on culture from 47% of the patients with complications vs. 19% of those without.

*Conclusions.*—Complications in patients with chronic suppurative otitis media are more likely in patients younger than 15 years with a short history of ear discharge, in patients with anaerobic organisms isolated on culture of ear discharge, and in patients with granulation tissue isolated at surgery. Ears with lytic lesions on radiographs are also more likely to have complications; however, the otoscopic findings cannot distinguish between patients with and without complications.

▶ These authors describe very interestingly the continuum of changes that may occur between childhood and adulthood in patients with chronic, suppurative otitis media. A history of ear discharge for a short duration in patients younger than 15 years who have anaerobes in the ear discharge, and especially granulation tissue at surgery, increases the probability of complications developing in these patients. What the authors are describing is the continuum that can and frequently does occur in children with otitis media with effusion, characterized by liquid pathologic findings, who subsequently have chronic otitis media and chronic mastoiditis, characterized by pathologic findings of granulation tissue that can occupy the middle ear cleft. If the child's condition does not resolve, as most of them do, with appropriate therapy such as medications and ventilation tubes, then a minority will develop the continuum, leading not only to chronic otitis media but to a variety of sequelae and potential complications, as these authors indicate.

**M.M. Paparella, M.D.**

---

**Bilateral Otogenic Temporal Lobe and Post-aural Abscesses**
Gupta AK, Nagarkar NM, Mann SBS, et al (Inst of Med Education and Research, Chandigarh, India)
*J Laryngol Otol* 111:284–285, 1997                                    6–28

---

*Background.*—Chronic suppurative otitis media (CSOM) of the unsafe type can result in postaural abscesses and sometimes life-threatening complications, such as meningitis or brain abscesses. A patient with an unusual presentation of CSOM was described.

> *Case Report.*—Woman, 24, came to the emergency department at a medical center in Chandigarh, India, reporting a history of fever, bilateral ear discharge, bilateral postaural swellings, and

headache of 3 days' duration. She also had nausea, vomiting, and vertigo. The patient had had bilateral intermittent, scanty, offensive discharge and bilateral reduced hearing since childhood. On clinical examination, she was found to be febrile with pallor. The bilateral postaural swellings were tender and fluctuant with erythematous overlying skin. The posterior canal walls of both external auditory canals sagged, with mucopurulent, offensive discharge. Findings of a nose and throat examination were normal. Intracranial involvement was suggested on neurosurgical consultation. A bilateral fundus assessment demonstrated papilloedema, which suggested increased intracranial tension. The patient was also found to be anemic and had leukocytosis. Bilateral radiographs of the mastoid showed lytic cavity suggesting unsafe CSOM (Fig 1). Bilateral temporal lobe abscesses were seen on a CT scan (Fig 2). Broad spectrum IV antibiotics and IV mannitol were begun. Bilateral postaural abscesses were drained, producing about 10 mL of thick pus. A microscopic examination showed cholesteatoma in the attic in both ears. The patient subsequently underwent excision of the temporal lobe abscesses and a left modified radical mastoidectomy. The disease was removed completely, and wide conchomeatoplaty was performed. Her recovery was uneventful.

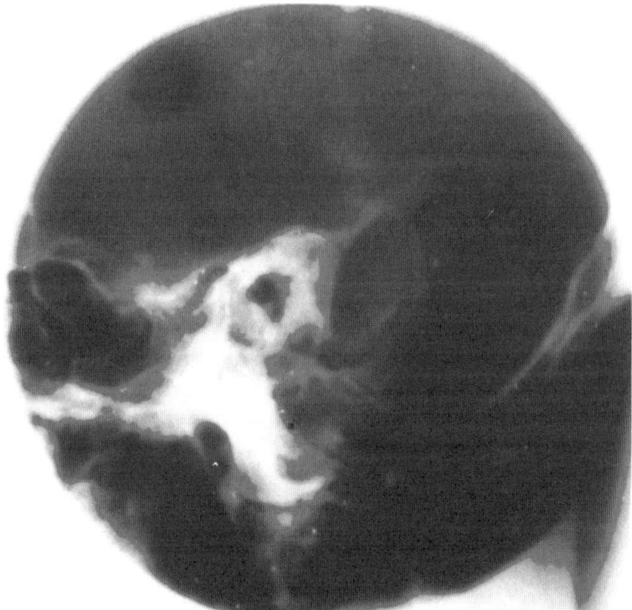

FIGURE 1.—X-ray mastoids. Law's lateral view, showing some posterosuperior erosion. (Courtesy of Gupta AK, Nagarkar NM, Mann SBS, et al: Bilateral otogenic temporal lobe and postaural abscesses. *J Laryngol Otol* 111:284–285, 1997.)

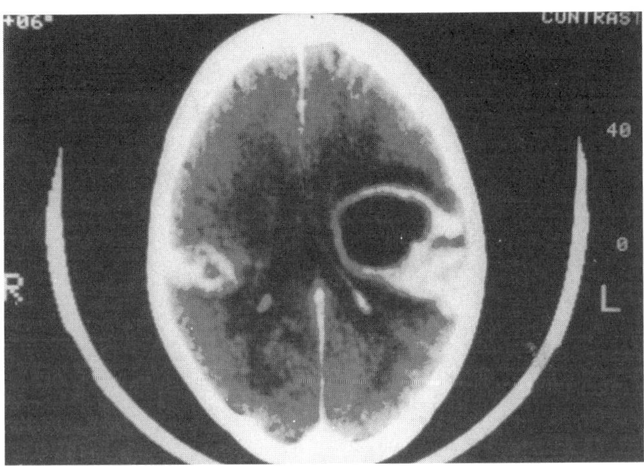

FIGURE 2.—Computed tomographic scan showing bilateral temporal lobe abscess. (Courtesy of Gupta AK, Nagarkar NM, Mann SBS, et al: Bilateral otogenic temporal lobe and postaural abscesses. *J Laryngol Otol* 111:284–285, 1997.)

*Conclusions.*—Clinical suspicion and brain CT scanning enabled detection of intracranial abscesses in this patient. Timely intervention was life-saving. Blockage of the aditus by the disease process in this patient may have caused obstruction of the free flow of pus into the middle ear and external auditory canal, which resulted in pus collecting under tension and extending through the periosteum, appearing clinically as a subperiosteal abscess.

▶ Brain abscesses as a result of CSOM continue to be seen occasionally in the United States. As this article would suggest, they are far more prevalent in developing countries. We know that complications can ensue from otitis media in the temporal bone, particularly involving the labyrinth, but certainly we cannot neglect the fact that intracranial complications still can and do happen with untreated cases of chronic otitis media, with or without cholesteatoma.

**M.M. Paparella, M.D.**

**SECTION 2**

# HEAD AND NECK SURGERY

———

## G. RICHARD HOLT, M.D., M.S.E., M.P.H.

# Introduction

Many exciting advances in head and neck surgery research are on the verge of translation into clinical settings. Identification of active tumor products that persist in causing posttherapy immunosuppression may be identifiable. If so, countermeasures to this product could be developed to allow the patient's intrinsic tumor surveillance/fighting capabilities to regain effectiveness. Additionally, an assay of circulating malignant cells originating in a solid head and neck tumor may be available in the future. Particularly important in tumors which exhibit hematogenous spread, an assay of such sentinel cells could allow for the early treatment with systemic anti-tumor drugs to prevent implantation and growth of metastatic disease.

We have recently seen an increasing interest in quality-of-life issues and outcome studies in head and neck surgery, providing us with some objective instruments for use in determining how patients view their tumor ablation/reconstruction aftermath and the effect on their lives. This year, we feature issues of cost-management analysis and perceived benefits in the treatment of allergic rhinitis—very important to consider because of the huge industry in the U.S. of such treatment. The role of antioxidants and herbal remedies in bolstering the immune system in rhinosinusitis is unknown but potentially promising. As more scientific data on alternative medications is sought and analyzed by the National Institutes of Health, perhaps this issue will become better clarified.

While autologous cartilage (septum, concha) and calvareal bone are still utilized by many surgeons for reconstruction of the orbit, new materials such as titanium mesh and polytetrafluoroethylene (Gore-Tex) are gaining increasing acceptance for this application. Rehabilitation of the paralyzed face now offers many options for the patient, including free innervated muscle transfer, pedicle muscle flaps, and static suspension using polytetrafluoroethylene (Gore-Tex). Further information on metallic bone implants hints that the surface design may actually enhance bone regeneration—biomechanical engineering is critical here.

Advances in laryngeal surgery continue to be exciting. Virtual imaging of the lower airway may someday be combined with virtual surgery to provide safe and high-tech capabilities in this special anatomy. It is proffered that Reinke's edema may be commonly associated with laryngeal hyperfunctioning. That possibility, as well as an association with reflux, should be considered in all patients. The controversy on whether to use a rigid or a flexible bronchoscope in the retrieval of airway foreign bodies is still active. As fewer general otolaryngologists take responsibility for these emergencies in the future ("age attrition"), the issue may be decided by our colleagues in pediatric otolaryngology.

While we are all familiar with the success of botulinum toxin injections into the larynx for laryngeal movement disorders, new information is being published on its efficacy in reducing hyperfunctional forehead and glabellar motion lines. The aesthetic utilizations have increased in frequency so much that the supply of toxin was severely limited for a time. Finally, as the plane of dissection of facial rhytidectomy becomes deeper and more extensive, there is an interest in studying the effects of resuspending the facial fat pads to achieve a more "preaging" position.

**G. Richard Holt, M.D. M.S.E., M.P.H.**

# 7 Advances in Head and Neck Surgery Research

**Suppressive Factor or Factors Derived From Head and Neck Squamous Cell Carcinoma Induce Apoptosis in Activated Lymphocytes**
Billings KR, Wang MB, Lichtenstein AK (Univ of California, Los Angeles; West Los Angeles Veterans Med Ctr; Jonsson Comprehensive Cancer Ctr, Los Angeles)
*Otolaryngol Head Neck Surg* 116:458–465, 1997                    7–1

*Introduction.*—In head and neck squamous cell carcinoma, the ability of tumors to produce soluble factors capable of suppressing the immune system of the host has been demonstrated. These cells produce a heterogenous group of factors with potent immunosuppressive capabilities, and their complexity plays an important role in the development and progression of tumors. A previous study showed how a 25-kD immunosuppressive factor obtained from an esophageal squamous cell carcinoma cell line inhibited the proliferation of peripheral blood T lymphocytes and T-cell lines, and induced apoptotic death in these target cells. The nature of the interaction between a soluble factor derived from head and neck squamous cell carcinoma that impairs lymphocyte proliferative responses in vitro and T lymphocytes was investigated.

*Methods.*—Tumors from patients having surgical resection of head and neck cancer were used. There was tumor supernatant preparation, maintenance of the Jurkat T-cell line, preparation of peripheral blood lymphocytes, proliferation assays, and gel electrophoresis of DNA.

*Results.*—The supernatants of 13 (41.9%) of 31 recently explanted head and neck squamous cell carcinoma samples significantly suppressed the proliferative activity of phytohemagglutinin-stimulated peripheral blood lymphocytes and the Jurkat T-cell line. The suppressive supernatants were inducing or predisposing T cells to apoptotic death according to a characteristic morphologic appearance of these suppressed cells and ladderlike pattern of DNA fragmentation on gel electrophoresis. This apoptosis-inducing activity may be similar to that demonstrated previously in a suppressive supernatant that was derived from an esophageal carcinoma cell line.

*Conclusions.*—These findings contribute to a better understanding of the mechanism that causes soluble immunosuppressive factors to be produced by head and neck squamous cell carcinoma. T-cell proliferation was inhibited by a soluble inhibitory factor derived from the supernatants of freshly explanted head and neck squamous cell carcinoma tumor cells. These soluble suppressive factors should be investigated further to better understand their function.

▶ I believe it is commonly held that the initial neoplasia of squamous cell carcinoma involves the failure of the immune surveillance and suppressive system to properly manage mutant cells. This study suggests that *after* the carcinoma develops, there is a continued immunosuppression that is effected by a product of the tumor itself. This is worrisome on the one hand, because it implies a kind of self-perpetuating existence that seems ominous and, well, malignant. On the other hand, if such a product can be identified and isolated, some chemical countermeasure might be developed to turn off this immune suppressant. That would be a valuable clinical tool for us.

**G.R. Holt, M.D., M.S.E., M.P.H.**

---

**A New Immunocompetent Murine Model for Oral Cancer**
O'Malley BW Jr, Cope KA, Johnson CS, et al (Johns Hopkins Univ, Baltimore, Md; Univ of Pittsburgh, Pa; Baylor College of Medicine, Houston)
*Arch Otolaryngol Head Neck Surg* 123:20–24, 1997                    7–2

---

*Background.*—Although animal models have long been used to study head and neck cancer in humans, no one has yet described a model of immunocompetent squamous cell cancer with tumors in a natural head and neck site. A new immunocompetent murine model developed to parallel the clinical and biological nature of head and neck cancer was reported.

*Methods.*—The growth rate and histologic features of the SCC VII/SF cell line were determined in tissue culture experiments. Subsequently, C3H/HeJ mice were directly injected with $5 \times 10^5$ SCC VII/SF cells in the floor of the mouth. The mice were killed after 1, 2, and 3 weeks for assessment of tumor growth, invasion, and regional and distant metastases.

*Findings.*—After 5 to 7 days, the mice had SCCs in the floor of the mouth that could be palpated and measured externally. There was also local invasion into the mylohyoid musculature and mandible. At between 2 and 3 weeks, cervical lymph node and pulmonary metastases were evident.

*Conclusion.*—This new murine model of oral cancer shows initial locoregional tumor invasion, direct extension into the neck, early cervical metastases, and pulmonary metastases. These features reflect the biological behavior and progression of oral tumors in humans. This model will, therefore, be useful for clinically applicable research in primary and metastatic head and neck cancer.

▶ If this model can provide a rigorous foundation for head and neck cancer research, it will be of potentially great impact. The model appears to provide the local and regional clinical processes that approximate the staging we see in humans. I am very excited about this advance and will monitor its application closely.

**G.R. Holt, M.D., M.S.E., M.P.H.**

## KTP Laser and Neutral Red Phototherapy of Human Squamous Cell Carcinoma

VanderWerf QM, Castro DJ, Nguyen RD, et al (Univ of California, Los Angeles)
*Laryngoscope* 107:316–320, 1997

7–3

*Objective.*—The cytotoxicity of certain anticancer drugs is enhanced when they are illuminated by visible laser light. Neutral red (NR), a weakly cationic, nontoxic vital dye used as a histologic stain for proliferating cells, is selectively taken up by proliferating cells. The usefulness of NR as a photosensitizer for human squamous cell carcinoma was examined.

*Methods.*—Neutral red uptake was tested in human squamous carcinoma cell line UCLA-SO-P3. The P3 cells were incubated with serial dilutions (0.05–50 µg/mL) of NR in phosphate buffer, pelleted, washed, and either placed in the dark or exposed to the potassium titanylphosphate 532 crystal laser at 5 W for 0–60 seconds. Cell viability was determined after 72 hours using the MTT assay.

*Results.*—Almost 100% cell death was observed at NR concentrations of 0.5 or more µg/mL. Cell toxicity was related to NR dose and light intensity.

*Conclusion.*—Neutral red is an extremely good photosensitizer that is rapidly concentrated by human cancer cells in vitro. It is nontoxic in the absence of light. Preclinical in vivo testing is being conducted to establish safety and efficacy.

▶ This research attempts to further understand the options in phototherapy against carcinomas using the combination of NR in cells excited by the KTP laser. This area of cell sensitization and photodestruction has been of interest for a number of years. With significant clinical applications and results, this research will be more accepted and utilized.

**G.R. Holt, M.D., M.S.E., M.P.H.**

## Detection of Circulating Thyroid Cells in Peripheral Blood

Ditkoff BA, Marvin MR, Yemul S, et al (Columbia Univ, New York)
*Surgery* 120:959–965, 1996

7–4

*Background.*—The detection of circulating malignant thyroid cells may be a useful method for identifying patients at risk for metastatic thyroid cancer after surgery. Thyroglobulin messenger RNA (mRNA) was identified in the circulating peripheral blood of such patients and compared with clinical staging.

*Methods.*—To detect thyroglobulin RNA transcripts, reverse transcriptase-polymerase chain reaction analysis was performed using primers for thyroglobulin on blood samples. Samples were obtained from 9 patients with known metastatic thyroid cancer, 78 with thyroid cancer and no evidence of current metastases, 6 with benign thyroid disease, and 7 healthy persons.

*Findings.*—Thyroglobulin transcripts were found in all the patients with metastatic thyroid cancer. Seven patients with thyroid cancer and no current metastases were shown to have thyroglobulin transcripts. Five of these patients had a history of metastatic disease previously treated surgically, 1 had a coexisting parathyroid cancer, and 1 had papillary and follicular thyroid cancers. No thyroglobulin transcripts were detected in any of the patients with benign thyroid disease or in the healthy persons.

*Conclusion.*—Reverse transcriptase-polymerase chain reaction can be used to detect thyroglobulin mRNA in peripheral blood. The presence of these transcripts is associated with that of extrathyroidal disease.

▶ What a great benefit it would be to be able to detect circulating malignant cells, not just of thyroid origin. Could this be the cancer advancement of the decade? Would it make a difference in survival if these cells could be detected and the appropriate chemotherapy initiated based on the malignant cell's early detection and determination of its susceptibility to drugs? Can other cell lines be detected, such as lung, breast and prostate? This is a potentially exciting development.

**G.R. Holt, M.D., M.S.E., M.P.H.**

## Survival of Normothermic Microvascular Flaps After Prolonged Secondary Ischemia: Effects of Hyperbaric Oxygen

Stevens DM, Weiss DD, Koller WA, et al (Natl Naval Med Ctr, Bethesda, Md; Naval Med Research Inst, Bethesda, Md)
*Otolaryngol Head Neck Surg* 115:360–364, 1996

7–5

*Background.*—Hyperbaric oxygen has been found to improve the survival rate of ischemic grafts and many types of flaps. However, its use in free-tissue transfer has not been studied extensively. The effect of hyperbaric oxygen on flap survival after exposure to critical combinations of primary ischemia, reperfusion, and secondary ischemia times was studied in Sprague-Dawley rats.

*Methods.*—Unilateral abdominal adipocutaneous island flaps based on the superficial inferior epigastric vessels were raised and primary normothermic ischemia induced by applying a microvascular clamp to the vascular pedicle for 6 hours. The clamp was removed for 2 hours of reperfusion, reapplied for 6, 10, or 14 hours for secondary ischemia, then removed again, and the rats were assigned randomly to 1 of 3 treatments. A control group was exposed to normobaric air and the other 2 groups to normobaric 100% or hyperbaric oxygen for 2 90-minute periods for 7 days. Flap survival was evaluated 7 days after surgery. Maximum likelihood-derived survival curves were used to calculate the secondary ischemic time at which 50% of the flaps survived (D50).

*Findings.*—The air and 100% oxygen groups had a D50 of 6 hours, compared with 10 hours in the hyperbaric oxygen group. This difference was significant. Further analysis of pooled data verified a significant increase in flap survival in the rats treated with hyperbaric oxygen compared with those treated with air or 100% oxygen.

*Conclusion.*—Hyperbaric oxygen increases the tolerance of normothermic microvascular flaps to prolonged secondary ischemia, suggesting that the additional expense and technology of a hyperbaric chamber system are justified.

▶ Hyperbaric oxygen therapy (HBO) has assisted us in head and neck surgical reconstruction for 2 decades. This new study indicates the potential of HBO for enhancing survival of free flaps after prolonged primary and secondary ischemic times. Because free-flap procedures are commonly performed at tertiary care centers, a protocol should be developed in conjunction with the closest HBO facility to handle such flaps if indicated, and if future clinical studies confirm its efficacy.

**G.R. Holt, M.D., M.S.E., M.P.H.**

---

## Age-related Changes of Elastic Fibers in the Superficial Layer of the Lamina Propria of Vocal Folds

Sato K, Hirano M (Kurume Univ, Japan)
*Ann Otol Rhinol Laryngol* 106:44–48, 1997                                    7–6

---

*Background.*—The precise mechanisms of the aging of the human voice have not been clearly determined. The age-related changes of elastic fibers in the superficial layer of the lamina propria of the aged vocal folds were investigated.

*Methods.*—Ten normal adult larynges obtained at autopsy were studied. Five were from persons aged 74 to 87 years, and 5 were from persons aged 34 to 39 years. Age-related morphologic changes of elastic fibers were studied by electron microscopy, and age-related metabolic changes in elastin and elastic fibers were assessed by elastase digestion study.

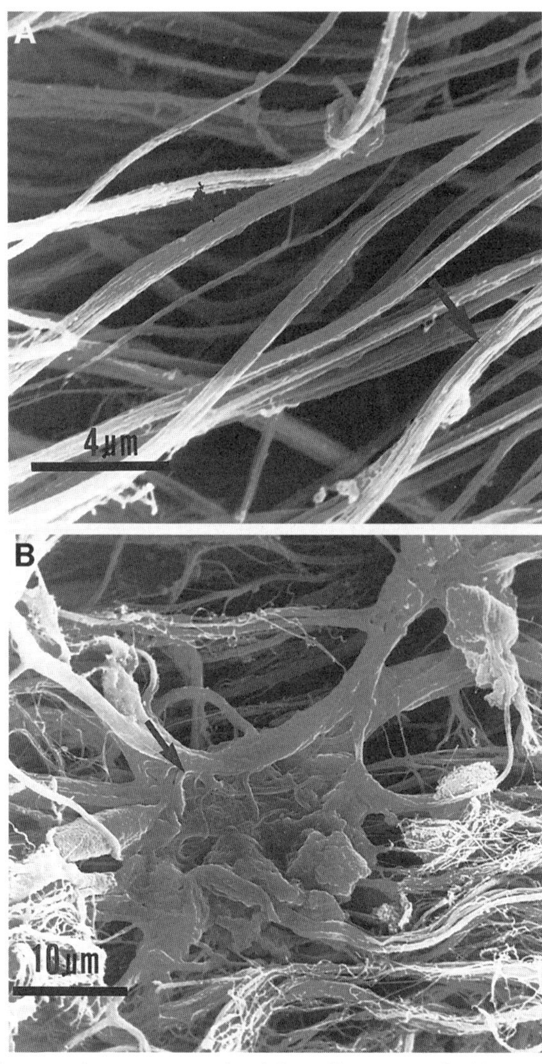

FIGURE 1.—Scanning electron micrographs of elastic fibers in superficial layer of lamina propria of vocal fold. **A**, younger adult. *Arrows* indicate elastic fibers. **B**, aged adult. *Arrow* indicates elastic fibers united to form sheet with rough surface. (Courtesy of Sato K, Hirano M: Age-related changes of elastic fibers in the superficial layer of the lamina propria of vocal folds. *Ann Otol Rhinol Laryngol* 106:44–48, 1997.)

*Findings.*—The elastic fibers of the aged vocal folds (EFAVFs) consisted of amorphous substances and microfibrils. The amount of amorphous substances was increased in the aged EFAVFs, and the microfibrils became less numerous. Also, EFAVFs ran in various directions, were branched, and formed a complicated network. The fiber surface was rough and the fibers appeared to vary in size. Some EFAVFs united, forming a sheet with a rough surface. Compared with EFAVFs from younger adults, those of elderly adults could not be easily digested by elastase (Fig 1).

*Conclusion.*—Elastic fibers in the superficial layer of the lamina propria of aged vocal folds are changed morphologically, and their metabolism is disturbed, resulting in slow turnover and repair. Also, newly synthesized elastic fibers are decreased. The elastic fibers apparently lose their function and provide inadequate resilience to the tissue. These changes partly contribute to the aging of the voice.

▶ Those who see aging patients concerned about their failing voices will be pleased to note these findings. The elastic fibers of the lamina propria may undergo degenerative changes over time that can affect the vibratory properties of the vocal fold. Given similar degenerative changes in other connective tissues of the aging body, it does seem reasonable that the vocal cord would be no exception. Our own studies comparing the larynges of young and old male and female baboons identified changing sex steroid receptor sites in the vocal cord lamina propria. These findings have led us to speculate that such receptor changes will affect the connective and muscular fibers of the vocal cords. The question now is, can we somehow stop or reverse these changes? Perhaps using receptor modulation could be the answer.

**G.R. Holt, M.D., M.S.E., M.P.H.**

---

**Cross-innervation of the Thyroarytenoid Muscle by a Branch From the External Division of the Superior Laryngeal Nerve**
Nasri S, Sercarz JA, Beizai P, et al (Stanford Med Ctr, Calif; Univ of California, Los Angeles; Wadsworth Veterans Administration Med Ctr, West Los Angeles)
*Ann Otol Rhinol Laryngol* 106:594–598, 1997                                    7–7

---

*Purpose.*—There is debate regarding the anatomy and physiology of the external division of the superior laryngeal nerve (ExSLN). Anatomic studies have suggested innervation of the ExSLN and the thyroarytenoid (TA) muscle; however, it is unknown whether this connection contains muscle fibers. The anatomy and function of the distal ExSLN were studied in vivo in dogs.

*Methods.*—Seven canine larynxes were studied by microanatomic dissection. After dissection, electrodes were placed on the nerves to see whether they produced muscular contraction. Muscle function was confirmed by electromyography and videostroboscopy.

*Results.*—Three of 7 larynxes showed motor innervation to the TA muscle from the ExSLN. When the ExSLN was electrically stimulated through microelectrodes, the TA muscle contracted; the motor function of the nerve was also confirmed by electromyographic recordings. On videostroboscopy, vocal fold vibration was seen to improve with stimulation of the ExSLN.

*Conclusions.*—In addition to the recurrent laryngeal nerve, the TA muscle appears to receive motor innervation from the ExSLN. This cross-innervation of an essential muscle may be relevant to the clinical treatment of adductor spasmodic dysphonia and other neurologic laryngeal disorders. Histologic studies to develop a detailed map of laryngeal motor centers within the nucleus ambiguus are ongoing.

▶ The possibility that the ExSLN provides limited (anterior) innervation to the TA muscle is intriguing. Is such innervation really present in some humans? Does it actually function in pitch control? Could it be a potential source of spontaneous partial reinnervation of a paralyzed hemilarynx? These questions should be addressed to further our clinically applied knowledge of laryngeal neurophysiology.

**G.R. Holt, M.D., M.S.E., M.P.H.**

---

**Physiologic Motion After Laryngeal Nerve Reinnervation: A New Method**
Sercarz JA, Nguyen LI, Nasri S, et al (Univ of California, Los Angeles; Harvard Med School, Boston)
*Otolaryngol Head Neck Surg* 116:466–474, 1997                    7–8

---

*Introduction.*—For the treatment of unilateral vocal fold paralysis, many approaches have been proposed that primarily involve reinnervation or vocal fold medialization. Restoration of physiologic abduction and adduction to the paralyzed vocal fold has not been possible with these methods. Reinnervation can be ansa reinnervation of the paralyzed recurrent laryngeal nerve, or phrenic nerve transfer to the posterior cricoarytenoid muscle to improve the airway in bilateral recurrent laryngeal nerve paralysis. The effectiveness of using the contralateral intact terminal adductor branch to reinnervate the paralyzed adductor muscles by direct anastomosis or ansa cervicalis cable graft was studied.

*Methods.*—Physiologic measures of phonation were performed 3 months after contralateral thyroarytenoid branch reinnervation of the anterior division of the recurrent laryngeal nerve. A control group of canines was used to compare the results. Two dogs had division of the left recurrent laryngeal nerve and immediate anastomosis of the right vocalis terminal nerve branch to the left distal stump, whereas the other 2 dogs had a similar anastomosis, but through an ansa cervicalis cable graft. The procedure involves division of the left anterior recurrent laryngeal nerve and reinnervation with axons from the thyroarytenoid branch of the contralateral recurrent laryngeal nerve. Then there is division of the posterior branch of the left recurrent laryngeal nerve. To maintain tone in the posterior cricoarytenoid muscle, the posterior branch of the left recurrent laryngeal nerve was sutured to the ansa cervicalis. The right dista vocalis stump was reinnervated with an ansa cervicalis nerve in all 4 animals.

*Results.*—During mechanical stimulation of the supraglottis (adduction) and during tracheostomy obstruction (abduction), physiologic vocal fold motion and electromyographic activity could be demonstrated after 3 months. The reinnervated animals showed improvement of jitter, shimmer, signal-to-noise ratio, and vocal efficiency, according to acoustic data, when compared with paralyzed canines before treatment. However, there was no statistical significance with these results.

*Conclusions.*—This method allows phonation after thyroarytenoid sacrifice on the donor side, and it allows the thyroarytenoid branch to remain active during vocal fold adduction. After reinnervation of the anterior recurrent laryngeal nerve by the use of the contralateral thyroarytenoid nerve, vocal fold synkinesis was avoided and physiologic fold motion was restored. The results may be improved with a longer period of reinnervation. It is not known how this procedure would work in humans.

▶ The authors have devised a selective reinnervation scheme that promotes reaxonitization of similar fibers, i.e., adductor nerve graft or anastomosis from the good side to the bad. This is similar to crossover reinnervation of the orbicularis oris or orbicularis oculi muscles in facial paralysis. The ansa cervicalis is hooked into the posterior cricoarytenoid muscle (PCA) to maintain tone. It would certainly be helpful to devise a crossover from PCA to PCA or to reinnervate that muscle by a nerve that is involved in respiration. It has been performed in electrical pacing, but not, to my knowledge, in a physiologic setting. Selective abductor/adductor reinnervation is an exciting concept.

**G.R. Holt, M.D., M.S.E., M.P.H.**

---

**Ovine Fetal Laryngeal Chemoreflex Thresholds and Respiratory Effects**
Chan K, Kullama LK, Day L, et al (Harbor–Univ of California at Los Angeles Med Ctr)
*Otolaryngol Head Neck Surg* 116:91–96, 1997                    7–9

---

*Introduction.*—During feeding and regurgitation, the laryngeal chemoreflex is thought to be a protective mechanism for the airway, but when it is poorly coordinated, such as is found in very young or premature newborns, bradycardia and prolonged apnea may be fatal. Concentration and volume thresholds for laryngeal fluid swallowing stimulation were defined. Also, whether a true laryngeal chemoreflex is present during fetal life was determined.

*Methods.*—Eight time-bred ewes were prepared with fetal electrocortical diaphragm and esophageal electrodes and a nasopharyngeal catheter to determine whether the laryngeal chemoreflex is present during fetal life. There was a 60-minute control period. Through the nasopharyngeal catheter, increasing volumes (0.1–1.0 mL/kg) of 0.15 mol/L of sodium chloride or distilled water (0.05–1.0 mL/kg), and decreasing concentrations of sodium chloride (0.15–0.02 mol/L) at a fixed volume (0.3 mL/kg) were sequentially administered after the control period.

*Results.*—Swallowing was stimulated by a minimum water volume that was significantly less than the minimum sodium chloride volume (0.10 mL/kg vs. 0.70 mL/kg). Swallowing was stimulated by a maximum sodium chloride concentration of 0.04 mol/L. Respiratory activity averaged 14.6 breaths/min during the control period. During absent swallow responses or isotonic saline–induced swallows, the respiratory activity did not change. During water and hypotonic saline–induced swallow responses, respiratory activity significantly decreased. During absent or stimulated swallows, fetal electrocortical activity did not change.

*Conclusions.*—Fetal swallowing may be stimulated and fetal respiratory activity may be suppressed by laryngeal water or hypotonic saline solution, similar to the newborn laryngeal chemoreflex. An exaggeration of the laryngeal chemoreflex apnea response in newborns may predispose them to sudden infant death syndrome.

▶ While the authors are investigating the laryngeal chemoreflex as a factor in sudden infant death syndrome, it struck me that this reflex might also be protective in children who have near-drowning events. In these cases, in addition to the "diving reflex" of bradycardia, this laryngeal reflex could prevent the flow of water into the lungs in favor of swallowing water, thus keeping the alveolar epithelium undamaged. Does this sound possible to you? Write or e-mail your comments.

**G.R. Holt, M.D., M.S.E., M.P.H.**

---

**Fatty Acid Modulation of K+ Channels in Taste Receptor Cells: Gustatory Cues for Dietary Fat**
Gilbertson TA, Fontenot DT, Liu L, et al (Louisiana State Univ, Baton Rouge)
*Am J Physiol* 272:C1203–C1210, 1997                                      7–10

---

*Introduction.*—The basic tastes of salty, sour, sweet, and bitter are detected by taste receptor cells in the oral cavity, which respond to a variety of sapid molecules. Comparatively little attention has been given to the sensory properties of fats, particularly free fatty acids. Fatty acids may have direct effects on ion channels, including several types of K+ channels, Na+ channels, and $Ca^{2+}$ channels. In a variety of systems, free fatty acids may be important regulators of signal transduction. Patch-clamp recordings were performed on isolated rat taste receptor cells during application of free fatty acids to determine the chemosensory cues, if any, provided by fats in the oral cavity.

*Methods.*—Fungiform taste buds were isolated from the tongues of 2- to 5-month old male rats. Electrophysiologic recordings were taken and analysis was conducted. The whole cell patch-clamp configuration was used to record voltage-activated currents from individual taste receptor cells maintained in the taste bud.

*Results.*—Delayed-rectifying K+ channels were inhibited with *Cis*-polyunsaturated fatty acids when they were applied extracellularly. These fatty acids also enhance inwardly rectifying K+ currents in a subset of cells. No significant effect on K+ currents was found with saturated, monounsaturated, or *trans*-polyunsaturated fatty acids. Activation of G protein–mediated pathways were not involved in these effects. They also did not involve protein kinase C or protein kinase A, lipoxygenase pathways, cyclooxygenase pathways, or cytochrome *P-450* pathways. This is consistent with the direct effects on these closely associated proteins or ion channels.

*Conclusions.*—Stimulus-induced depolarizations of taste receptors are prolonged by fatty acids. The mechanism by which fats are detected by receptor cells in the oral cavity is by their effects on K+ channels. To design acceptable fat alternatives, an understanding of both the textural and gustatory cues that fats provide is required.

▶ I thought this was an interesting study because it made me consider whether taste receptor cells could be tricked, trained, or taunted to cause a preference for good triglycerides such as monounsaturated oils, which could have a positive effect on lipid metabolism. Much like any aversion-drug therapy, if one could block or cause dysgeusia with saturated fatty acids, a patient could potentially be trained to prefer or select healthier foods. Sounds good, right?

**G.R. Holt, M.D., M.S.E., M.P.H.**

---

**Cartilage Viability With Interpolated Skin Flaps: An Experimental Study**
Park SS, White GJ, Cook TA, et al (Oregon Health Sciences Univ, Portland)
*Otolaryngol Head Neck Surg* 116:483–488, 1997                          7–11

---

*Introduction.*—Reconstructive surgeons commonly encounter nasal problems. The most challenging are full-thickness defects because they require replacement of skin, cartilage, and inner lining. The carrier flap can survive through ingrowth of vessels from the recipient site after an unknown critical period and pedicle division. The blood supply to the flap is partially compromised in the immediate period after pedicle division, and this could affect cartilage survival. It is unknown whether prolonging the time of pedicle division would offer any additional benefit to the cartilage component. The timing of pedicle division was investigated in a rabbit model to optimize cartilage viability for a midline forehead flap and repair of full-thickness nasal defects.

*Methods.*—In each of 5 groups of 5 rabbits, the skin flap pedicle was divided at 0 days, 4 days, 3 weeks, 6 weeks, and 10 weeks. The animals had a full-thickness skin defect created on the dorsum of the left nose. They had a nasal defect, paramedian forehead flap, and contralateral composite auricular graft (Fig 2, A). A pedicled vessel was demonstrated after composite graft was in position for nasal repair. The animals had

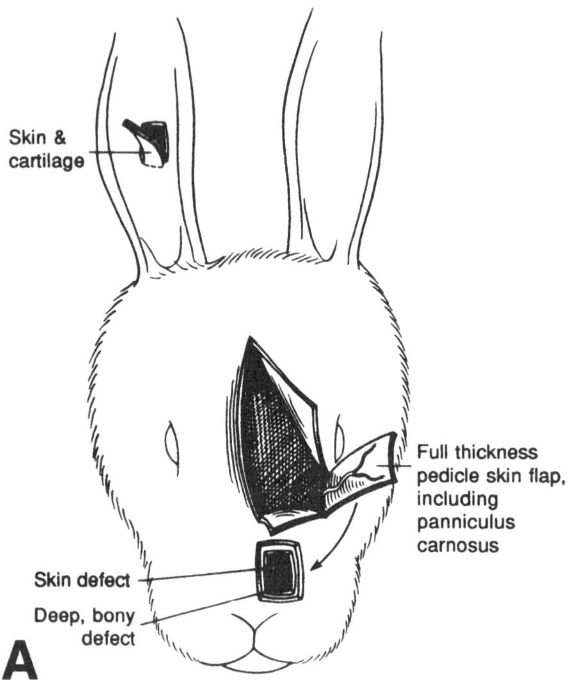



**FIGURE 2, A.**—Nasal defect, paramedian forehead flap, and contralateral composite auricular graft. (Courtesy of Park SS, White GJ, Cook TA, et al: Cartilage viability with interpolated skin flaps: An experimental study. *Otolaryngol Head Neck Surg* 116:483–488, 1997.)

pedicle division after a designated interval. Skin flap viability was quantified according to no hair growth, partial hair growth, or full hair growth.

*Results.*—Partial skin flap necrosis resulted from early pedicle division, but the cartilage grafts tolerate this ischemic period better. Between the 5 groups, there was not a significant difference and cartilage viability was about 70%. The preliminary study showed that the critical period for flap survival was around 4 days, and those divided at 4 days had obvious necrosis. Those divided at 7 and 10 days had no necrosis with partial hair loss.

*Conclusions.*—The timing of pedicle division in the carrier skin flap did not affect cartilage composite graft viability, but there were clear effects on skin flap viability. Cartilage grafts survived based on their peripheral revascularization alone and were not dependent on skin flap viability. To determine optimum timing for pedicle division in this animal model, a larger composite graft and better definition of the skin flap's critical period are needed.

▶ Because of the peculiar (and incompletely understood) parameters of the viability of cartilage grafts, this study was constructed, in my opinion, to provide additional information helpful to the reconstructive surgeon. We all worry about necrosis of a transferred cartilage graft, and when it is designed for structural support, we would like to ensure survival as best possible. Although further studies are indicated, the results give us some notion that the short-term viability is good, in spite of vascular insult with early pedicle division. Perhaps cartilage is tougher than we give it credit.

**G.R. Holt, M.D., M.S.E., M.P.H.**

## Torsion-Axial Force Characteristics of SR-PLLA Screws

Shetty V, Caputo AA, Kelso I, et al (Univ of California, Los Angeles)
*J Craniomaxillofac Surg* 25:19–23, 1997                    7–12

*Introduction.*—Biodegradable polymers appear to be attractive alternatives to the traditional metals used for fabricating internal fixation devices for maxillofacial trauma and orthognathic surgery, especially poly-L-lactide. Plates and screws of this material could provide stability and stress transfer functions during osseous healing and gradually degrade as the bone regains its structural integrity. Currently, titanium alloys and stainless steel devices are used for stabilizing osseous segments. The torsion-axial force characteristics of prototype self-reinforced poly-L-lactide screws were compared with those of conventional titanium screws.

*Methods.*—A test apparatus incorporating an Instron machine was used to measure axial forces developed by incremental increases in the torque applied to the individual screws. The self-reinforced poly-L-lactide screws used were made by Bioscience, and 40-mm screws as well as 20-mm screws were investigated. Eight screws of each type were tested.

*Results.*—There was a nonlinear relationship with a marked relaxation throughout the test range for the self-reinforced poly-L-lactide screws in the relationship between applied torque and axial force development. A maximum was reached in the axial forces with increasing torque, and then there was failure of the screws. There was a steeper slope in the response curve for titanium screws of the same length. With the titanium screws, no failures or force relaxation were seen.

*Conclusions.*—The use of self-reinforced poly-L-lactide screws should be restricted to low–stress-bearing areas at this time. The larger heads of the biodegradable screws may cause problems where there is limited soft-tissue coverage. The shorter length biodegradable screws are similar in torque-axial force to the titanium screws up to a certain point, and may be used for stabilizing lamellar mandibular fractures and osteotomies.

▶ Because of their molecular framework structure, polymers are more likely to slip, as opposed to metals, where movement of the molecular boxes or plates is not so slippery. Metal will fatigue, of course, but it takes time; acute fatigue will cause shearing of the metal. Inherently, metals are considerably tougher than biodegradable polymers, and will resist indentation or deformation to a higher degree. This study demonstrates that the biological polymer studied would not tolerate torsion-axial forces (screw tightening) as did titanium. Thus, one cannot expect to get away with using them where such forces are important, such as distracting fragments.

**G.R. Holt, M.D., M.S.E., M.P.H.**

**The Effect of Insulin-Like Growth Factor 1 on Craniofacial Bone Healing**
Kobayashi K, Agrawal K, Jackson IT, et al (Inst for Craniofacial and Reconstructive Surgery, Southfield, Mich)
*Plast Reconstr Surg* 97:1129–1135, 1996                                    7–13

*Background.*—Insulin-like growth factor 1, one of a group of local factors believed to influence bone healing, plays an important role in controlling differentiation and growth rates of chondrocytes and bone-forming cells. The effects of insulin-like growth factor 1 on formation of bone, and on healing of full-thickness defects of calvarian bone, were determined in this study.

*Methods.*—Full-thickness, 10 mm $\times$ 10 mm bone defects were created in the calvarium of 40, 8- to 10-week-old rats. Recombinant human insulin-like growth factor 1 was delivered between the dura mater and the periosteum of the defect, by osmotic minipumps, in 20 rats at a dose of 100 µg every 2 weeks. The remaining 20 animals received injections of vehicle at the same volume. Five animals from each group were killed after 3, 6, 9, and 12 weeks, and the operative sites were examined histologically for indications of bone healing.

*Results.*—In rats treated with insulin-like growth factor, bone defects filled rapidly with thick fibrous tissue, and bone formation occurred from both the edges of the bone defects and from the center, resulting in the presence of both trabecular and lamellar bone throughout the site by 12 weeks. In control animals, defects filled with fibrous tissue, with bone growth occurring later and only from the perimeter of the lesions. There was no indication of trabecular or cartilage formation by 12 weeks in these animals. The mean area of newly formed bone was 2.8 and 1.7 mm$^2$ in the treated and control groups, respectively ($P < 0.05$).

*Conclusions.*—Exposure of calvarial bone defects to insulin-like growth factor 1 stimulates osteogenesis from both the center and the margin of the lesion. Further research is needed to optimize the dosage protocol and to explore the effect on osteogenesis of combining insulin-like growth factor 1 with other growth factors.

▶ Much of the bulk of bone-healing research has been in the region of the axial skeleton, with particular reference to enhancing fixation or closure of long-bone fractures. This study could have implications in our own field, for example, in developing a relatively easy method of introducing insulin-like growth factor into a calvarial defect of traumatic or reconstructive origin. My method of choice to fill a calvarial bone graft donor site is to use hydroxyapatite and blood, but growth factor could make a nice addition to the mix.

I would feel better about the safety of the donor site if new bone could be formed in the outer table.

**G.R. Holt, M.D., M.S.E., M.P.H.**

---

**Antithrombotic and Platelet Activating Effects of Heparin in Prevention of Microarterial Thrombosis**
Arnljots B, Dougan P, Bergqvist D (Univ Hosp, Uppsala, Sweden)
*Plast Reconstr Surg* 99:1122–1128, 1997        7–14

---

*Background.*—Heparin is an anticoagulant used to prevent venous thrombosis. Its use in the prevention of arterial thrombosis has not been as successful. It has been proposed that this relative inefficacy of heparin in the prevention of arterial thrombosis is due to the platelet-activating properties of standard heparin preparations. This study investigated the platelet-activating properties of heparin in vivo with a rabbit model.

*Methods.*—An established rabbit model of microarterial thrombosis involving monitoring labeled platelet accumulation at trauma sites was employed to examine the platelet-activating properties of heparin in vivo. Six rabbits received isotonic saline solution, 6 received heparin, and 6 received heparin that had been prepared on affinity columns to have low affinity for antithrombin III (low-affinity heparin). Low-affinity heparin has low anticoagulant properties but has a similar molecular weight distribution to standard heparin.

*Results.*—Platelet accumulation at the trauma sites was significantly increased in the rabbits treated with low-affinity heparin compared with those treated with saline solution, revealing an in vivo platelet-activating activity of heparin. The antithrombic effect of heparin was expressed incompletely in these rabbits; only 2 of 3 treated vessels remained patent.

*Conclusions.*—These results demonstrate heparin-induced platelet activation in vivo under conditions of platelet-mediated thrombus formation. This platelet-activation property of heparin may help to explain the limited efficacy of heparin treatment in the prevention of arterial thrombosis.

▶ It is interesting that the effects of heparin appear to be different (at least in vivo) in the artery and in the vein. The authors postulate that the anti-thrombin effect in the vein counteracts the platelet-activation effect of the heparin at that site. This countereffect does not seem to take place in the arterial model. This information is not only of potential clinical importance with free flaps, but perhaps also with pedicle flaps such as the latissimus or pectoralis. Presumably, the maintenance of adequate vascular fluid volume is also an important factor for vessel patency.

**G.R. Holt, M.D., M.S.E., M.P.H.**

## Rapid Prototyping Techniques for Anatomical Modelling in Medicine

McGurk M, Amis AA, Potamianos P, et al (Guy's Hosp, London; Imperial College of Science Technology and Medicine, London)
*Ann R Coll Surg Engl* 79:169–174, 1997                                    7–15

*Objective.*—The revolution in CT and MRI techniques has made it possible to provide detailed soft tissue 3 dimensional images that improve surgical planning and describe tumor margins. Rapid prototyping techniques (RPT) can reproduce a computer image as an acrylic model in a few hours to aid surgeons in understanding the complex geometry of the underlying pathology. The development and current technologies available in RPT and the applications of this advance in surgery are discussed and illustrated with 2 case reports.

*Methods.*—The various RPT techniques include the leading technology, sterolithography, and selective laser sintering, solid process, fused deposition modelling, laminated object manufacturing, 3-D printing, and multiphase jet solidification.

> *Case 1.*—A girl, 9, with progressive facial deformity resulting from hemifacial microsomia, had reduced growth potential in her left mandible. Treatment to lengthen the mandible involved the attachment of an intraoral screw device to the ramus posteriorly through a bone plate and to the body of the mandible anteriorly through an acrylic plate cemented to the teeth. A model of the facial skeleton generated from CT data made possible the design and accurate placement of the device.
>
> *Case 2.*—A patient needing secondary reconstruction after a traffic accident had complete disruption of the maxillary skeleton, a fracture of the mandible, and loss of an eye and nose. Three-dimensional computer images of hard and soft tissue allowed the construction of models that restored the normal proportions of the face and allowed correct positioning and alignment of the mandible and maxilla and bone fragments (Fig 4).

*Conclusion.*—RPT is a useful aid for surgical planning. It is an expensive tool, but its cost can be offset by savings in operating time and perhaps by cutting down the number of operations required.

▶ Two aspects of this prototype modeling struck me as exciting. First, inexpensive models of the patient's face and head could be rendered for use in actually practicing the reconstructive techniques we propose in a surgical plan. Otherwise, we rely upon our spatial intelligence capabilities to produce an image of a defect or abnormality in our mind's eye—and we know that some surgeons are better than others at applying their right brain to these challenges. A model levels the playing field for surgeons. Second, the manufacturing of a prosthesis can be developed such that the optimal choice

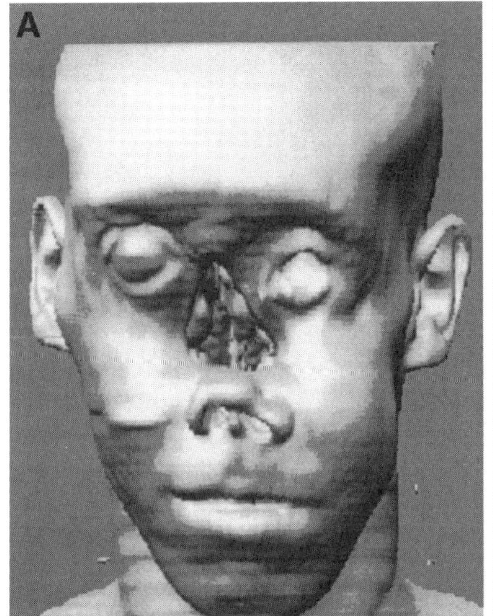
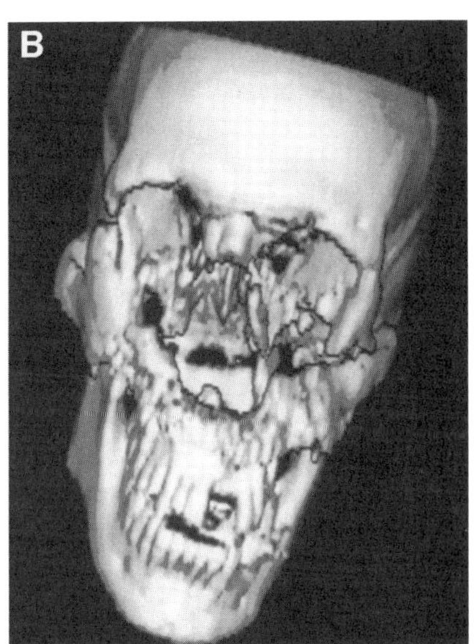
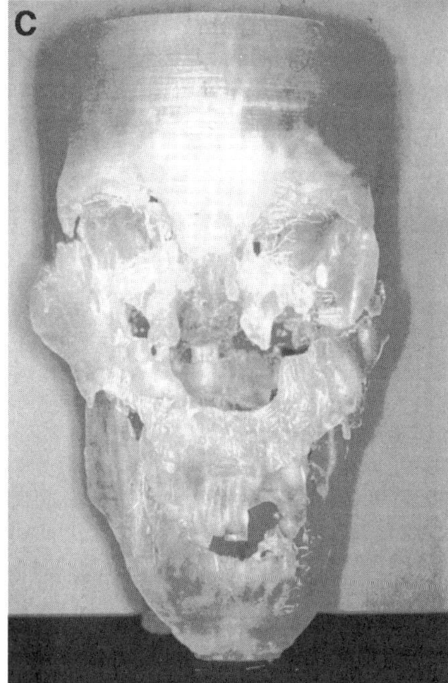

FIGURE 4.—Case 2 showing (**A**) 3-D MRI of the facial soft tissues (**B**) 3-D CT scan showing the bony facial skeleton and (**C**) the SLA model. (Courtesy of McGurk M, Amis AA, Potamianos P, et al: Rapid prototyping techniques for anatomical modeling in medicine. *Ann R Coll Surg Engl* 79:169–174, 1997).

of an implant biomaterial can be made—say a composite or alloy—to fit the mechanical stresses or strains required by the defect. I'm excited about the possibilities for this technology.

**G.R. Holt, M.D., M.S.E., M.P.H.**

# 8 Rhinology and Paranasal Sinuses

**Cost of Therapy for Allergic Rhinitis**
Wessels F, Green R, Luyt D (Parklane Clinic, Johannesburg, South Africa)
*S Afr Med J* 87:141–145, 1997                                    8–1

*Introduction.*—Allergic rhinitis is common and has significant potential morbidity. Allergic rhinitis is a perennial problem in South Africa with its long pollen season. Cost-effective therapy is needed. An assessment of the rand value of a therapy in association with its documented efficacy can help define an "adjusted" cost per treatment period. This makes it possible to compare the cost of 2 agents so that the physician can make an informed choice. This study evaluates the cost of each drug registered for allergic rhinitis in South Africa. Using documented efficacy, the cost of each agent is assessed.

*Methods.*—There were no attempts made to suggest how or for how long individual agents should be used in the treatment of allergic rhinitis. Two treatment periods were examined to help distinguish between acute and chronic treatment: a treatment course and a month of treatment, 10 and 30 days, respectively. A measure of efficacy was used to make the transition from price to cost.

*Results.*—Intranasal corticosteroids were the least costly treatments for allergic rhinitis and sodium cromoglycate was the most costly (20 times more expensive than nasal steroids). Anticholinergic sprays, topical decongestants, and antihistamines were more costly than nasal steroids. Ketotifen, an older-generation antihistamine, was more costly and had greater sedative side effects than 3 newer-generation oral agents in the same class. Levocabastine, a new topical antihistamine, outperformed all oral antihistamines.

*Conclusion.*—Topical steroids are the least costly antihistamine, have no systemic side effects, and can be applied topically in adults and children. These findings enable physicians to compare costs when they are choosing a drug regimen for patients with allergic rhinitis.

▶ When you consider the issue of quality of life in treating allergic rhinitis, together with the cost of various therapies, you almost have to develop a matrix of choices on your spreadsheet program. We must all be cognizant of these 2 factors when treating this common disorder and not trivialize their impact. We are talking about millions of patients and billions of health care dollars spent on this therapy (and industry) that, if wisely spent, could attain our goals and yet have some money left over for other efforts, such as research and raising the standard of health care in America.

**G.R. Holt, M.D., M.S.E., M.P.H.**

## Measuring Health-related Quality of Life in Rhinitis

Juniper EF (McMaster Univ, Hamilton, Ont, Canada)
*J Allergy Clin Immunol* 99:S742–S749, 1997                     8–2

*Background.*—Including health-related quality of life (HRQL) evaluations in clinical assessments is becoming more and more common. Assessment of HRQL in patients with rhinitis was discussed in the current paper.

*Discussion.*—Patients with rhinitis are affected by troublesome symptoms, such as headache and fatigue, as well as the nasal symptoms. This combination of symptoms can severely impair daily physical, emotional, occupational, and social functioning. The breadth of HRQL impairment associated with rhinitis is often not appreciated and is sometimes trivialized by health care workers.

> In the management of rhinitis, all individual problems must be recognized and treated appropriately. Studies have shown that conventional nasal symptom severity diaries and HRQL are only weakly to moderately correlated. Thus quality of life must be measured to get an overview of a patient's health status. Burden of illness across different medical conditions can be assessed by generic health status questionnaires, but such questionnaires are often not responsive enough to the small but clinically important changes in a patient's quality of life. Disease-specific instruments for rhinitis with strong measurement properties, which are much more sensitive to these changes, have been developed recently. Performing an HRQL assessment in clinical practice seems to be beneficial. However, whether clinical practice is altered by the results of such assessments has yet to be determined.

▶ At first glance, taking seriously an article on "quality of life" in rhinitis might be debated or trivialized. Can the issue really be comparable to that involved in, say, head and neck cancer? My answer is, yes we should take it seriously. Rhinitis is one of the most common self-generated complaints that patients have, and has a functional effect to some degree on the many millions of patients who suffer from it. Patients go home from work with a headache and "sinus pressure," can be asocial when feeling poorly, and try all sorts of remedies to feel better. The author helps us understand that we must look at the discomfort the patient with rhinitis feels, and make sure it is taken into account when prescribing or testing treatment modalities.

**G.R. Holt, M.D., M.S.E., M.P.H.**

**Sedation in Allergic Rhinitis Is Caused by the Condition and not by Antihistamine Treatment**

Spaeth J, Klimek L, Mösges R (Technical Univ of Aachen, Germany; Univ of Mainz, Germany; Univ of Cologne, Germany)

*Allergy* 51:893–906, 1996　　　　　　　　　　　　　　　　　　　8–3

*Background.*—Sedation is considered to be a common adverse effect of most $H_1$-antihistamines. However, central sedative potency is difficult to assess. The result of the different components of the central interaction in 5 clinical studies conducted between 1989 and 1994 was assessed.

*Methods and Findings.*—A total of 1,070 patients were included in the trials. A visual analogue scale was used. In a double-blind, placebo-controlled study conducted in 1989, the vigilance of patients with seasonal allergic rhinitis increased significantly more when treated by an antihistamine compared with placebo. Between 1992 and 1994, azelastine nasal spray was compared by the double-dummy technique with oral antihistamines (cetrizine, loratadine, and astemizole) and by the double-dummy or placebo-controlled design with monotherapy or combined treatment with azelastine tablets. With all compounds, vigilance was markedly or significantly improved. Even when taking azelastine orally, patients reported a similar increase in vigilance.

*Conclusion.*—In all 5 studies, the baseline values of vigilance of untreated symptomatic patients were far below physiologic condition, improving with treatment to the upper range of healthy persons. Thus, the sedation reported by patients with allergic rhinitis appears to be caused by the disorder itself rather than by antihistamine treatment.

▶ In South Texas, we have what is called "cedar fever"—sensitivity to red mountain cedar antigen. It is given the moniker "fever" because those who have it feel as though they have a cold: headache, sore throat, nasal stuffiness and rhinorrhea, and even a feeling of malaise and somnolence. Indeed, if untreated, many patients simply want to go to bed and sleep. When adequately treated, these same individuals will get out of bed, go to work, and be productive. That is why this article intrigued me. Is sedation a symptom of allergic upper airway disease? What do you think?

**G.R. Holt, M.D., M.S.E., M.P.H.**

## Adenoid Bacteriology and Sinonasal Symptoms in Children

Lee D, Rosenfeld RM (State Univ of New York, Brooklyn)
*Otolaryngol Head Neck Surg* 116:301–307, 1997                    8–4

*Background.*—In children with sinonasal symptoms refractory to medical treatment, the adenoid may act as a reservoir of pathogenic bacteria, as in otitis media. More studies of the relationship between adenoid bacteriology and sinonasal symptoms are needed urgently. The correlation of sinonasal symptoms in children with the prevalence of bacterial pathogens in the adenoid core was studied.

*Methods.*—Eighty-four consecutive children, aged 2 to 12 years, were included in the prospective survey. The children underwent adenoidectomy between July and November 1995.

*Findings.*—At least 1 bacterial pathogen was isolated from the core samples of all adenoids. In 26% of the specimens, the concentration was >105 colony-forming units (CFUs). The most common pathogens were *Haemophilus influenzae*, group A β-hemolytic streptococcus, and *Staphylococcus aureus*. In a multivariate analysis, sinonasal infection symptom scores were significantly associated with CFUs of adenoid core pathogens, after adjustment for the confounding effects of nasal obstructive symptoms and adenoid size.

*Conclusions.*—Nearly half of the variability in quantitative bacteriology of the adenoid core is explained by sinonasal infectious symptoms, independent of adenoid size. These findings suggest that adenoidectomy may have a role in the treatment of refractory sinusitis in children. Longitudinal studies are needed to verify these observations.

▶ This complex but forthright study was well-designed to investigate the association, if any, between adenoid bacteriology and sinonasal symptoms in children. The authors felt that their data indicated a relationship of some sort in roughly half of the children. Obviously, there is more to do to further identify the strength of this relationship over time, and the authors intend to do so. I have been intrigued for some time by the notion of an "adenoiditis" in children, which could cause infection of the nose, sinuses, ears and tonsils. Since the adenoids are a focused area of microbial surveillance and response, it seems reasonable that they could also be a potential site of swelling and infection as well. Perhaps they get infected simultaneously with the other areas, not as the cause of the spreading infection.

**G.R. Holt, M.D., M.S.E., M.P.H.**

**Antioxidant Levels in the Nasal Mucosa of Patients With Chronic Sinusitis and Healthy Controls**

Westerveld G-J, Dekker I, Voss H-P, et al (Vrije Universiteit, Amsterdam)
*Arch Otolaryngol Head Neck Surg* 123:201–204, 1997                8–5

---

*Introduction.*—When the delicate balance between oxidant production and local antioxidant defense (oxidative stress) is upset, pathologic conditions may occur. The importance of sufficient mucosal antioxidant defense has been repeatedly stressed. The antioxidant defense systems (glutathione, uric acid, and vitamin E) in the nasal mucosa were examined in patients with chronic sinusitis and healthy controls to determine whether patients with compromised tissues had diminished antioxidant tissue status.

*Methods.*—Nine patients with chronic sinusitis underwent functional endoscopic sinus surgery and 10 healthy controls underwent surgical procedures for complaints of nasal obstruction caused by either a nasal septum deviation or hypertrophy of the inferior turbinate. Mucosal specimens of the osteomeatal area or the uncinate process were collected during surgery in both groups. Antioxidant assays were performed in tissue samples from both groups. They included the reduced glutathione and oxidized glutathione assay, uric acid assay, vitamin E assay, and xanthione oxidase assay.

*Results.*—A significant reduction is reduced glutathione levels and uric acid levels was observed in the mucosal samples taken from patients with chronic sinusitis, compared with controls. There were no between-group differences in levels of oxidized glutathione or vitamin E.

*Conclusion.*—Patients with chronic sinusitis had impaired antioxidant defense, as evidenced by decreased levels of reduced glutathione and uric acid. The vitamin E level was of lesser importance. These findings may be associated with the pathogenesis of sinusitis. Pharmacotherapeutic intervention with antioxidants may be worthwhile.

▶ As one who believes in antioxidant therapy, I was pleased to see this article. However, I was surprised that one of my favorite antioxidants, vitamin E, did not seem to be a big player in the maintenance of healthy sinus mucosa. But, I am more inclined to think that vitamin C in hefty doses could help maintain the nasal passages free of infections. Other possible therapies might include echinacea and zinc. I regularly use them all myself and recommend these supplements for my patients  I have the body of a 54-year-old but the sinus mucosa of a 23-year-old.

**G.R. Holt, M.D., M.S.E., M.P.H.**

## Analysis of Pain and Endoscopic Sinus Surgery for Sinusitis

Acquadro MA, Salman SD, Joseph MP (Harvard Med School, Boston)
*Ann Otol Rhinol Laryngol* 106:305–309, 1997                    8–6

*Introduction.*—There is skepticism regarding the need for sinus surgery for treatment of headache or facial pain, particularly when imaging studies show normal sinuses. Patients who underwent endoscopic sinus surgery for sinusitis were evaluated to determine whether they had pain relief from the surgery and whether they had new pain postoperatively.

*Methods.*—A series of 252 consecutive patients with inflammatory sinus disorders meeting specific clinical definitions of sinusitis and criteria for surgically treatable sinus disorders were prospectively assessed for their experience of presurgical and postsurgical pain.

*Result.*—Preoperatively, 146 patients (58%) had preoperative sinus pain and 106 patients (42%) had no preoperative pain. At a 6– 12-month follow-up, none of the patients with no preoperative pain developed pain. Of 146 patients with preoperative pain, 82 (56%) had no pain, residual symptoms, or further sequelae and were considered cured; 42 (29%) reported marked improvement in pain or discomfort; 9 (6%) had the same degree of pain or discomfort as before; 3 (2%) reported worse pain or discomfort; and 10 (7%) reported new pain or discomfort.

*Conclusion.*—There is an unlikely risk of the development of new pain or discomfort after endoscopic sinus surgery in patients with no preoperative pain or discomfort. There was a less than 10% risk of worsening pain or new pain in patients with preoperative sinus pain. These findings provide preliminary information for a new trial that should address what types of pain can be attributed to specific sinuses when there is no infection.

▶ Early in my surgical career, I was admonished by a wise and senior clinician not to operate on patients for pain symptoms alone; it is hard to cure pain. This study, however, indicates that if specific and definitive criteria are used to identify a patient with sinusitis who is a candidate for surgery, improvement or alleviation of preoperative pain could be a pleasant side benefit. However, one should not promise a patient that any operation can relieve their pain totally, but that it is "hoped" that the pain might be reduced. Then, if the pain goes away, you're a hero! If not, you're an honest surgeon.

**G.R. Holt, M.D., M.S.E., M.P.H.**

## Antrochoanal Polyps in Children

Woolley AL, Clary RA, Lusk RP (Children's Hosp of Alabama, Birmingham;
Washington Univ, St Louis)
*Am J Otolaryngol* 17:368–373, 1996                                       8–7

*Background.*—Antrochoanal polyps, representing 4% to 6% of all nasal polyps in the general population, have a much higher prevalence among children. The diagnosis and management of these polyps in children were discussed, and 1 series was presented.

*Methods and Findings.*—The cases of 7 children, aged 7 to 16 years, diagnosed as having antrochoanal polyps between 1993 and 1995 were reviewed. The most common initial symptoms were nasal obstruction and nasal drainage, followed by snoring with obstructive sleep apnea, cheek pain, headaches, recurrent epistaxis, hemotympanum, and weight loss. All 7 patients underwent endoscopic removal of the polyp while under general anesthesia. The polyps were located in different positions in the maxillary sinus. Only 1 patient had a recurrence during a mean 15 months of follow-up.

*Discussion.*—Antrochoanal polyps should be considered in the differential diagnosis of a child with nasal obstruction and a nasal mass (Table 2). Because a variety of conditions have similar symptoms and physical findings, a careful history, nasal endoscopy, and a radiologic workup are required. Endoscopic surgery ensures complete removal of the antral part of the polyp and treatment of any associated sinus disease while preserving normal mucosa.

▶ This paper takes a common sense approach to diagnosing and treating a polypoid mass in the nasal cavity of a child. The real key, of course, is adequate diagnosis, for if one encounters an angiofibroma when a presumptive diagnosis of antrochoanal polyp has been made, a risky encounter can occur. The nasal endoscope has greatly improved the surgical morbidity of sinus surgery in children and can be effectively used to safely remove antrochoanal polyps.

**G.R. Holt, M.D., M.S.E., M.P.H.**

TABLE 2.—Differential Diagnosis of Pediatric Polypoid Nasal Masses

Juvenile angiofibroma
Encephalocele
Nasopharyngeal malignancies
Grossly enlarged adenoids
Hypertrophy of turbinates
Cystic fibrosis/nasal polyposis
Allergic fungal sinusitis

(Courtesy of Woolley AL, Clary RA, Lusk RP: Antrochoanal polyps in children. *Am J Otolaryngol* 17:368–373, 1996.)

## Prevalence of Sinusitis Signs in a Non-ENT Population

Gordts F, Clement PAR, Buisseret T (Free Univ Brussels, Belgium)
*ORL J Otorhinolaryngol* 58:315–319, 1996                                    8–8

*Introduction.*—In patients with suspected intracranial neurologic pathologic conditions who can be considered as representative of the general population, MR imaging is a well-suited instrument for visualizing all sinuses and minute inflammatory changes. A better insight into the prevalence of sinusitis was obtained in the general population by correlating sinus complaints with MR images.

*Methods.*—From 58 men and 41 women who were referred for MR imaging of the brain, 107 images were gathered. The patients, ranging in age from 21 to 73 years, also filled out a questionnaire that asked whether they had nasal obstruction, nasal discharge, sneezing, or surgery. An axial imaging plane parallel with the canthomeatal plan was used, and T2-weighted images were used for sinus evaluation.

*Results.*—Nearly 60% of sinuses were affected on MR imaging. By excluding a maxillary polyp or cyst, the most common lesion, which could be considered nonpathologic, about 40% of the sinuses of this group were affected. The maxillary sinuses comprised 40% of the abnormal images, followed by the anterior ethmoidal sinuses with 14% of the abnormal images. Other sinuses that had abnormal images were the sphenoidal (2.5%), the frontal (2%), and the posterior ethmoidal (1.5%).

*Conclusion.*—The 40% prevalence of sinusitis signs on MR imaging is high, even among a non–ear-nose-and-throat population, particularly for the maxillary and anterior ethmoidal sinuses, but it is comparable to a previous study. Polyps were considered nonpathologic in this study. Magnetic resonance imaging should not be considered the gold standard for detecting sinusitis. The gold standard should be histology. Before lesions can be attributed to sinusitis, clinical correlation and thorough physical examination are necessary.

▶ This study utilized MR scanning performed for suspected CNS lesions to identify the basal level of sinus abnormalities in a "general" population. It was retrospective and not correlated with a detailed history and physical examination. However, in spite of these deficiencies, I felt there were 2 messages to be had from this article. It has been my experience that MR scans *overestimate* the degree of sinus disease, and in order to have sufficient "practical" assistance to me, a CT scan must be performed. Second, there undoubtedly is a certain level of clinically insignificant but radiologically apparent sinus disease in the population. Our *ethical* responsibility is to address those who require our care clinically, and *not* to bother patients with asymptomatic disease.

**G.R. Hold, M.D., M.S.E., M.P.H.**

**Effectiveness of Surgical Management of Epistaxis at a Tertiary Care Center**
Barlow DW, Deleyiannis FWB, Pinczower EF (Univ of Washington, Seattle)
*Laryngoscope* 107:21–24, 1997                                    8–9

*Background.*—Severe epistaxis can be life-threatening and often requires more intensive care and surgical treatment in a tertiary care facility. Surgical procedures include arterial ligation, endoscopic cautery, and angiographic embolization. However, the best surgical treatment has not been definitively established. The current study identified predictors of surgical treatment and compared the efficacy of different surgical treatments.

*Methods and Findings.*—Charts for 44 consecutive patients hospitalized with epistaxis at a tertiary care center were reviewed. Costs were also analyzed. Nonsurgical treatment was successful in 18 patients, and surgery was necessary in 26. The need for surgery was significantly predicted by posterior site of bleeding, an admission hematocrit <38%, and blood transfusion. The rate of rebleeding after initial surgery was 33% with embolization, 33% with endoscopic cautery, and 20% with ligation.

*Conclusions.*—Because the failure rates associated with embolization, ligation, and endoscopic cautery appear to be comparable, other factors such as cost and institutional expertise should be considered in the choice of surgical procedure in patients with epistaxis. A randomized, prospective, multicenter study of the surgical treatment of epistaxis may be warranted.

▶ This is an important topic to evaluate, as epistaxis continues to be problematic in our clinical practices. Successful angiographic embolization is really dependent upon the skill and experience of the radiologist, which might vary considerably in a community. Similarly, not all current and recently graduated otolaryngology residents are familiar with a Caldwell-Luc approach to the pterygomaxillary space or to finding the ethmoid arteries via an external approach. Sometimes whether the patient is a candidate for surgery will determine which method to choose. My own preference has been (and still is) surgical ligation, and my own rebleed rate is considerably <20%. I've probably just been lucky.

**G.R. Holt, M.D., M.S.E., M.P.H.**

**Influence of Age on the 'Nasal Cycle'**
Mirza N, Kroger H, Doty RL (Univ of Pennsylvania, Philadelphia)
*Laryngoscope* 107:62–66, 1997                                    8–10

*Background.*—The regular left-to-right fluctuation in engorgement of the nasal mucosa and in airflow, the "nasal cycle," is correlated with several body function indices, including performance of tasks requiring visual/spatial ability and electroencephalographic (EEG) activity. The pacemaker for the nasal cycle appears to be located in the suprachiasmatic nucleus within the hypothalamus, an area that participates in the control of other ultradian and circadian rhythms and which is known to degenerate with increasing age. This study explored the effect of age on the nasal cycle and the association between nasal cycle quality and cognitive state.

*Methods.*—Twenty-nine men and 31 women were administered the Mini-Mental State Examination (MMSE), an indicator of cognitive state, and were evaluated for nasal patency every 15 minutes for 6 hours by use of a liquid crystal thermography exhalation monitor. Periodicity of the cyclical trends for each nostril, and the relationship between exhalation patterns of the right and left nostrils were established.

*Results.*—Only 25% of participants aged 18 to 29 years exhibited alternating rhythmicity typical of a "normal" nasal cycle. This proportion was negatively and significantly associated with age, decreasing to 20%, 15% and 5% in the 30- to 49-year, 50- to 69-year, and 70- to 85-year age groups, respectively. Performance on the MMSE was not associated with nasal cycle parameters.

*Conclusions.*—There is a clear decrease with age in the proportion of subjects with the alternating rhythmicity of nasal airflow typical of the classical nasal cycle. Although there appears to be no consistent relationship between nasal cycle parameters and performance on the MMSE test, nasal cycle parameters may be a marker for CNS changes associated with increasing age.

▶ This article suggests that the slowly progressive diminishment in my nasal airway as I get older is not just related to ptosis of the nasal tip! Clearly, the nasal cycle is a very complex arrangement, and neural degeneration could affect it. Older persons also tend to be chronically dehydrated, are often taking vasoactive medications or CNS-suppressive or stimulant drugs, and may have pulmonary compensating airflow disturbances (oral breathing rather than nasal). Certainly worth some clinical observations in our own practices.

**G.R. Holt, M.D., M.S.E., M.P.H.**

---

**Nasal Mucociliary Transport Is Impaired at Altitude**
Barry PW, Mason NP, O'Callaghan C (Univ of Leicester, England; Hôpital Henri Mondor, Paris; British Mount Everest Med Expedition, Hyssington, Powys, Wales)
*Eur Respir J* 10:35–37, 1997                                        8–11

---

*Objective.*—Although high altitudes increase the amount of work the nasal passages have to do to condition inspired air and to recover heat and moisture from expired air, no studies of nasal mucociliary function at high altitudes have been conducted. Partial nasal blockage can lead to mouth breathing which increases heat and water loss. Subjective feelings of nasal blockage and nasal mucociliary function were measured in a group of lowlanders traveling to an altitude of 5,300 meters.

*Methods.*—Members of the British Mount Everest Medical Expedition (n = 54) were studied in the UK before leaving, after arriving at base camp, and after 2 weeks of acclimatization at altitudes greater than or equal to 5,000 meters. With 1 nostril occluded, volunteers rated their inhalation as 0 (fully open), 1 (partially blocked), or 2 (blocked). The test was repeated with the other nostril giving a possible total score of 4. Time to perceive the sweetness of saccharin placed in the anterior nose was recorded and repeated in 26 volunteers after the expedition. Results were compared statistically.

*Results.*—Median nasal obstruction scores measured before beginning the expedition and at altitude were 0 and 1. The score increased for 23 people and decreased for 7 making the increase in score on ascent significant. The saccharin test time was 11 minutes at sea level and 60 minutes at 5,300 meters. Test time increased for 25 of the individuals and decreased for 5 making the decrease in nasal mucociliary transport at a high altitude significant. After acclimatization, median saccharin time remained at 60 minutes but increased in 5 volunteers and decreased in 2. Upper respiratory symptoms were reported by 15 volunteers in the month before testing at altitude.

*Conclusion.*—High altitude increases nasal obstruction and nasal mucociliary transport times. Because these problems can interfere with an individual's ability to climb, additional studies need to be conducted to study the impact of the physiological changes and of controlling environmental conditions.

▶ While few of us will ever experience the Mount Everest Base Camp in Nepal, a good number will regularly visit ski resorts and ski at 2800–3000 meters. This presents a common need, then, to better understand nasal and pulmonary physiology and their interaction at high altitudes. The patient and physician should bear in mind that both oral and topical hydration may improve mucociliary transport time as well as reduce reflexive vasodilation. Additionally, the use of oral decongestants (not topical, which might further adversely affect ciliary function) and steam inhalations (showers, vaporizers, etc.) can provide symptomatic relief. Progressive dyspnea must be watched for the development of altitude sickness, which requires prompt medical treatment.

**G.R. Holt, M.D., M.S.E., M.P.H.**

## Image-guided Endoscopic Surgery: Results of Accuracy and Performance in a Multicenter Clinical Study Using an Electromagnetic Tracking System

Fried MP, Kleefield J, Gopal H, et al (Harvard Med School, Boston; Joint Ctr for Otolaryngology, Boston; Brigham & Women's Hosp, Boston; et al)
*Laryngoscope* 107:594–601, 1997

8–12

*Background.*—The use of image-guided surgery appears to improve functional endoscopic sinus surgery localization. It enables accurate identification of the surgical field boundaries, permitting safer, more thorough sinus surgery. One experience with the InstaTrak, a device for image-guided endoscopic sinus surgery, was reviewed.

*Methods and Findings.*—The InstaTrak System has a simple headset and instrumentation solution that compensates for arbitrary head movement, which is critical for maintaining accuracy during surgery. The device provides a simple automated registration method that eliminates the time-consuming setup process. Also, the device incorporates the localizing probe onto interchangeable suction tips to improve manipulation and access in the surgical field. The InstaTrak System (Figs 1, 2, and 3) was used during functional endoscopic sinus surgery in 55 patients, aged 15 to 73 years. It was found to be easy to use and accurate. It consistently localized structures in surgically critical sites. Also, the need for a second CT scan for image guidance was obviated; the initial CT scan was useful for intraoperative localization.

*Conclusions.*—The InstaTrak was found to be accurate and easy to implement during functional endoscopic sinus surgery. The use of image guidance may decrease complications and the number of revisions needed, thereby lowering costs.

▶ In the U.S. Army Armor Corps, tank drivers and gunners are trained on virtual simulators. These young people take to the use of this aiming and guidance technology very well. Why? Most of them have grown up with video games and simulators and feel right at home with them. I predict that our students and residents at this time and in the future will take to using technology such as this very well indeed. It just might be harder for the "older" otolaryngologist whose main technology recollection as a child was a Dick Tracy decoding ring. Perhaps I'll be around long enough to see the surgeon performing this surgery through remotely controlled instrument arms using virtual reality technology! It is not out of the realm of possibility.

**G.R. Holt, M.D., M.S.E., M.P.H.**

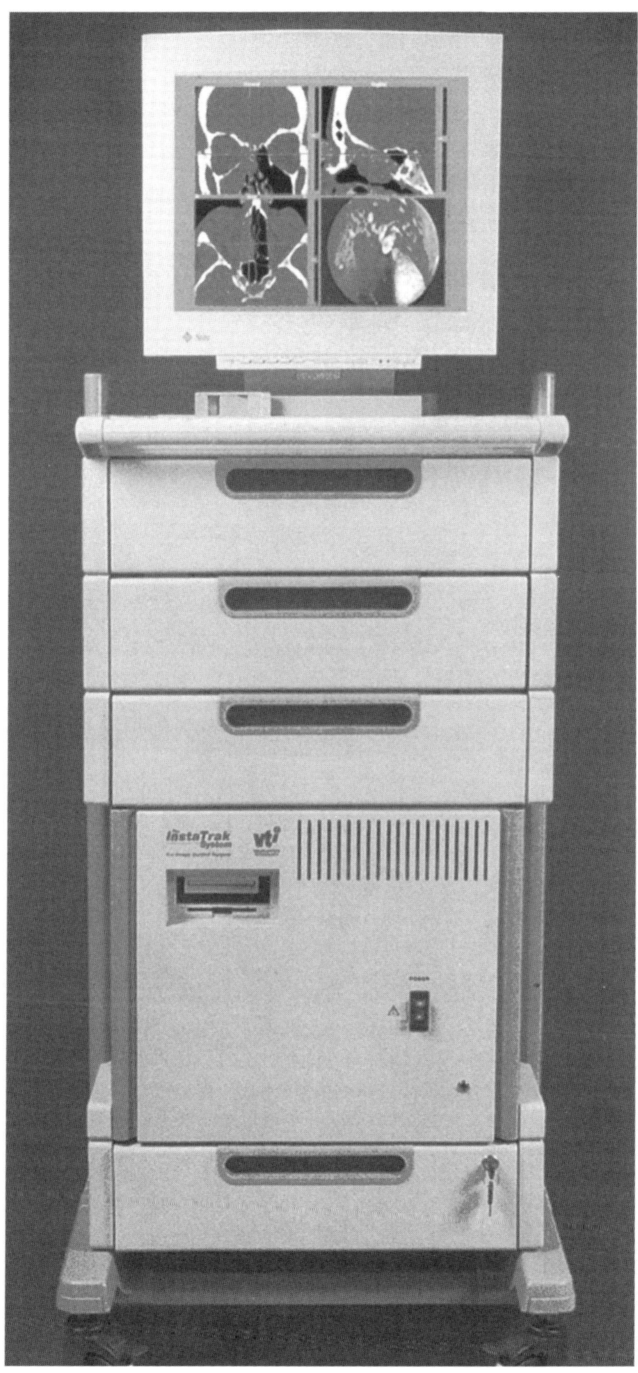

FIGURE 1.—The InstaTrak System. (Courtesy of Fried MP, Kleefield J, Gopal H, et al: Image-guided endoscopic surgery: Results of accuracy and performance in a multicenter clinical study using an electro-magnetic tracking system. *Laryngoscope* 107:594–601, 1997. Copyright Triological Society.)

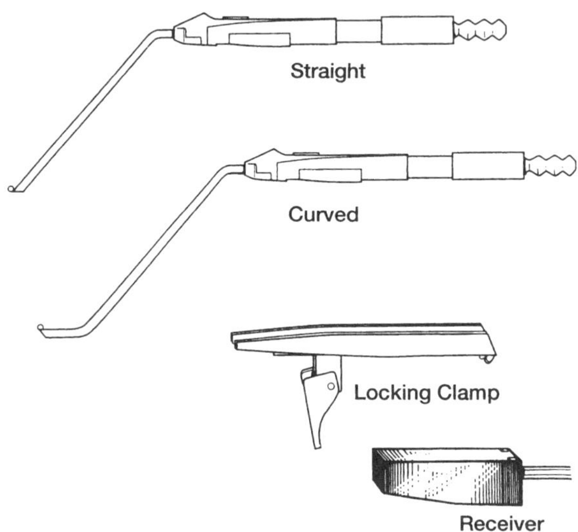



FIGURE 2.—Straight and curved sensors incorporated into suction tips. (Courtesy of Fried MP, Kleefield J, Gopal H, et al: Image-guided endoscopic surgery: Results of accuracy and performance in a multicenter clinical study using an electromagnetic tracking system. *Laryngoscope* 107:594–601, 1997. Copyright Triological Society.)

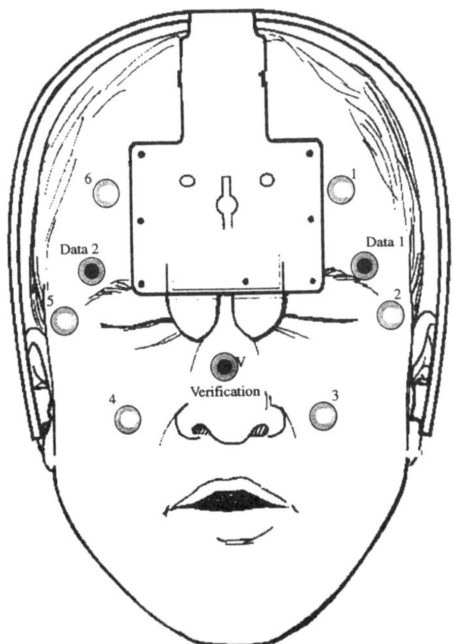



FIGURE 3.—Headset in place for automatic registration. Fiducials (numbered 1 to 6 and 2 data points) used in this study for conventional registration. Verification point on nasal dorsum. (Courtesy of Fried MP, Kleefield J, Gopal H, et al: Image-guided endoscopic surgery: Results of accuracy and performance in a multicenter clinical study using an electromagnetic tracking system. *Laryngoscope* 107:594–601, 1997. Copyright Triological Society.)

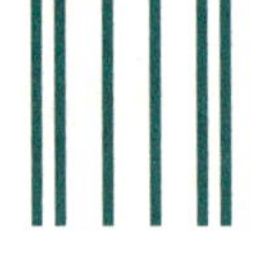

# BUSINESS REPLY MAIL
FIRST-CLASS MAIL    PERMIT NO 135    ST LOUIS  MO

POSTAGE WILL BE PAID BY ADDRESSEE

SUBSCRIPTION SERVICES
MOSBY–YEAR BOOK, INC.
11830 WESTLINE INDUSTRIAL DRIVE
ST. LOUIS    MO 63146-9988

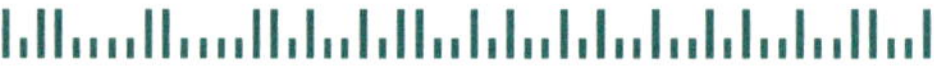

# BUSINESS REPLY MAIL
FIRST-CLASS MAIL    PERMIT NO 135    ST LOUIS  MO

POSTAGE WILL BE PAID BY ADDRESSEE

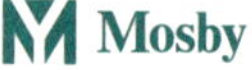 Mosby

PAT NEWMAN
11830 WESTLINE INDUSTRIAL DRIVE
PO BOX 46908
ST. LOUIS    MO 63146-9934

## *Want to speed up the process?*

**To order the *Year Book*,
you also may call 1-800-426-4545**

**To subscribe to the journal today,
call toll-free in the U.S.:
1-800-453-4351
or fax 314-432-1158
Outside the U.S., call:  314-453-4351**

Visit us at:
*www.mosby.com/Mosby/Periodicals*

**Mosby–Year Book, Inc.**
Subscription Services
11830 Westline Industrial Drive
St. Louis, MO   63146  U.S.A.

Mosby

## Minimally Invasive Head Holder to Improve the Performance of Frameless Stereotactic Surgery

Bale RJ, Vogele M, Freysinger W, et al (Univ ENT Dept, Innsbruck, Australia)
*Laryngoscope* 107:373–377, 1997                    8–13

*Objective.*—Conventional stereotactic head frames make imaging difficult and can obscure part of the surgical field. Other navigations systems are inconvenient because they require periodic realignment. The newly developed Vogele-Bale-Hohner (VBH) head holder and registration device is easy to use, easy to fix, and results in exact positioning.

*Methods.*—The VBH head holder consists of an iron base plate, headrest, hydraulic arms, a carbon-fiber mouthpiece (MP) with connecting tube, and a countersupport. It uses a dental cast of the patient's upper teeth squeezed to the upper jaw to position the MP precisely. A viewing wand uses CT to visualize probe positions.

*Technique.*—The awake patient is placed in the supine position on the CT table, scans are performed, and the MP is inserted and fixed to the upper teeth and hard palate under pressure (Fig 4). Anesthesia is induced, and the 3 hydraulic arms are mounted on the base plate and fixed. The MP is connected to the hydraulic arms (Fig 5). Anatomic landmarks and skin surface are checked to assure no deviation has occurred, and surgery is begun.

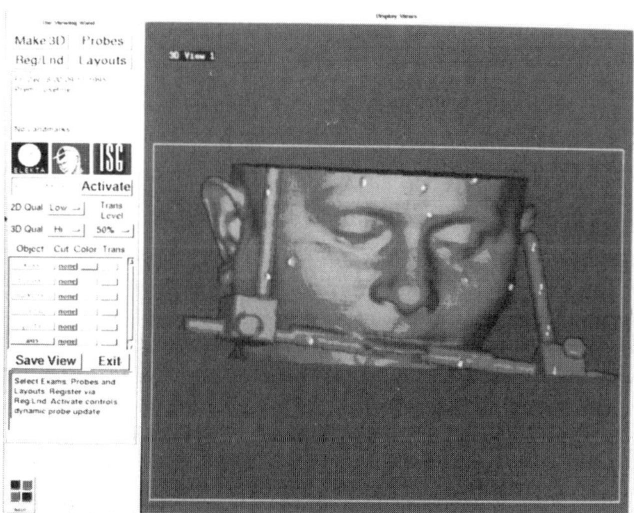

FIGURE 4.—Intraoperative view of three-dimensional reconstruction of a patient and the registration device. The MP with the registration device does not produce metallic artifacts in the CT. (Courtesy of Bales RJ, Vogele M, Freysinger W, et al: Minimally invasive head holder to improve the performance of frameless stereotactic surgery. *Laryngoscope* 107:373–377, 1997, copyright Triological Society.)

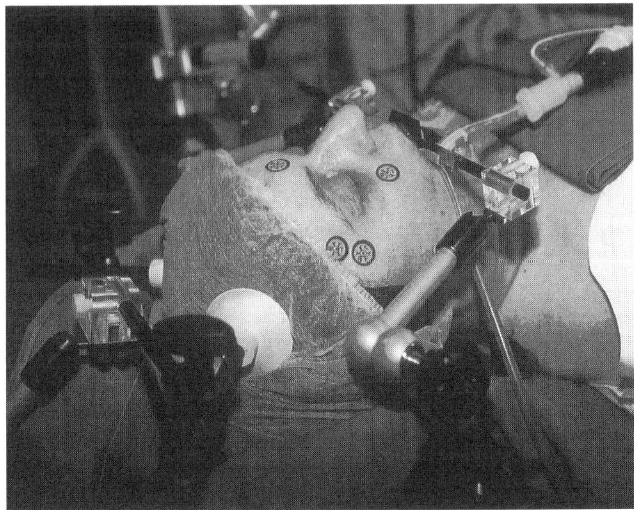

FIGURE 5.—Preoperative setup. The anesthetized and intubated patient is immobilized in the head holder. For backup reasons, we have used fiducial markers attached to the skin; for details see text. Note that the surgical area remains fully accessible. (Courtesy of Bales RJ, Vogele M, Freysinger W, et al: Minimally invasive head holder to improve the performance of frameless stereotactic surgery. *Laryngoscope* 107:373–377, 1997, copyright Triological Society.)

*Results.*—Between August and November 1995, 15 patients (14 with polyposis and 1 with adenocarcinoma) were successfully treated and tolerated the process well. The registration device does not produce CT artifacts and was stable throughout the procedure. There were 6 air leaks. The device was unsatisfactory in 2 toothless patients. Intraoperative accuracy was in the 1–2 mm range.

*Conclusion.*—The minimally invasive VBH head holder performed satisfactorily in this small study, did not produce CT artifacts, and was well tolerated by patients.

▶ The development of an easy-to-apply, reliable, and safe head holder will greatly facilitate advancements in stereotactic otolaryngic surgery. Computer assistance to orient the surgeon in delicate areas at the skull base is analogous to the global positioning systems which assist terrain navigators. Those who doubt this technology will be clinically significant within ten years—please see me at that time.

**G.R. Holt, M.D., M.S.E., M.P.H.**

**Effect of Sinus Surgery on Pulmonary Function in Patients With Cystic Fibrosis**
Madonna D, Isaacson G, Rosenfeld RM, et al (Temple Univ, Philadelphia; St Christopher's Hosp for Children, Philadelphia; State Univ of New York, Brooklyn)
*Laryngoscope* 107:328–331, 1997                                    8–14

*Objective.*—Patients with cystic fibrosis (CF) experience significant pulmonary and gastrointestinal morbidity. The impact and timing of medical and surgical treatment for nasal obstruction, recurrent sinusitis, and nasal polyposis are unknown. Objective measures of pulmonary function were used to explore the effect of endoscopic sinus surgery on lung disease in patients with CF.

*Methods.*—Between 1992 and 1995, 15 patients (6 males) aged 5–24 years with CF in The Cystic Fibrosis Program at St. Christopher's Hospital for Children in Philadelphia underwent endoscopic ethmoidectomy and antrostomy. Preoperative and postoperative forced vital capacity (FVC), forced expiratory volume (FEV), and flow between 25% and 75% of the vital capacity ($FEF_{25-75}$) were recorded. Spirograms were obtained preoperatively and postoperatively at 2–3 weeks and 6 months. Data were compared using the Student's *t* test.

*Results.*—Lung function ranged from normal to moderate obstruction ($FEV_1$ 58% to 135% and FVC 83% to 134% of predicted). The $FEV_1$ at the first second declined from a preoperative value of 2.01 to 1.88 at 6 months. Similarly, FVC declined from 2.66 to 2.48, $FEF_{25-75}$ decreased from 1.90 to 1.84, and $FEV_1$/FVC (%) declined from 78.03 to 77.22.

*Conclusion.*—Sinus surgery does not appear to improve pulmonary function in patients with CF.

▶ I felt that the findings in this study were particularly germane to current practice concepts, i.e., that the control of sinusitis in patients with CF is beneficial to both their upper and lower respiratory passages. Although the study group was small, the authors performed a well-run study, and their results should be critically reviewed. A larger study might show different trends, but this one certainly calls for the presentation of other series in the literature for comparison. Until then, sinusitis care in patients with CF should continue to be based on clinical indicators to improve their quality of life and to prevent complications.

**G.R. Holt, M.D., M.S.E., M.P.H.**

# 9 Trauma and Reconstructive Surgery

---

**Early and Delayed Repair of Orbitozygomatic Complex Fractures**
Carr RM, Mathog RH (Wayne State Univ, Detroit; Dearborn, Mich)
*J Oral Maxillofac Surg* 55:253–258, 1997                    9–1

---

*Objective.*—There are numerous strategies for management of zygomatic fractures. Whereas early diagnosis and repair offer the best outcome, early treatment is sometimes not possible or not done. A treatment plan should be based on a thorough knowledge of anatomic and physiologic factors that are affected by the various types of structures. The long-term results of primary and delayed repair of orbitozygomatic complex (OZC) fractures and guidelines for treatment planning are presented.

*Methods.*—Records of 78 patients (12 females), aged 11 to 68, with 80 OZC fractures (and 81 surgical procedures) sustained between 1982 and 1992 were reviewed retrospectively. Forty patients (43 repairs) were available for follow-up 6 months to 10 years later. Functional ophthalmologic problems, esthetics problems, neurosensory deficits, and masticatory problems were assessed.

*Results.*—Injuries were the result of a fight (n = 45), motor vehicle accident (n = 20), sports (n = 6), falls (n = 4), or industrial accident (n = 3). There were 42 monofragment injuries, 33 comminuted, and 5 incomplete. There were 49 primary and 32 delayed repairs including 10 osteotomies (21 days to 5 months delay) and 22 onlay bone grafts (4 months to 16 years delay). Of the 43 repairs available for follow-up, there were 25 primary repairs, including 5 osteotomies, and 13 onlay bone grafts. In patients receiving primary repair, 4% had malar depression, 48% had hypoesthesia, 4% had enophthalmos/hypophthalmos, 4% had diplopia, and 4% had trismus. In patients receiving late repair, the respective percentages were 22%, 72%, 22%, 11%, and 6%.

*Conclusion.*—Patients who received early surgery for orbitozygomatic fractures had substantially better functional and esthetics results. After 21 days post-injury, delayed repair techniques such as osteotomy and onlay bone grafting are required.

▶ The authors present their views on how orbitozygomatic fractures should be handled; of course, different practitioners will have varying opinions, but Drs. Carr and Mathog present some basic points to consider. The very best time to obtain optimal reduction and fixation of these fractures is in the acute post-trauma period, optimally after the soft tissue swelling has receded. Late repair, at least in my experience, never really achieves optimal results. It is also very important to have a complete ophthalmological evaluation *preoperatively*, as an injury to the globe might be detected which would require postponing any osseous repair until resolved. Finally, one must have definitive criteria in one's mind as to the indications for exploring the orbit.

**G.R. Holt, M.D., M.S.E., M.P.H.**

## Supraorbital Roof Fractures: A Formidable Entity With Which to Contend

Martello JY, Vasconez HC (Univ of Kentucky, Lexington)
*Ann Plast Surg* 38:223–227, 1997

9–2

*Background.*—Supraorbital roof fractures are uncommon, but are usually associated with extensive craniofacial, ophthalmologic, and other bodily injuries. The reported incidence of supraorbital roof fractures is between 1% and 5%, although in 1 study, orbital roof fractures were not isolated from adjacent glabellar fractures. The incidence of and morbidity from supraorbital roof fractures may be higher than previously thought. The incidence and treatment of these fractures, as well as associated complications, were investigated.

*Methods.*—The medical records of 621 patients with facial fractures were reviewed. Of those, there were 58 patients with 64 supraorbital roof fractures. An analysis was done of method of injury; accident details; patient characteristics; associated clinical, CT, and operative findings;

TABLE 1.—Associated Clinical Findings

| Clinical Findings | No. of Patients |
|---|---|
| Periorbital edema and ecchymosis | 52 (90%) |
| Restriction of extraocular movements | 10 (17%) |
| No light perception | 5 (9%) |
| Rhinorrhea | 5 (9%) |
| Pulsatile proptosis | 3 (5%) |
| Otorrhea | 3 (5%) |
| Telecanthus | 2 (3%) |
| Diplopia | 2 (3%) |
| Lateral canthus CSF leak | 1 (2%) |

(Reprinted from Martello JY, Vasconez, HC: Supraorbital roof fractures: A formidable entity with which to contend. *Ann Plast Surg* 38:223–227, 1997 by permission of Little, Brown and Company, Inc.)

**TABLE 2.**—Neurologic Injuries

| Neurologic Injuries | No. of Patients |
| --- | --- |
| Frontal contusions | 25 (43%) |
| Closed-head injuries | 10 (17%) |
| Epidural hematomas | 10 (17%) |
| Subarachnoid hemorrhages | 8 (14%) |
| Temporal contusions | 7 (12%) |
| Cranial nerve VI injuries | 6 (10%) |
| Seizures | 5 (9%) |
| Cranial nerve VII injuries | 3 (5%) |
| Decreased hearing | 1 (2%) |

(Reprinted from Martello JY, Vasconez, HC: Supraorbital roof fractures: A formidable entity with which to contend. *Ann Plast Surg* 38:223–227, 1997 by permission of Little, Brown and Company, Inc.)

other bodily injury; fracture characteristics; associated facial, frontal sinus, and skull fractures; neurologic and ophthalmologic injuries; treatment; and complications.

*Results.*—Of the 58 patients, 47 were male and 11 were female. The average patient age was 31 years. Motor vehicle accidents were the most common reason for injury. Periorbital edema and ecchymosis were present in 90% of patients (Table 1). Neurologic injuries included frontal contusions in 43% of patients, closed-head injuries in 17% of patients, and epidural hematomas in 17% of patients (Table 2). Associated skull fractures occurred in 69% of patients and frontal sinus fractures occurred in 54% of patients. Thirty-two patients were treated operatively and in 31 patients, open treatment was used. There were dural tears in 14 patients, traumatic encephalocele in 3 patients, proptosis in 6, pulsatile proptosis in 3, orbital apex syndrome in 1, persistent CSF leak in 3, and meningitis in 5 patients. Associated intracranial bleeds occurred in the majority of patients.

*Discussion.*—These results suggest that the incidence of and morbidity from supraorbital roof fractures are greater than previously thought. The incidence in this study was 9.3%. Treatment of such patients should be individualized and should take factors such as displacement, associated skull and frontal sinus fractures, dural tears, and intracranial hemorrhage into account. In general, operative intervention should be considered in cases of a CSF leak, or neurologic or ophthalmologic injury.

▶ Unfortunately, orbital roof fractures ("supraorbital" seems redundant) usually involve significant damage to the structures of the anterior cranial fossa or the neuromuscular structures in the superior orbit. Craniotomy is often required to repair the damage intracranially. Diplopia and decreased vision may also persist. Normally, the repair of the roof is best managed from above, although an uncomplicated fracture may only require exploration and reinforcement of the roof with some sturdy material such as temporalis fascia. An interdisciplinary team approach with neurosurgery and ophthalmology departments is best.

**G.R. Holt, M.D., M.S.E., M.P.H.**

## Repair of Traumatic Orbital Wall Defects With Nasal Septal Cartilage: Report of Five Cases

Li KK (Univ of California, Irvine)
*J Oral Maxillofac Surg* 55:1098–1102, 1997                    9–3

*Background.*—Restoration of orbital wall defects after facial fractures is often recommended because unrepaired defects can be followed by enophthalmos and diplopia because of increased orbital volume, herniation of orbital contents, and atrophy of herniated fat and muscle. Autogenous bone is still the preferred grafting material for orbital reconstruction. Donor sites such as the ilium, rib, and calvarium are associated with a certain amount of morbidity. Cartilage from the nasal septum is an excellent alternative. The use of such autogenous tissue has received little attention compared to bone grafts.

*Methods.*—The records of 5 patients with disruption of the orbital wall after facial trauma were reviewed. Four of the patients were men, and the mean patient age was 25 years. Open reduction with internal fixation of the fractures, and repair of the orbital wall defect with autogenous septal cartilage were performed.

*Results.*—There were 4 cases of orbital floor defect and 1 case of orbital roof defect. All patients were treated successfully with nasal septal cartilage and restoration of the orbital wall continuity. In 1 patient with a supraorbital rim fracture, an existing laceration was used. In 2 patients with pure blowout fractures, a transconjunctival (preseptal) approach without lateral canthotomy was used (Fig 3). In 2 patients with zygomatic complex fractures, a transconjunctival (preseptal) approach with lateral canthotomy was used.

*Discussion.*—Nasal septal cartilage is easier to harvest than cranial bone and is readily accessible by the standard submucous resection technique. When meticulous surgical technique is used, the harvesting is associated with minimal risk, although complications can occur. However, the complications are minor compared to the potential complications of autogenous bone harvest. Nasal septal cartilage is also easily manipulated and can be used for firm support or contouring.

▶ I have used nasal septal cartilage successfully for 2 decades to repair orbital defects. In that time, I have learned a few lessons. One, it is very difficult to leave perichondrium on one side of the cartilage, as the mucosa and perichondrium do not separate easily. Two, you have to figure on a fair amount of absorption over time of the cartilage—therefore, one needs to consider stacking 2 or 3 layers of cartilage. This may initially overcorrect a hypophthalmos, but in the long term will be better. Three, I will occasionally wrap the cartilage in a covering of temporalis fascia, which I think (haven't "proved" yet) may reduce cartilage absorption. For the medial wall, especially when a telescoping nasoethmoid fracture is present, thinned-out con-

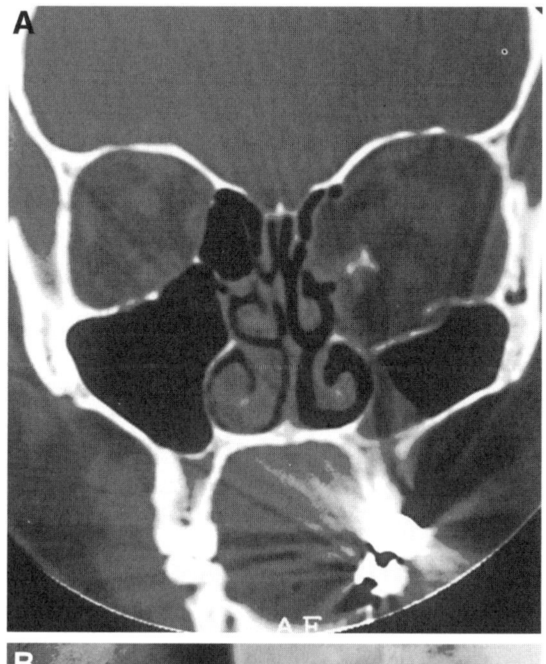

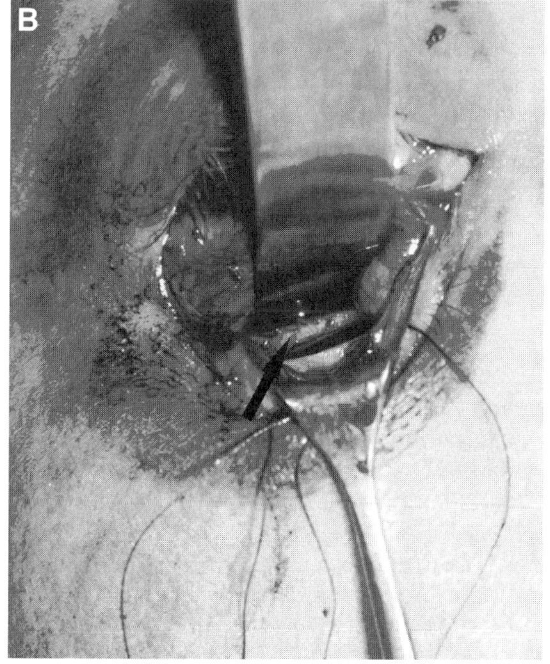

(*Continued*)

FIGURE 3 (cont.)

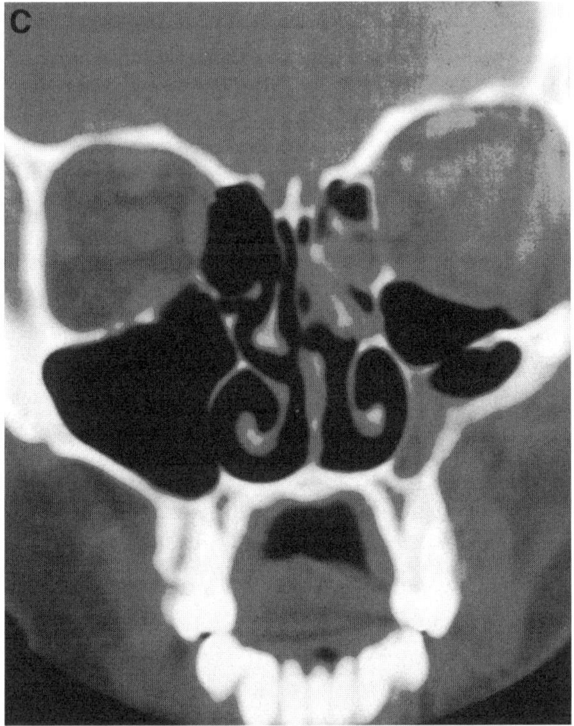

FIGURE 3.—**A,** coronal CT scan showing disruption of the orbital floor (*arrow*). **B,** orbital floor exposed by a transconjunctival (preseptal) approach. The nasal septal cartilage graft has been placed (*arrow*). **C,** postoperative CT scan. (Courtesy of Li KK: Repair of traumatic orbital wall defects with nasal septal cartilage: Report of five cases. *J Oral Maxillofac Surg* 55:1098–1102, 1997.)

chal bowl cartilage with attached perichondrium or temporalis fascia can be used as alternatives, and they fit the curvature well.

**G.R. Holt, M.D., M.S.E., M.P.H.**

## Factors Predictive of Poor Compliance With Follow-up Care After Facial Trauma: A Prospective Study

Stewart MG, Chen AY (Baylor College of Medicine, Houston)
*Otolaryngol Head Neck Surg* 117:72–75, 1997                    9–4

*Background.*—Facial trauma is a common problem treated by otolaryngologist-head and neck surgeons at trauma centers and urban hospitals. Compliance with follow-up care in this patient population was assessed prospectively.

*Study Design.*—From January to July 1995, 59 patients with isolated facial trauma who were treated by the Otolaryngology-Head and Neck Surgery service at Ben Taub General Hospital, Houston, were prospectively studied. The treating physicians interviewed patients at the initial evaluation and recorded demographic, social, and clinical information. Compliance with clinic follow-up care was evaluated.

*Findings.*—Young, minority, male victims of assault with blunt injury mechanisms predominated in this urban population. Midface fractures and soft-tissue injuries were the most common. Of the 59 patients, 31 were admitted and the rest were treated as outpatients. Although 66% of patients made it to their initial follow-up appointment, only 46% completed follow-up treatment. Multivariate analysis identified orbital injury site, white race, and not having a home telephone as predictive of poor compliance with the initial follow-up. Failure to keep the initial appointment and treatment with observation, suture, or open reduction internal fixation only were associated with poor compliance with follow-up completion. Age, marital status, employment, education, and hospital admission were not predictive of compliance with follow-up care.

*Conclusions.*—In this series of urban patients with isolated facial trauma, there was a 66% rate of compliance for initial follow-up, but only a 46% rate of compliance with completion of follow-up care. As compliance with follow-up care may not be complete in this population, especially for patients with orbital fractures and those treated with watchful waiting, patients with facial trauma should initially be managed aggressively.

▶ I was surprised to see that patients with orbital trauma were among the least compliant for follow-up appointments. Perhaps a trick I learned might help other physicians with this problem. If I suspect a patient could be noncompliant, I tell them the following on discharge: "If you don't come back to keep your appointment to see us, you might go blind." Not surprisingly, they come back. It's a true statement when you consider the possibilities of retinal detachment, hyphema development, and retrobulbar hematoma. If they fear they could miss out on Monday night football forever, they'll come back.

**G.R. Holt, M.D., M.S.E., M.P.H.**

---

**Orbital Floor Reconstruction With Autogenous Mandibular Symphyseal Bone Grafts**

Krishnan V, Johnson JV (Univ of Detroit Mercy; Detroit Receiving Hosp)
*J Oral Maxillofac Surg* 55:327–330, 1997                                     9–5

---

*Background.*—Many types of material are used to repair orbital floor defects. The most well tolerated grafts are autogenous bone grafts. Use of the mandibular symphyseal bone as a graft for reconstruction of the orbital floor was assessed.

*Study Design.*—From June 1990 to June 1993, 16 patients with orbital fractures or defects of less than 2 cm in diameter who were seen at the Oral and Maxillofacial Surgery service at the University of Texas, Houston,

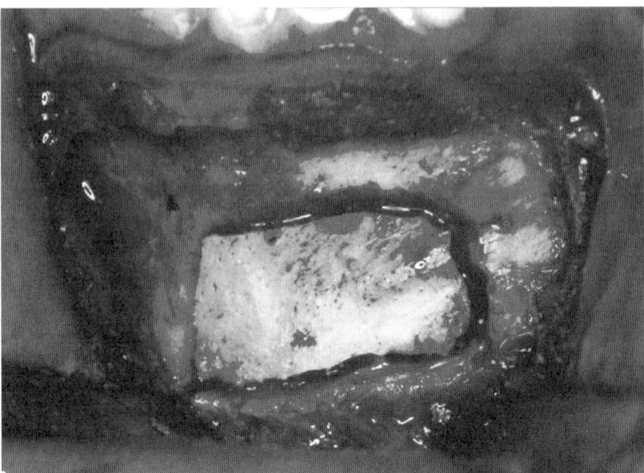

FIGURE 1.—Mandibular symphysis with osteotomies performed for graft harvest. (Courtesy of Krishnan V, Johnson JV: Orbital floor reconstruction with autogenous mandibular symphyseal bone grafts. *J Oral Maxillofac Surg* 55:327–330, 1997.)

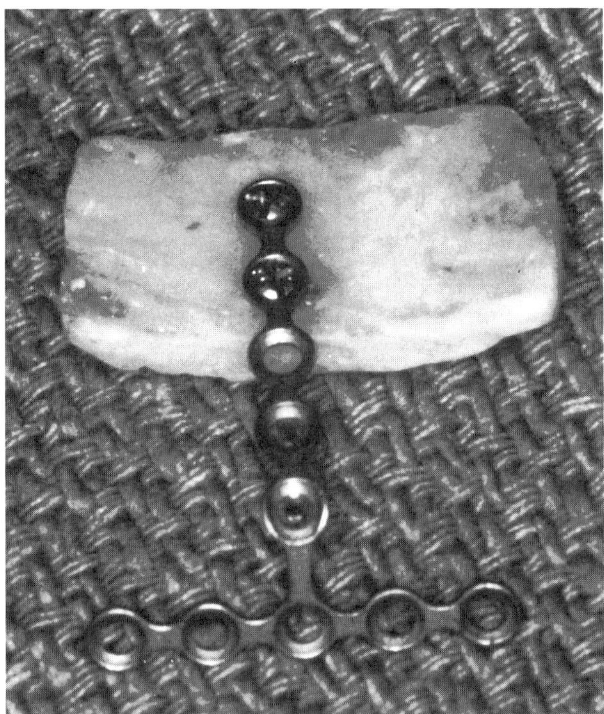

FIGURE 2.—Bone plate fixated to the bone graft on the side table. (Courtesy of Krishnan V, Johnson JV: Orbital floor reconstruction with autogenous mandibular symphyseal bone grafts. *J Oral Maxillofac Surg* 55:327–330, 1997.)

underwent reconstruction with mandibular symphyseal bone grafts. Indications for operation included diplopia, infraorbital nerve paresthesia, enophthalmos by clinical examination, and radiologic evidence of an orbital floor defect. After orbital floor exploration, the bone graft was harvested from the symphysis (Fig 1). When screws were used for fixation, the bone graft was held while the screw-hole was drilled. When bone plate fixation was used, it was attached on the side table (Fig 2). The graft and attached bone plate were placed in the orbital floor and the bone plate was adapted and fixed. The patients in the study group were followed up from 9 to 36 months.

*Findings.*—No postoperative complaints were recorded. There was no clinical evidence of enophthalmos or diplopia. Extraocular movements were preserved. There were no infections. None of the grafts were lost or extruded. Normal chin contour was maintained. There were no sensory defects. Postoperative radiographs demonstrated that the contour of the orbital floor was restored in all cases.

*Conclusions.*—The mandibular symphysis appears to be a useful source of bone for reconstruction of the orbital floor. It can be harvested easily and can be readily adapted for reconstruction. These grafts can be used successfully to repair defects measuring up to 2 cm in diameter and should be considered by the maxillofacial surgeon when reconstructing the orbital floor.

▶ I thought this was a clever method of obtaining a bone graft for small orbital rim defects or minimal floor elevation. If one elects to use this site, one must be *very* careful not to damage the underlying dental roots or their neurovascular pedicles with osteotomes or drill bits. This could be particularly useful in a patient with a protruding chin and less useful where a thin symphyseal cortex is found. Considering what's underneath the donor site, it may be less risky than a calvarial graft, especially when just a small piece of bone is required.

**G.R. Holt, M.D., M.S.E., M.P.H.**

---

**Analysis of 100 Cases of Free-muscle Transplantation for Facial Paralysis**
Terzis JK, Noah ME (Internatl Inst of Reconstructive Microsurgery, Norfolk, Va)
*Plast Reconstr Surg* 99:1905–1921, 1997                                      9–6

---

*Introduction.*—Several procedures have been used to restore facial function in patients with unilateral facial paralysis. Microneurovascular transfer of a free-muscle transplant is the procedure of choice for long-standing facial paralysis, because it can restore facial movement and some emotional animation. Preoperative and intraoperative factors of 100 free-muscle transplantations used in the treatment of facial paralysis were assessed.

*Methods.*—Seven of 93 patients with facial paralysis underwent 2 muscle transplantations. Factors evaluated included age, sex, cause of paralysis, choice of muscles, number of nerve coaptations, and ischemia time of the muscle. Preoperative and postoperative videos were judged for functional and aesthetic outcomes by 4 independent raters not involved in the care of the patients evaluated.

*Results.*—There were 33 male and 60 female patients, with an age range of 3 to 57 years (average, 22.2 years). Muscles used for transplantation were the gracilis (n = 63), pectoralis (n = 34), segment of the rectus abdominis (n = 2), and segment of the latissimus dorsi (n = 1). In 89 patients for whom data was recorded, the onset of muscle function ranged from 6 to 48 weeks (average, 21.6 weeks). Young female patients tended to have earlier onset of function and higher aesthetic rating. There was no correlation between onset of muscle function and intraoperative ischemia of the free muscle. A higher postoperative rating was observed for 94% of patients using a 5-step scale of judgments. A moderate or better result was seen in 80% of all patients.

*Conclusion.*—Age, sex, and intraoperative ischemia had no significant effect on patient outcome. During surgery, the insetting of the muscle transfer and the tension used are adjusted by constantly referring to the preoperative videos. This can produce a better smile, but never a normal smile.

▶ I respect the results obtained in this series of free-muscle transplantations for facial paralysis. The authors are honest about their reporting and analysis of the results as well as their understanding of the procedure's inherent limitations. I was particularly struck that the results displayed in children were particularly good. Perhaps that is where the best results can be obtained, as the younger patient may be more "plastic" regarding healing and regeneration. On the other hand, some older patients may opt for the immediate results of a static suspension procedure rather than the more delayed results from the free transfer.

**G.R. Holt, M.D., M.S.E., M.P.H.**

## A New Flap for Nasal Tip Reconstruction

Wheatley MJ, Smith JK, Cohen IAJ (Oregon Health Sciences Univ, Portland, Ore; Univ of Pittsburgh, Pa)
*Plast Reconstr Surg* 99:220–224, 1997                                9–7

*Background.*—Many of the current options for aesthetic reconstruction of tumor defects of the nasal tip are not satisfactory. A new flap for the management of nasal tip and supratip defects is described.

*Technique.*—With the patient under local anesthesia, the skin tumor is excised with frozen-section margins. After excision, the surgeon makes an incision in the superior alar sulcus extending to the nasojugal fold and makes a backcut in the nasojugal fold parallel to the nasolabial fold. The surgeon then completely elevates the transposition flap, including the nasalis muscle and an interpositional flap from the lateral alae, at the perichondrial and deep subcutaneous levels, respectively. The arterial branches to the nasalis muscle are identified and preserved during transposition flap elevation. Transposition of the nasalis flap in an anterior and caudal direction creates a midline dog-ear that requires resection. The surgeon rotates the interpositional flap in an opposite, cephalad direction to fill the advancement defect in the nasojugal fold. Inset of the flap leaves incisions in the natural skin lines of the superior alar sulcus and nasojugal fold. The interpositional flap maintains the definition of the nasojugal fold. Peripheral undermining is essential for easy rotation of the flaps to cover tip defects. Bilateral flaps can be used to cover large central tip defects.

*Discussion.*—This flap, used in 18 patients with nasal tip and supratip tumor defects, has resulted in well-concealed donor scars and minimal changes in nasal contour. Color and texture matches have been excellent. Also, the pincushion deformity is eliminated. Thus the modified nasalis flap is ideal for nasal tip reconstruction.

▶ The authors present a modification of a transposition flap that appears to work well on a convex surface such as the tip of the nose. It utilizes a small triangular flap above the alar rim to reduce the lateral distortional pull of the cheek, had it been undermined in the usual fashion. We must always recall that for some patients other options can be considered and offered—healing by secondary intent, primary closure, and full thickness skin graft. Remember to assure that the patient has ceased taking aspirin or other potential anti-platelet medications at least a week preoperatively. We give our patients a list of over-the-counter medications that contain aspirin.

**G.R. Holt, M.D., M.S.E., M.P.H.**

---

## A Comparison of Resource Costs for Head and Neck Reconstruction With Free and Pectoralis Major Flaps

Kroll SS, Evans GRD, Goldberg D, et al (Univ of Texas, Houston)
*Plast Reconstr Surg* 99:1282–1286, 1997                                    9–8

---

*Introduction.*—The high cost of medical care is under scrutiny, and some have wondered about the costs related to complex surgical procedures such as free tissue transfer. Because free flaps result in fewer complications, have more rapid patient recovery, and better quality results, free flaps have been used for repair of oropharyngeal defects more often than reconstruction with regional myocutaneous flaps at one institution. To determine whether reconstruction with free flaps was less or more expensive than reconstructions with regional myocutaneous flaps, a series of immediate reconstructions with regional or distant tissue for repair of oropharyngeal defects caused by treatment of head and neck cancer was reviewed.

*Methods.*—There were 178 patients included in this study, and of these 89 had the radial forearm free flap, 56 had the rectus abdominis free flap, and 33 had the pectoralis major myocutaneous flap. By adding all the costs to the institution providing each service studied using salaried employees, resource costs were determined. To compare free flaps with the pectoralis major myocutaneous flap, a regional myocutaneous flap, the 2 free flap groups were combined.

*Results.*—There were similar failure rates in the 2 groups with 3.4 % for the free flaps and 3% for the pectoralis major myocutaneous flap. The free flaps had slightly higher surgical costs, but there were lower subsequent hospital stay costs. The total mean resource cost for the myocutaneous flap group was higher at $40,992 than it was for the free flap group at $28,460. More patients with advanced disease and systemic medical problems may have been selected for the pectoralis major myocutaneous flap, which may have contributed to the longer hospitalization and added cost.

*Conclusion.*—Free flaps may provide cost-savings for selected patients and are not necessarily more expensive than other methods. Although the use of free flaps is supported by this study, there is still not sufficient proof that they are generically less expensive than myocutaneous flaps for head and neck reconstruction.

▶ It appears from this study that the use of major free flaps to reconstruct head and neck defects was cost-effective when compared with the pectoralis major myocutaneous flap. It was also interesting to note that the free and pedicled flaps had comparably low failure rates (3.0% to 3.4%). When I first began utilizing the regional myocutaneous flap, it seemed like a giant leap forward in our reconstructive efforts. However, it was just a step along the continuum of innovation and progress in applied technology. Who knows what the next step will be? At any rate, the patient is well-served when the *best* flap for his or her defect is chosen. In many institutions, interdisciplinary collaboration is necessary for reconstructive decision-making.

**G.R. Holt, M.D., M.S.E., M.P.H.**

---

**Further Experiences With the Sternocleidomastoid Myocutaneous Flap: A Clinical Appraisal of 31 Cases**
Ariyan S (Yale Univ, New Haven, Conn)
*Plast Reconstr Surg* 99:61–69, 1997                    9–9

---

*Background.*—The success rate of the sternocleidomastoid myocutaneous flap for reconstruction of surgical wounds after resection of head and neck cancers has been variable, causing most surgeons to abandon this procedure as their primary choice. The experience of 1 surgeon with the use of these flaps was presented.

*Methods and Findings.*—The outcomes of 31 consecutive reconstructions with the sternocleidomastoid myocutaneous flap in the oropharyngeal area were reviewed. Although the complication rate was high (52%), essentially all complications were partial epidermal losses. All flaps healed with no need for additional surgery. The impact of previous radiation therapy, blood supply location, and concomitant neck dissection was analyzed and revealed no differences in outcomes among groups.

*Conclusion.*—Although a number of other reliable myocutaneous flaps and free flaps are available for reconstructions, the sternocleidomastoid myocutaneous flap should still be considered for selected patients. This flap provides for a small skin paddle that is available locally, and it is readily within the reach of many sites in the oropharyngeal area. The partial epithelial loss noted in this series appears to be a reflection of the tenuous blood supply from the muscle to the overlying skin.

▶ Dr. Ariyan should be credited with promulgating the clinical use of myocutaneous flaps, especially the pectoralis major. Here he reiterates his support for the sternocleidomastoid flap. This flap remains in my own personal repertoire (to which my fellows can attest) for a fairly wide range of applications. In my hands, it is quite helpful for defects around the mandible, tongue and floor of mouth, and tonsil. As long as the vascular supply is identified and protected, this flap can fill an approximately 3-cm defect in the areas noted. For posterior oral cavity defects, placement of the flap is best performed after a radical neck dissection in which the great vessels are visualized and securing of the flap in the proper position can be achieved.

**G.R. Holt, M.D., M.S.E., M.P.H.**

---

**Experience With the Osteocutaneous Fibula Flap: An Analysis of 24 Consecutive Reconstructions of Composite Mandibular Defects**
Wolff K-D, Ervens J, Herzog K, et al (Free Univ of Berlin)
*J Craniomaxillofac Surg* 24:330–338, 1996                    9–10

---

*Objective.*—Patients with squamous cell carcinoma of the floor of the mouth infiltrating bone may need mandibular resection. In reconstructing the mandible and floor of the mouth, the bone must be stable enough for insertion of endosseous implants and the skin thin enough for an anatomical reshaping of the mucosal contours. Until recently, there have been few reports of use of the osteocutaneous fibula flap for this purpose. The authors report their experience with the osteocutaneous fibula flap for combined replacement of the mandible and floor of the mouth.

> *Technique.*—The authors' clinical use of this flap was based on the results of anatomical dissections of the skin supply of the peroneal artery. Because of variation in the skin perforators and large lower leg vessels and the risk of atherosclerotic damage, preoperative angiography and Doppler ultrasound were essential.

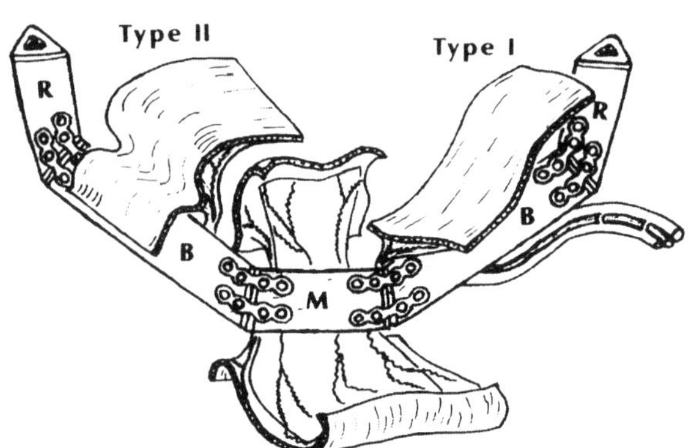



FIGURE 3.—Schematic illustration of reconstruction possibilities for osteocutaneous fibula transplants. (Courtesy of Wolff K-D, Ervens J, Herzog K, et al: Experience with the osteocutaneous fibula flap: An analysis of 24 consecutive reconstructions of composite mandibular defects. *J Craniomaxillofac Surg* 24:330–338, copyright 1996 by permission of the publisher, Churchill Livingston.)

The flap was raised by a lateral approach at the same time as tumor resection. Care was taken to preserve the blood supply to the skin and bone. The skin islands were raised from the distal third of the lower leg, with blood supply from a single perforating vessel. At all times, at least 7 cm was left between the distal osteotomy and the lateral malleolus. A split-thickness skin graft was used to cover the donor site.

*Experience.*—The technique was used in 24 patients, including 22 primary and 2 secondary reconstructions. The fibular segments ranged from 5.5 to 18 cm in length, and the skin component from 3 × 5 to 6 × 15 cm. With an average vascular pedicle length of 11 cm, just 1 patient required a vein graft. Titanium miniplates were used for fibular osteosynthesis, with endosseous implants inserted secondarily (Figs 3 and 4).

The approach had a success rate of 96%, with 1 case of transplant loss and 1 of pseudarthrosis. All patients had satisfactory reconstruction of the mandibular shape, even though the width of the fibula was limited. The skin was thin and pliable enough for intraoral coverage, with little surplus volume left over. Two patients had chronic wound healing problems at the donor site, although neither had impaired walking ability.

*Conclusion.*—The success rate of use of the osteocutaneous fibula flap for reconstruction of composite mandibular defects is 95%, with low donor site morbidity. This flap avoids the need for a 2-step reconstruction or concomitant application of 2 microsurgical flaps. Even for patients with a reduced life expectancy, the immediate complete reconstruction provides valuable improvement in quality of life.

► This article nicely summarizes the clinical use of the fibular flap for mandibular reconstruction. Except for smaller, isolated defects or when a free flap is not possible, a flap such as this must be the first consideration.

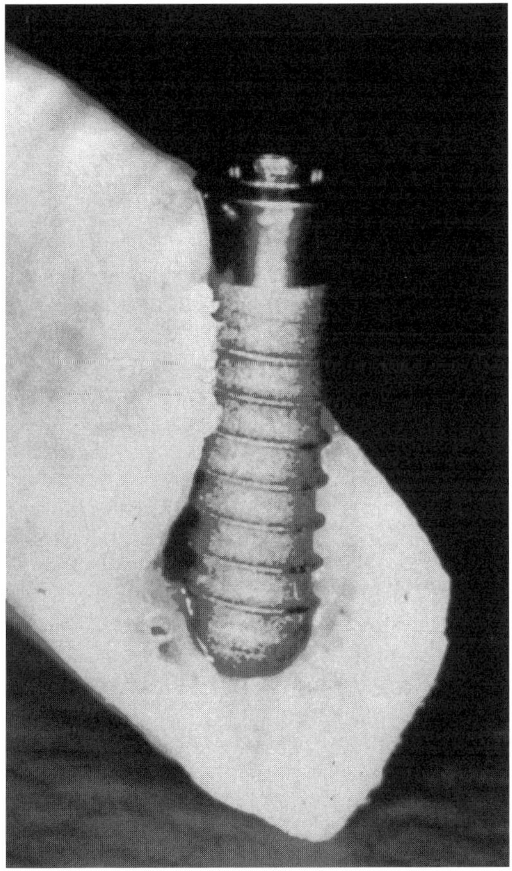

**FIGURE 4.**—The width of the fibula is sufficient for the inclusion of endosseous implants, and the cortical bone component ensures high primary stability. (Courtesy of Wolff K-D, Ervens J, Herzog K, et al: Experience with the osteocutaneous fibula flap: An analysis of 24 consecutive reconstructions of composite mandibular defects. *J Craniomaxillofac Surg* 24:330–338, copyright 1996 by permission of the publisher, Churchill Livingstone.)

Adequate soft-tissue coverage must be provided by either a pedicled muscular flap, a skin paddle on the osseous free flap, or both.

**G.R. Holt, M.D., M.S.E., M.P.H.**

---

**Success and Failure Rates Osseointegrated Implants in Function in Regenerated Bone for 6 to 51 Months: A Preliminary Report**
Fugazzotto PA (Milton, Mass)
*Int J Oral Maxillofac Implants* 12:17–24, 1997                    9–11

---

*Objective.*—Whereas the short-term success of guided bone regeneration (GBR), utilizing immediate placement of an implant into an extraction socket, is well known, the long-term clinical success has not been documented. Preliminary statistics related to implants functioning in regenerated bone from 6 to 51 months are presented.

*Methods.*—IMZ titanium plasma-sprayed implants of various lengths and 3.3, 4.0, or 4.25 mm in diameter were placed in demineralized freeze-dried bone allograft-filled residual sockets or in augmented bony ridges in 331 patients (146 male), aged 17 to 82. There were 341 maxillary implants and 285 mandibular implants. Patients were not allowed to use the implants for 6 weeks. Fenestration and dehiscence dimensions were documented. Prostheses were removed at least every 6 months and examined for implant mobility, pain/and or suppuration, peri-implant radiolucency, and vertical bone loss.

*Results.*—Two maxillary single-tooth replacements were lost after 5 and 7 months, and 5 mandibular implants were lost, 3 supporting a fixed prosthesis after 14 months (in a chemotherapy patient) and 2 supporting a 3-unit fixed prosthesis after 17 months. Two maxillary implants failed because of bone loss ≥0.2 mm annually. After 51 months, the success rate was 94.9% for the maxilla and 91.9% for the mandible. If the chemotherapy patient is excluded, the success rates become 96.7% for the mandible, and 95.8% overall, but the rate for the maxilla remains unchanged.

*Conclusion.*—Up to 51 months, regenerated bone functioned effectively and supported titanium plasma-sprayed cylindrical implants placed in individual residual sockets or in augmented bony ridges.

▶ Although research in the area of the biomechanics of regenerated bone is extensive, much is still not known about its capabilities, vis-à-vis its response to implant loading, particularly over time. The mandible apparently relies heavily upon axial and shear forces to maintain its strength and integrity. Evidence such as presented in this article indicates that titanium-sputtered implants may actually enhance bone regeneration, perhaps due to the re-establishment of properly aligned (i.e., similar to tooth) forces in the bone. There must be a lesson in here somewhere about treating or preventing osteoporosis of the spine.

**G.R. Holt, M.D., M.S.E., M.P.H.**

---

**Cutaneous Nasal Malignancies: Is Primary Reconstruction Safe?**
Evans GRD, Williams JZ, Ainslie NB (Univ of Texas MD Anderson Cancer Ctr, Houston)
*Head Neck* 19:182–187, 1997                                               9–12

---

*Introduction.*—The most common tumor in the United States is skin cancer, with up to 50% of the white population older than 65 years having some form of skin cancer. The nose is the most common site for cutaneous malignancies. Because the nose is perceived to be associated with an individual's character, ethnicity, and familial identity, nasal reconstruction takes on an added importance. However, nasal reconstruction is often hampered by local recurrence after surgical extirpation. Patients at high risk for cutaneous nasal recurrence should be identified. Most initial reconstructive timing recommendations have been made on patients who have not had reconstruction. The safety of primary nasal reconstruction in selected patients was examined.

*Methods.*—A total of 71 patients, 35 men and 36 women with an average age of 60 years, who had nasal reconstruction in an 8-year period were retrospectively reviewed. Defects secondary to malignancies were the causes for nasal reconstructions. The most common lesion was basal cell carcinoma, followed by squamous cell carcinoma and melanoma.

*Results.*—The nasal dorsum was the most common location of the cutaneous lesions. The most common adjacent tissue used for reconstruction was the forehead flap. For 42 of 49 basal cell carcinomas, 6 of 10 squamous cell carcinomas, 6 of 7 melanomas, and 3 of 5 other lesions, immediate reconstruction was performed. For 7 of 49 basal cell carcinomas, 4 of 10 squamous cell carcinomas, 1 of 7 melanomas, and 2 of 5 additional lesions, delayed restoration was performed. There was an average time of 8.2 months between surgical extirpation and the start of nasal reconstruction for basal cell carcinoma. For squamous cell carcinoma, the average time was 29 months, and for melanoma, the average time was 10 months. At an average of 36 months after extirpation, 26 recurrent lesions were identified. There was an average follow-up of 41 months. No evidence of disease was seen in several patients who are still alive.

*Conclusions.*—In selected patients, primary reconstruction is safe. If margins are questionable, if there is perineural or deep bony invasion, if postoperative radiotherapy is to be initiated, or if the pathology is determined to be aggressive, surgical delay in reconstruction should be considered. In an effort to restore self-image, nasal reconstruction can be performed with few complications.

▶ This study supports immediate reconstruction of nasal defects after cancer resection. However, when there is a concern about margins or if the cancer is particularly aggressive, it is wise to apply a skin graft and revisit a full-thickness reconstruction up to a year later. When resected using a Mohs' fresh tissue method, one can perhaps be more comfortable with reconstructing the defect primarily than when frozen-section margins are obtained. Don't forget that it is also acceptable to wait for permanent sections, having dressed the wound appropriately, and then reconstruct after clear permanent section margins are reported. For small defects, healing by secondary intent obviates the concern over immediate reconstruction.

**G.R. Holt, M.D., M.S.E., M.P.H.**

## Penetrating Injuries of the Face

Chen AY, Stewart MG, Raup G (Baylor College of Medicine, Houston; Ben Taub Gen Hosp, Houston)
*Otolaryngol Head Neck Surg* 115:464–470, 1996                    9–13

*Introduction.*—There is a plethora of reports concerning the injury patterns and treatment algorithms for penetrating injuries to the neck, chest, and abdomen, but little is published about penetrating injuries to the face. A retrospective review of gunshot, shotgun, and stab wounds to the face was conducted and a classification scheme was created, with respect to site of entry and weapon type.

*Methods.*—Medical records of all patients with penetrating trauma to the face from gunshot, shotgun, or stab wounds were reviewed for the 3-year period 1992–1994. The site of entry was categorized into 1 of 2 zones: midface or mandible (Fig 1). Because shotgun wounds invariably penetrated every facial zone, these injuries were analyzed as separate injuries.

*Results.*—Seventy-eight patients (63 male, 15 female) with a median age of 26 years (range, 15–67 years) were identified. Emergent airway establishment was significantly more likely to be needed for patients with gunshot wounds. A significantly higher prevalence of globe injury was

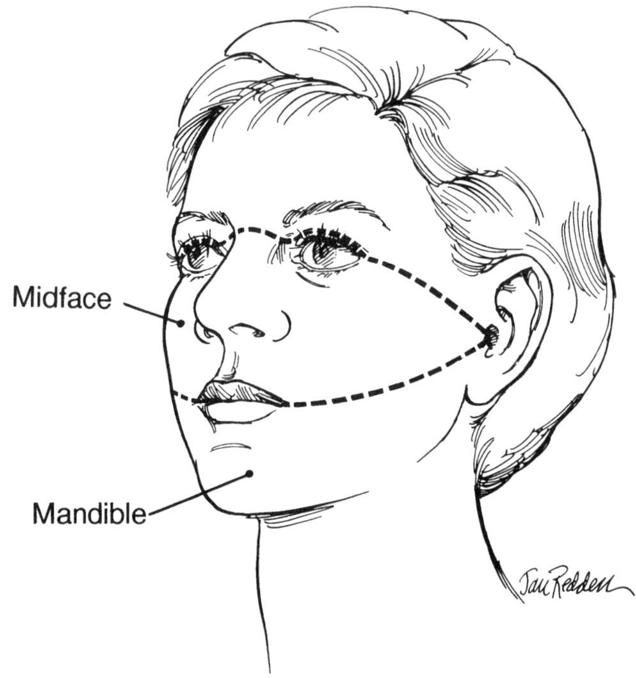


FIGURE 1.—Midface and mandible zones. (Courtesy of Chen AY, Stewart MG, Raup G: Penetrating injuries of the face. *Otolaryngol Head Neck Surg* 115:464–470, 1996.)

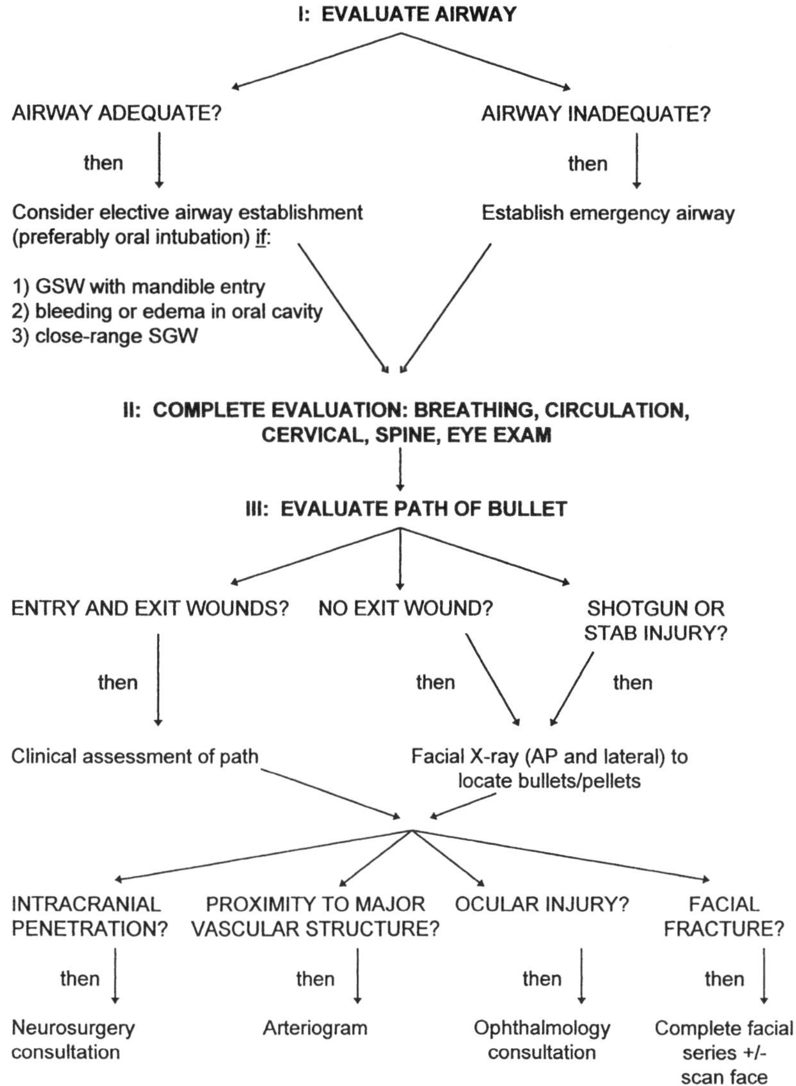


FIGURE 2.—Algorithm for penetrating facial trauma. *Abbreviations: GSW*, gunshot wound; *SGW*, shotgun wound; *AP*, anteroposterior. (Courtesy of Chen AY, Stewart MG, Raup G: Penetrating injuries of the face. *Otolaryngol Head Neck Surg* 115:464–470, 1996.)

observed in patients with shotgun compared with gunshot wounds. Intracranial penetration occurred in 9 patients with a bullet or gunshot pellet (12%). Patients with gunshot wounds required open reduction and internal fixation of facial bone fractures significantly more often, compared with patients with shotgun wounds. Of 30 patients who underwent arteriograms, there were 10 positive findings. There were 3 deaths. Twenty-nine patients (37%) had some complication from their penetrating facial trauma. Twelve patients were blinded by their injury. There were no between-group differences in the prevalence of complications and cause of injury. An algorithm for the evaluation and management of penetrating injuries to the face was created (Fig 2).

*Conclusion.*—Penetrating wounds to the face are seldom fatal, but they can involve multiple organ systems and may cause significant morbidity. Systematic evaluation and treatment of patients can be performed, using site of entry and type of weapon as guides. Patients should be carefully assessed for secondary complications, even if these are not obvious.

▶ The authors present a simple and common sense approach to civilian penetrating wounds. Military/paramilitary wounds can be somewhat more problematic, as the irregular shape of shrapnel and the "tumbling" effect of very high velocity military rounds makes tracking the path similar to following a tornado. For the most part, I am inclined to err on the side of obtaining an arteriogram if there is any question at all; the positive yield may be low, but I prefer that to an undiagnosed vascular injury. Because the face and neck are so vascular (remember all those blood vessels we memorized in anatomy?), there is a good chance the penetration got one of them or was very close. Also, stab wounds do not show up well on a CT scan unless a hematoma is present.

**G.R. Holt, M.D., M.S.E., M.P.H.**

---

**A Study of Primary Closure of Human Bite Injuries to the Face**
Donkor P, Bankas DO (Univ of Science and Technology, Kumasi, Ghana)
*J Oral Maxillofac Surg* 55:479–481, 1997                                9–14

---

*Introduction.*—Management of human bites to the face typically means closure of the wound after a period of delay during which the wound is packed open. The Maxillofacial Unit of the Komfo Anokye Teaching Hospital serves the whole of the northern sector of Ghana. Patients must travel long distances to use the service, and economic considerations must be addressed. Conventional treatment adds considerably to cost of care because patients must either be admitted or find a place to live while undergoing treatment. Since 1995, the defects resulting from human bites have undergone primary closure after debridement of the wound. The management of primary closure of human bite injuries to the face was assessed over 12 months at the Komfo Anokye Teaching Hospital.

*Methods.*—Data regarding patient age, sex, assailant, site of injury, duration of injury, previous treatment, surgical repair, and treatment outcome were collected in 30 patients treated for human bite injury to the face. Wounds were thoroughly debrided, then closed by either direct suturing, a local flap, or skin grafting on the day the patient was seen. In most patients, only local anesthesia was necessary. Tetanus prophylaxis was administered, and a 1-week course of antibiotic therapy was given.

Sutures were removed after 1 week, and skin grafts were uncovered 10 days after surgery.

*Results.*—Of 30 patients, 21 were males and 9 were females. Age range was 17 to 55 years (mean age, 31.8 years). The lips were involved in 66% of patients. The time between injury and evaluation was 1 to 4 days. At the time of suture removal, healing was complete in 27 patients (90%). Two of the remaining 3 wounds healed without further complications after wound cleansing and a course of antibiotic therapy.

*Conclusion.*—Immediate closure of human bite injuries to the face may be considered safe, even when there is a delay. With thorough wound debridement, appropriate antibiotic therapy, and clear postoperative instructions, this approach may be considered a convenient and cost-saving approach to these injuries.

▶ In a rising country such as Ghana, advanced medical technology, health insurance coverage, and rapid arrival to a trauma center are not necessarily accepted as the standard of care, as we have grown to expect in America. Practical considerations in patient care may well take precedence over the extensive use of highly sophisticated and readily available resources. For avulsion injuries, where tissue punctures by teeth are not present, comprehensive wound care and primary closure has an excellent chance for success. However, the clinician must be aware of high-risk wounds, which may be better managed by local wound care, parenteral antibiotics, and delayed primary closure. In America we have the benefit (at least in most areas) of accessibility to close follow-up, readily available transportation, and accessibility to surgery centers, which facilitate delayed closure when required.

**G.R. Holt, M.D., M.S.E., M.P.H.**

# 10 Facial Plastic Surgery

**Cosmetic Upper-Facial Rejuvenation With Botulinum**
Ellis DAF, Tan AKW (Univ of Toronto)
*J Otolaryngol* 26:92–96, 1997

10–1

*Background.*—Repetitive muscle actions result in the hyperfunctional facial animation lines that occur with aging. Current methods used by plastic surgeons to correct such hyperfunctional animation lines—including surgical and nonsurgical techniques—do not address the underlying cause of wrinkles: hyperfunctional facial animation. The observation that patients with Bell's palsy have no hyperfunctional lines on the involved side of the face prompted the study of botulinum toxin A in the treatment of 1 group of patients with hyperfunctional facial lines. Botulinum toxin A blocks the release of acetylcholine at the presynaptic neuromuscular junction.

*Methods.*—Twenty-three patients recruited during a 15-month period were injected in a total of 72 anatomical areas. Twenty-three injections were at the lateral aspects of the lateral canthal lines, 23 at the inferior aspects of the lateral canthal lines, and 26 at the glabellar frown lines.

*Findings.*—The mean depth and length of the glabellar frown lines were significantly improved. Patients reported significant improvement subjectively. The lateral canthal lines showed more improvement than the inferior lateral canthal lines in patients receiving injections for crow's feet because the latter have a larger component of zygomaticus major and minor muscle, which contributes to the inferior lateral squint line.

*Conclusion.*—Botulinum toxin A injection is a safe, simple, effective treatment for hyperfunctional upper facial muscle action, which causes wrinkling. This treatment also retards the development of intradermal creasing and increases the duration of collagen injection.

▶ The observation of the effects on wrinkles in patients who underwent botulinum toxin injections for blepharospasm was instrumental in the hypothesis that perhaps botulinum could be helpful in reducing such wrinkles. The periorbital beneficial (relaxing) effects extended to the interbrow muscles, thus reducing their pull on the skin. That said, I am not sure how much success can be achieved with very deep wrinkles without the use of some other method as well, such as laser resurfacing or dermal augmentation. The method described here is a good alternative to endoscopic brow lift but may be nearly as expensive in the long term.

**G.R. Holt, M.D., M.S.E., M.P.H.**

## The Effect of Blepharoplasty on Eyebrow Position

Frankel AS, Kamer FM (Univ of California, Los Angeles)
*Arch Otolaryngol Head Neck Surg* 123:393–396, 1997    10–2

*Introduction.*—It is generally thought that more significant postoperative eyebrow ptosis occurs with patients with pre-existing eyebrow ptosis who have upper eyelid blepharoplasty performed. This is thought to be the case because the excision of skin and soft tissue brings the eyebrow closer to the eyelid margin, and the correction of blepharochalasis alleviates the patient's need to keep the eyebrows elevated. Nevertheless, no scientific evidence is available to support these theories. Eyebrow height was examined before and after upper eyelid blepharoplasty in a cosmetic surgery population.

*Methods.*—The study included 82 patients who were divided into 2 groups: 54 had blepharoplasty performed and 28 did not. The treatment group included patients who had preoperative and postoperative photographs and who had upper eyelid blepharoplasty by the senior surgeon. The control group had no procedure performed that could have altered eyebrow height. The height of the eyebrow was measured before and after treatment.

*Results.*—No significant difference was found in eyebrow height between patients who had a blepharoplasty and those who did not. There were no significant differences between patients younger than 40 years, 40–50 years, or older than 50 years. There were no differences between men and women. In a subgroup of patients who had eyebrow drop, there was still no significant change in eyebrow position in the treatment group when compared to the group that did not have surgery.

*Conclusion.*—A lowering of the eyebrow is not caused by upper eyelid blepharoplasty in a cosmetic surgery population.

▶ The authors report their evaluation of only a subgroup of their original study and control patients, but explain why they did so. I was glad to see that blepharoplasty of the upper eyelid did not appear to have some biomechanical impact on brow position. One might worry that fat excision and resection of skin and muscle could create an inferior traction. But, the forces would be small compared to the actions of the larger forehead muscles, and the frontalis/orbicularis interface that helps control brow position.

**G.R. Holt, M.D., M.S.E., M.P.H.**

## Aesthetic Analysis of the Eyebrows

Gunter JP, Antrobus SD (Univ of Texas, Dallas)
*Plast Reconstr Surg* 99:1808–1816, 1997                    10–3

*Objective.*—The possibility of achieving the perfect brow after browlift has been enhanced by new techniques and instrumentation. For the purpose of defining the ideal brow, brow aesthetics were evaluated by reviewing photographs of a group of fashion models and before-and-after photographs of a group of patients who underwent facial rejuvenation.

*Methods.*—Computer imaging was used to alter the shape and position of models' eyebrows and produce 4 different shapes. Aesthetic results were evaluated by groups of plastic surgeons attending a symposium. The shape and position of the eyebrows of 7 patients are discussed.

*Results.*—Brows need to be evaluated while considering the entire periorbital area, including the eyelids. Criteria for attractive eyes were developed (Figs 10 and 11). Common surgical mistakes include overelevating brows, placing the brow peak medially, creating too high a lateral peak, making large asymmetric differences in brow height, overresectioning of the medial brow depressors, and unmasking deep hollowing of the eyes.

*Conclusion.*—Simply performing a brow lift will not necessarily improve the patient's appearance. The eyebrow must be repositioned and/or

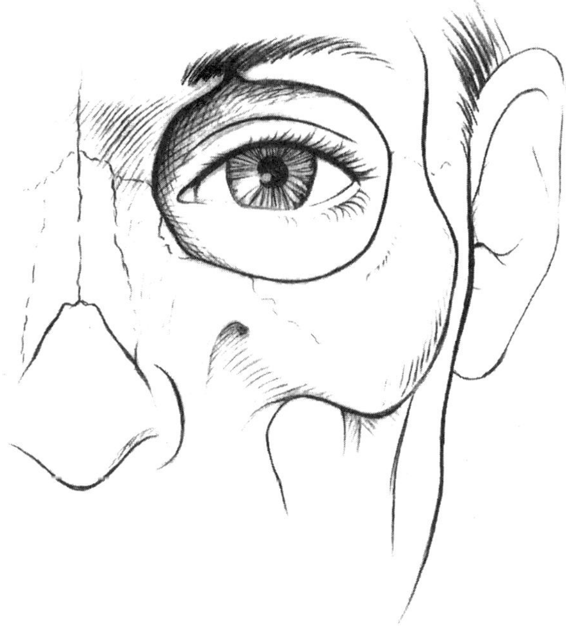

FIGURE 10.—Relationship of supraorbital ridge to eyebrow in females. (Illustration courtesy of Lisa Clark, from Gunter JP, Antrobus SD: Aesthetic analysis of the eyebrows. *Plast Reconstr Surg* 99:1808–1816, 1997.)

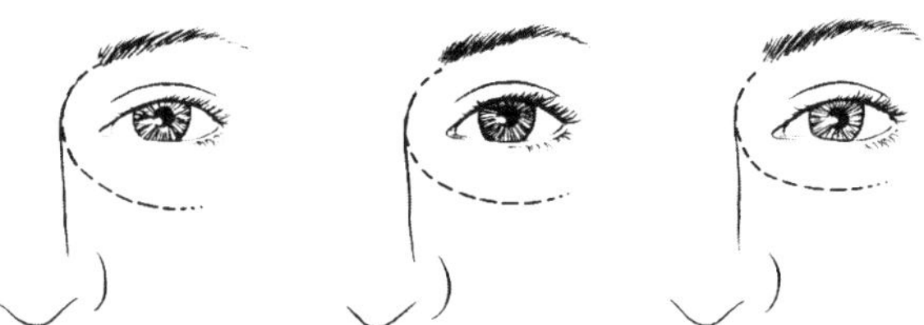

FIGURE 11.—The periorbital oval. (Illustration courtesy of Lisa Clark, from Gunter JP, Antrobus SD: Aesthetic analysis of the eyebrows. *Plast Reconstr Surg* 99:1808–1816, 1997.)

reshaped to suit the individual and to harmonize with the shape of the periorbital area.

▶ The authors have presented an excellent treatise on the goals of brow lift and the real difficulties in achieving what is planned preoperatively. Although it is important to look toward the "ideal" as a standard against which any given results are measured, I believe we must keep at least two practicalities in mind. First, most of us do not operate on models, nor do our patients all have the capability to look like a model postoperatively. Second, we must be careful *not* to lose the appearance of the patient's face that is uniquely that person. As paraphrased from a famous sailor, "we are what we are, and that's what we are."

**G.R. Holt, M.D., M.S.E., M.P.H.**

---

**Fibrin Glue Fixation in Forehead Endoscopy: Evaluation of Our Experience With 206 Cases**
Marchac D, Ascherman J, Arnaud E (Columbia Presbyterian Med Ctr, NY; Hosp Necker, Paris)
*Plast Reconstr Surg* 100:704–712, 1997                          10–4

---

*Background.*—Endoscopic surgery has become popular over the last decade. Fibrin glue has increasingly been used in surgical procedures. Results of 206 endoscopic forehead rejuvenation procedures performed with fibrin glue since 1983 were reviewed.

*Technique.*—The patient's face was evaluated before surgery. Two temporal and 2 paramedial incisions were used for the approach. The periosteum was elevated and undermined posteriorly in proportion to the planned eyebrow elevation. The endoscope was then introduced. The periosteum was incised. The procerus muscles were transected with a curved cutting instrument (Fig 3). A mixture of fibrin and thrombin was distributed in the undermined areas with a long cannula (Fig 4). Gluing in this manner allowed selective positioning. The incisions were then closed. The forehead could not be cleaned or rubbed for 24 hours to allow the glue to set completely.

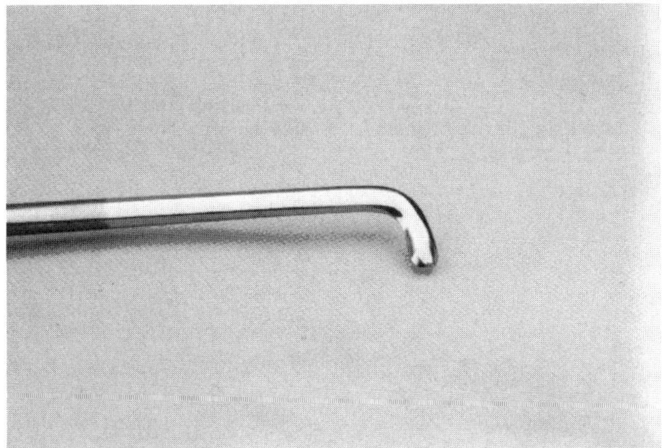

FIGURE 3.—The curved hook has a slightly cutting edge. It allows dissection and cutting of the muscles without damaging the nerves and vessels (Micro-France, Bourl on L'Archambault, France. (Courtesy of Marchac D, Ascherman J, Arnaud E: Fibrin glue fixation in forehead endoscopy: Evaluation of our experience with 206 cases. *Plast Reconstr Surg* 100:704–712, 1997.)

*Study Design.*—Between November 1993 and May 1996, 206 endo-forehead procedures were performed on 196 patients by 1 surgeon. Among the 163 patients with at least 6 months of follow-up, 97 had a full evaluation. Evaluation included quality of results, secondary procedures, and complications.

*Findings.*—A comparison of the results of 28 patients treated during the first 6 months and 69 patients treated later demonstrated a significant improvement in results. Satisfactory results increased from 71% to 86%

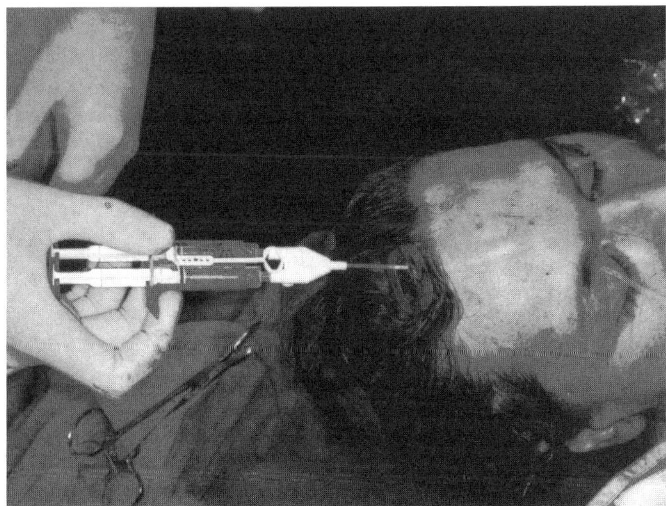

FIGURE 4.—Fixation is achieved by gluing the periosteum to the bone with fibrin glue. A special long cannula is used to distribute 2 or 4 cc of fibrin glue. (Courtesy of Marchac D, Ascherman J, Arnaud E: Fibrin glue fixation in forehead endoscopy: Evaluation of our experience with 206 cases. *Plast Reconstr Surg* 100:704–712, 1997.)

after the first 6 months of experience with this technique. Overall, there was a 6% rate of secondary procedures, with none required in the later group of patients. There were no permanent complications.

*Conclusions.*—Fixation of the endoscopically lifted forehead with fibrin glue is simple, effective, and flexible, and is not associated with adverse effects.

▶ The authors propose an alternative method of fixation of the endoscopically lifted forehead to suture or cortical screw. Their results (in only the short-term) appear quite acceptable. Longer follow-up, of course, will be required to better compare fixation options. They also admit that they got better with time as they used the adhesive. If the lift is performed in an office surgery center, the patient will need to be sent to a laboratory with hematology capabilility well in advance of the surgical date to have the fibrin component of the adhesive concocted. The thrombin will be readily available in the surgery suite.

**G.R. Holt, M.D., M.S.E., M.P.H.**

---

**The Contribution of the SMAS to the Blood Supply in the Lateral Face Lift Flap**
Whetzel TP, Stevenson TR (Univ of California, Sacramento)
*Plast Reconstr Surg* 100:1011–1018, 1997                                    10–5

---

*Background.*—The facelift literature reports a lower incidence of skin sloughing with subsuperficial musculoaponeurotic system (SMAS) techniques than with subcutaneous techniques. No anatomical explanation has been offered to explain this difference. The primary direct vascular flow into this region is from the transverse facial artery. The SMAS layer has not been reported to be vascular. The contribution of the SMAS layer to the arterial blood supply of the lateral cheek portion of the facelift flap was investigated in a cadaveric facelift model.

*Methods.*—Nine fresh cadavers underwent bilateral cervicofacial rhytidectomy, with 1 side undermined beneath the SMAS plane and the other side undermined in the subcutaneous plane above the SMAS layer. The transverse facial artery perforator was identified and either preserved or dissected. The transverse facial artery was then injected with ink and the cutaneous staining pattern observed.

*Results.*—In every case where the transverse facial artery perforator was preserved, the entire transverse facial artery lateral facial area was stained with ink after injection into the transverse facial artery. When the transverse artery perforator was transected, there was no cutaneous staining. The depth of dissection (SMAS or subcutaneous) had no effect on the cutaneous staining pattern.

*Conclusions.*—Study of the contribution of the superficial musculoaponeurotic system to the arterial blood supply of the surgically elevated facelift flap in a cadaveric facelift model demonstrates that lateral facelift flap circulation is dependent on preservation of the transverse facial artery and not on dissection depth. This suggests that the SMAS layer does not play an important role in flap viability.

▶ This simple, but well-done study provides an anatomical basis for the common technique of elevating the skin flap and SMAS separately to perform an "SMAS-pexy." More important to flap viability, as it appears to be in most flaps of the face and neck, is the protection of the subdermal arterial arcade, by leaving a few millimeters of hypodermal fat on the undersurface of the flap. If you see the shiny dermis, the flap is likely too thin. A little fat on the flap can be a good thing.

**G.R. Holt, M.D., M.S.E., M.P.H.**

---

**Update: Lifting the Malar Fat Pad for Correction of Prominent Nasolabial Folds**
Owsley JQ, Fiala TGS (Univ of California, San Francisco)
*Plast Reconstr Surg* 100:715–722, 1997                                    10–6

---

*Introduction.*—Plastic surgical correction of prominent nasolabial folds can be a difficult procedure. This problem may be addressed by surgical dissection beneath the midface malar fat pad, which is repositioned using a suspension suture to the superficial fascia underlying the malar prominence. The surgical technique and results of malar fat pad lift for correction of prominent nasolabial folds were reviewed.

*Technique.*—Facial aging is addressed in a 2-layer, 2-step operation, starting with a superficial musculoaponeurotic system (SMAS)-platysma rotation flap to correct the neck and lower face (Fig 3). Dissection of the malar fat pad begins at the fibers of the orbicularis oculi muscle in the lateral orbital region, anterosuperior to the transverse SMAS suture line. The dissection is carried caudally down to the origin of the zygomaticus muscle, where the malar fat pad becomes thicker (Fig 4). The malar fat pad is carefully dissected free using fingers and scissors. A 4-0 PDS suture is placed from the apex of the fat pad to the underlying SMAS fascia in the area of the malar eminence. Lateral tension is applied to stretch and tighten the superior edge of the fat pad and elevate it over the orbital rim. An appropriate vector perpendicular to the nasolabial crease is created to lift the fat pad and flatten the nasolabial fold. The suspension suture, which provides greater cephalad lift than is possible with skin flap traction alone, holds the fat pad in place until scar adherence. A more laterally directed vector is used for skin flap closure to avoid excessive elevation of the temporal hairline.

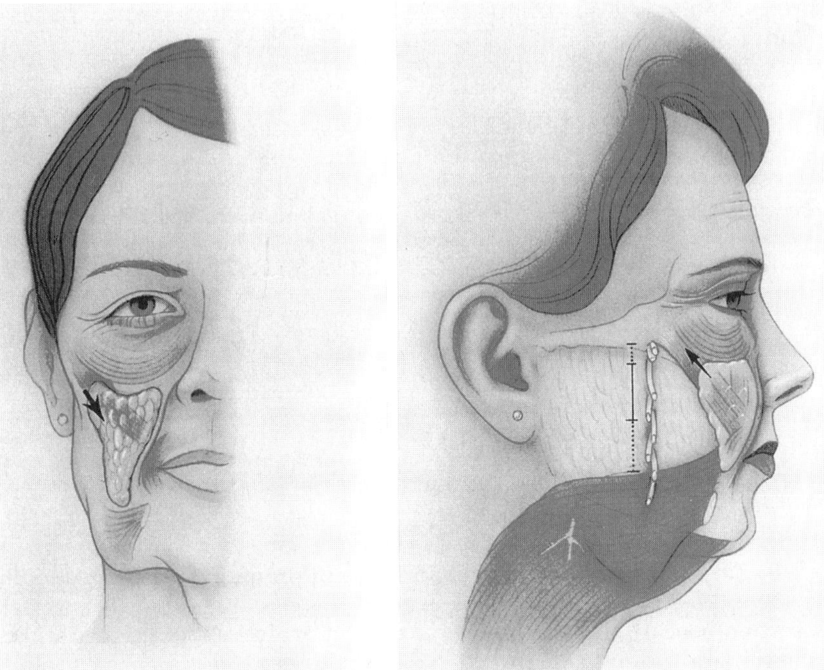

FIGURE 3.—*Left,* with advancing age, the malar fat pad descends further in the midface, and becomes attenuated at its superolateral aspect. The nasolabial fold continues to lengthen and deepen in appearance. *Right,* as the superficial musculoaponeurotic system and masseteric ligaments further lengthen, midmandibular jowls become prominent. The malar fat pad continues to shift anteriorly, with resultant anterior bulging. (Courtesy of Owsley JQ, Fiala TGS: Update: Lifting the malar fat pad for correction of prominent nasolabial folds. *Plast Reconstr Surg* 100:715–722, 1997.)

*Experience.*—Six of 25 patients who underwent elevation of the malar fat pad with suspension suture fixation were studied. All patients were pleased with their results, and believed that the areas of the cheek, neck, and nasolabial crease looked more youthful. They continued to be pleased with the results at 5-year follow-up. Standardized photographs taken at baseline and at 1- and 5-year follow-up were analyzed. The 1-year results showed improvement in all 4 areas evaluated: the upper third of the nasolabial crease, the area of the crease bordering the lip and oral commissure, the area between the commissure and mandibular angle, and the infraorbital area. In 92% of zones, the improvement was maintained at 5 years.

*Discussion.*—For patients seeking rejuvenation of the aging midface, malar fat pad suspension is an effective technique. It can be combined with SMAS-platysma rotation flap for a multivector approach to most of the anatomical changes of facial aging. With careful tensioning and positioning of the suspension suture, this procedure can not only enhance the improvement of intraorbital flattening but also correct prominent nasolabial folds.

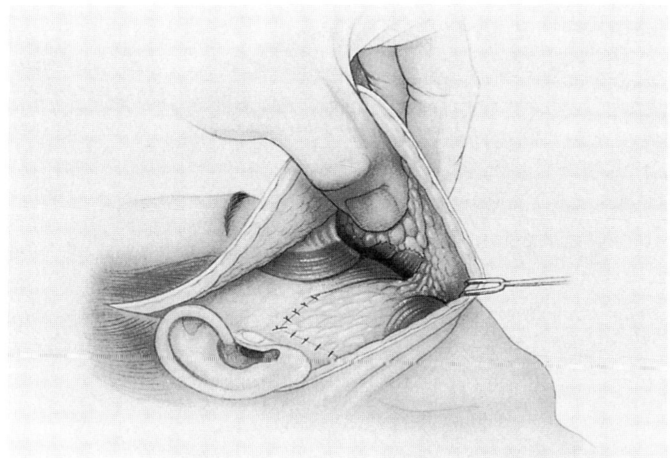

FIGURE 4.—An intraoperative illustration of the malar fat pad dissection. Elevation of the malar fat pad is performed after the correct plane of dissection has been identified immediately superficial to the orbicularis muscle. The zygomaticus and levator muscles are "tented" up. (Courtesy of Owsley JQ, Fiala TGS: Update: Lifting the malar fat pad for correction of prominent nasolabial folds. *Plast Reconstr Surg* 100:715–722, 1997.)

▶ For those who strive to achieve a major improvement in appearance with the facelift, this article will be of interest. As extended or deep-plane face-lifts are more widely used, access to parts of the face that contribute to the aging look is improved. In theory, the sagging fat pad can be a part of the appearance of the aging face—resuspending this structure should achieve a shifting of the ptotic components back superiorly and posteriorly to a more premorbid (read "younger") position. Because the facial nerve is close by, one must know the anatomy cold and, preferably, practice on a cadaver first.

**G.R. Holt, M.D., M.S.E., M.P.H.**

## Camouflaging Techniques and Dermatologic Surgery
Draelos ZD (Wake Forest Univ, Winston-Salem, NC)
*Dermatol Surg* 22:1023–1027, 1996                                                10–7

*Background.*—Dermatologic surgery may result in temporary or permanent cosmetic defects. Basic camouflaging cosmetic techniques can restore patients' self-confidence, allowing them to resume social contact. The principles and techniques of cosmetic camouflaging are discussed.

*Discussion.*—Contour and/or pigmentation defects can result from various dermatologic surgical procedures. Contour defects are areas of hypertrophy or atrophy. Pigmentation defects are the result of color blending from melanin, vascular structures, hemosiderin, and other metabolic byproducts (Table 1). The principles of cosmetic camouflaging are taken from stage makeup texts. For contour defects, the goal is to create the illusion of a flat surface. Dark colors make surfaces appear to recede, and

TABLE 1.—Postsurgical Pigment Alterations

| Pigment Defect | Postsurgical Etiology | Color Correction |
|---|---|---|
| Red | New blood vessel formation, post-laser erythema | Green |
| Blue | Acute hematoma, vascular malformation | Orange |
| Yellow | Resolving hematoma, residual solar elastosis | Purple |
| Hyperpigmentation | Postinflammatory, residual melasma, hemosiderin | White |
| Hypopigmentation, Depigmentation | Postinflammatory, melanocyte destruction | Brown |

(Reprinted by permission of the publisher from Draelos ZD: Camouflaging techniques and dermatologic surgery. *Dermatol Surg* 22:1023–1027, 1996, copyright by Elsevier Science Inc.)

light colors make surfaces appear to project. Recreating appendageal structures is also important, because the unaffected skin surface is not smooth; it is punctuated with terminal and vellus hair shafts, follicular ostia, and eccrine duct structures. Contour camouflaging techniques must aim to artistically recreate a patient's skin surface characteristics.

Changes in pigmentation can be altered by applying an opaque cosmetic that permits none of the abnormal underlying skin tones to be seen and by applying complementary cosmetic colors. The effective use of undercover colored cosmetics relies on an understanding of the artist's color wheel. Complementary colors, the combination of which makes brown, are the colors opposite one another on the color wheel (Table 1). The correct blending of undercover cosmetics permits the patient to continue wearing her usual facial cosmetics. Skin areas with postinflammatory hypopigmentation or depigmentation may be camouflaged by using facial foundations with the appropriate amount of brown pigment. Hyperpigmented areas can be lightened with a white cosmetic under the patient's usual cosmetic foundation.

*Conclusion.*—Erythema resulting from laser resurfacing, dermabrasion, and face peeling can be hidden by cosmetic camouflaging. Permanent scarring may also be managed by such techniques. An understanding of the principles and techniques of cosmetic camouflaging is essential for effective management of such changes in skin appearance.

▶ In both cosmetic and reconstructive surgery of the face, there is often an important need to camouflage the tissue with a cosmetic application that is not detrimental to the tissue or to continued healing. This gives the patient some immediate security regarding appearance, as well as providing a long-term camouflage, if needed. I think this article is a good review of cosmetic camouflage. If you wish to know where to obtain specific products, obtain the full article for the information in Table 2.

**G.R. Holt, M.D., M.S.E., M.P.H.**

**Gender and Racial Variations in Cephalometric Analysis**
Lee JJ, Ramirez SG, Will MJ (Brooke Army Med Ctr, Fort Sam Houston, Tex)
*Otolaryngol Head Neck Surg* 117:326–329, 1997                    10–8

*Background.*—The evaluation of obstructive sleep apnea is complex, and identifying the site of obstruction is key to selecting an appropriate surgical procedure. Cephalometric analysis is used with other examinations to assess craniofacial form and growth. There are established cephalometric skeletal norms for different ethnic populations. However, differences in soft-tissue measurements among different ethnic populations have not been recognized. The current norms for cephalometric analysis are based on white subjects between 18 and 65 years of age. Whether gender and racial differences exist in soft-tissue measurements was investigated.

*Methods.*—A sample of 89 volunteers completed a questionnaire about snoring, constant awakening episodes, daytime somnolence, witnessed apnea, ethnic classification, height, and weight. Volunteers with obstructive sleep apnea were excluded. Dental records were used to confirm the information, obtain cephalometric data, and rule out craniofacial abnormalities. Cephalometric landmarks were analyzed using standard cephalometric measurements of the posterior airway space, sella, nasion, posterior nasal spine, subspinale, supramentale, gnathion, gonion, hyoid, and palate.

*Results.*—Analysis was done in 42 men and 47 women, and in 36 black, 36 white, and 17 Hispanic subjects. The resulting data support the hypothesis of significant differences (1) in the sella-nasion-subspinale angle between black men and white men and between black men and Hispanic men; (2) in the sella-nasion-supramentale angle between black men and white men; (3) in the posterior airway space between white men and women; (4) and in the mandibular plane to hyoid distance between white men and women.

*Discussion.*—These findings indicate that only the sella-nasion-subspinale angle and the sella-nasion-supramentale angle are racially specific. There do not appear to be differences in anatomical measurements among women of different ethnic backgrounds. A separate set of normal values are needed for white women and white men, especially for the posterior airway space and mandibular plane to hyoid bone. These findings need to be confirmed in larger studies.

▶ The authors have given us important information that appeals to common sense—just as we cannot (or should not) apply Anglo facial proportions universally to non-Anglo patients. In my own practice, I try to work with patients to maintain their ethnic-specific features while discussing changing only a few aspects (i.e., broad nasal tip, hump deformity) of their choice. For the evaluation of sleep apnea, the cephalometric data standards appear to be in need of expansion.

**G.R. Holt, M.D., M.S.E., M.P.H.**

### Lateral Crural Strut Graft: Technique and Clinical Applications in Rhinoplasty

Gunter JP, Friedman RM (Univ of Texas, Dallas)
*Plast Reconstr Surg* 99:943–952, 1997

10–9

*Objective.*—Standard correction of the deformed lateral crura has to be tailored to each reconstruction problem. A new versatile technique using the lateral crural strut graft makes it possible to correct the boxy nasal tip, malpositioned lateral crura, alar rim retraction, alar rim collapse, and concave lateral crura.

*Methods.*—Strips of autogenous cartilage sutured to the deep surface of the lateral crura were used to correct crural deformities and deficiencies in 118 patients (Fig 1). Of the 88 patients followed at least 3 months, 33 had primary rhinoplasties and 55 had secondary rhinoplasties. Struts were used from autogenous septal cartilage in 78 patients, from auricular cartilage in 7, and from rib cartilage in 3.

*Technique.*—Using the open rhinoplasty approach, the lateral crura was trimmed, and the vestibular skin was undermined but left attached to the caudal border. Autogenous grafts, 3–4 mm by

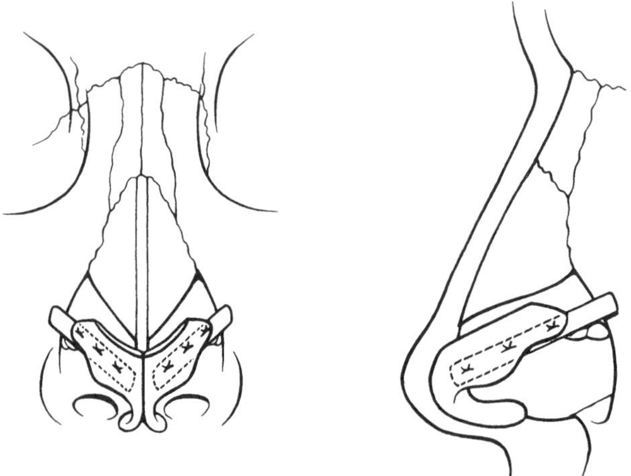

FIGURE 1.—The lateral crural strut graft. The graft is sutured to the deep surface of the lateral crus. (Courtesy of Gunter JP, Friedman RM: Lateral crural strut graft: Technique and clinical applications in rhinoplasty. *Plast Reconstr Surg* 99:943–952, 1997.)

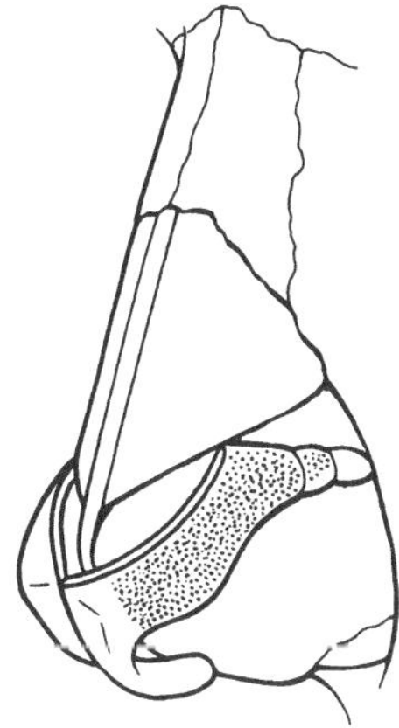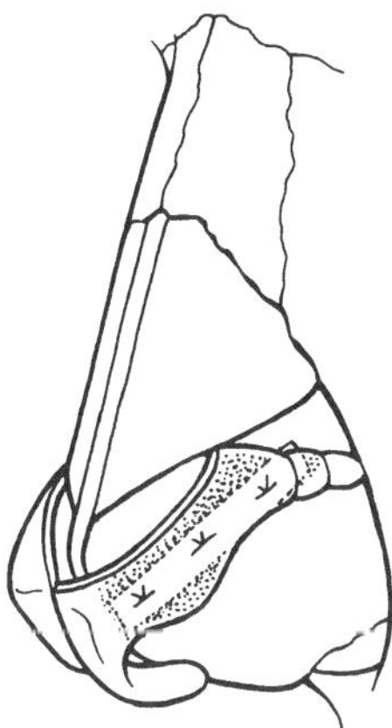

**FIGURE 2.**—*Left,* area of vestibular skin undermining for placement of the lateral crural strut graft. *Right,* relationship of graft to undermined region. (Courtesy of Gunter JP, Friedman RM: Lateral crural strut graft: Technique and clinical applications in rhinoplasty. *Plast Reconstr Surg* 99:943–952, 1997.)

15–25 mm, were secured in the pocket by 2 or 3 Vicryl (5–0) sutures (Fig 2).

*Results.*—The boxy nasal tip can be corrected without infringing the nasal airway. The strut eliminates the parentheses deformity of a malpositioned lateral crura and improves support of the alar rims. The strut allows correction of alar retraction and hanging columella. The graft can be used to correct alar rim collapse by strengthening the alar rim and removing the depression of the alar grooves. Complications included 3 undercorrections and 1 reoperation for nostril asymmetry.

*Conclusion.*—The lateral strut graft can be used to correct a number of problems resulting from the deformed lateral crus.

▶ This interesting technique comes from a master rhinoplastic surgeon and introduces us to still another form of "structural engineering" for problems with the nasal skeleton. Essentially used as an "underlay" graft, the strut can provide support and repositioning for a variety of lower lateral cartilage difficulties, including alar collapse and excessive resection. It is obvious that an open approach for the placement of these grafts is required—even so, the technique appears challenging.

**G.R. Holt, M.D., M.S.E., M.P.H.**

---

**Conservative Subtraction-addition Rhinoplasty**

Younger RAL (Univ of British Columbia, Vancouver, Canada)

*Otolaryngol Head Neck Surg* 117:330–337, 1997                    10–10

---

*Purpose.*—A very common and difficult plastic surgical procedure is realignment of the deviated external and internal nose. The classic approach to this problem is septorhinoplasty; however, a reoperation rate of about 10% has been reported with this approach. A conservative subtraction-addition rhinoplasty (CSAR) approach to the deviated nose was developed and the results in 304 patients were evaluated.

> *Technique.*—The CSAR approach was developed gradually over a 2-year period. Aggressive septal surgery was avoided. Rather, the approach focused on asymmetric turbinate volume reduction to equalize and enhance the airway. Bony and upper lateral work was minimized, using rasping, soft-tissue removal, and/or cartilage grafting techniques to achieve external nasal alignment.

*Results.*—The results of the CSAR approach in 304 patients were analyzed. A total of 1,119 procedures were performed. The most common subtraction procedures were bony rasping of a volume excess area of the upper bony nose and unilateral greenstick medialization of a bone. Free autogenous cartilage grafting into the upper lateral cartilage area was commonly performed. Cases of moderate septal deviation were managed by turbinate volume reduction to decrease airflow resistance on the low flow rate side. Sutures for shape shifting were commonly used for addition to the lower laterals. The most frequent approach to distal septal and columellar deviation was asymmetric soft-tissue subtraction from between the crural feet and nasal spine. With the CSAR approach, the reoperation rate was reduced to 1.3%. Nine patients still had some deviation postoperatively, but only 2 requested further surgery. Further surgery was performed to equalize air flow in 2 patients with airway asymmetry. Just 2 patients had epistaxis requiring additional packing after turbinate volume reduction.

*Conclusions.*—Through the use of both internal and external components, the technique of CSAR for the deviated nose maximizes structural stability and long-term nasal symmetry. The reliable, long-lasting results offered by the CSAR approach represent the state of the art in nasal realignment.

► The author presents a rather significant deviation from the classic approach to the crooked nose, one where indirect (and conservative) changes are made to achieve either the appearance of drastic change or to deceive the observer. Although this approach is too big a leap for me to make without a lot of thought and additional information, there are parts of it that I can understand. Adding cartilage grafts to fill out an external concavity is fine. Some of his proposals are based on suggestions of the past that have worked well. To put it together as he has may herald an entirely new approach to nasal surgery and may be revolutionary in a positive sense.

**G.R. Holt, M.D., M.S.E., M.P.H.**

## CO$_2$ Laser Safety Considerations in Facial Skin Resurfacing

Rohrich RJ, Gyimesi IM, Clark P, et al (Univ of Texas, Dallas)
*Plast Reconstr Surg* 100:1285–1290, 1997                    10–11

*Background.*—Carbon dioxide lasers are being used more frequently in plastic surgery. Laser safety during surgery is essential. Proper understanding of basic laser principles, hands-on training, and experience are needed to use the CO$_2$ laser safely. The energy delivered is controlled by the fixed spot size, high pulsed energy, and rapid scanning of tissue. Manufacturers achieve the appropriate energy delivery by varying these 3 factors. The surgeon must be familiar with the appropriate laser settings for a given procedure to prevent tissue damage.

*Methods.*—Flammability and safety margins were evaluated by subjecting several common objects found in the operative field during facial skin resurfacing to multiple passes of the Coherent 5000 C laser and the Laser Industries (Sharplan) model 150XJ laser Silktouch.

*Results.*—Polyvinyl chloride endotracheal tubes, wet and dry towels, wet and dry gauze sponges, cottonoids, eye protectors, and ophthalmic ointments were tested. The moistened objects were saturated with normal saline and wrung out; these wet objects did not flame or burn. The dry objects produced flame. By the third laser pass, the plastic corneal protectors began to melt and produce substantial heat. The ophthalmic ointments Lacrilube and Bacitracin began to vaporize after 3 laser passes.

*Discussion.*—On the basis of these findings, guidelines should be developed for the safe use of CO$_2$ lasers in facial skin resurfacing and for minimizing fire hazards in the operating room.

▶ I believe this article (and others cited in its references) should be kept in a bound cover in the laser suite for all new personnel to read and commit to memory. The recommendations given to protect the patient and personnel are excellent. With so much at stake in laser injury (vision, airway), there is no such thing as too much preparation.

**G.R. Holt, M.D., M.S.E., M.P.H.**

## Complications and Toxicities of Implantable Biomaterials Used in Facial Reconstructive and Aesthetic Surgery: A Comprehensive Review of the Literature

Rubin JP, Yaremchuk MJ (Harvard Med School, Boston)
*Plast Reconstr Surg* 100:1336–1353, 1997                    10–12

*Introduction.*—Implantable biomaterials are essential to many reconstructive and aesthetic facial procedures. The ideal biomaterial would be cost-effective; inert in body fluids; easily shaped during surgery; maintain its desired form in situ; and be nontoxic, nonantigenic, and noncarcinogenic. No one material can satisfy all these criteria in every situation. The most common implantable biomaterials currently used include metals, polymers, and ceramics.

*Toxicity.*—As implantable devices are in place for long periods in the body, the risk of malignancy is a concern. Clinical observations suggest that the risk of malignancy with either metal or polymer implants is very low. The risk of systemic disease developing over time is also of concern. Corrosion of metal implants will lead to metal ion release within the body. Despite documentation of metal ion spread, no direct association has been made between implant corrosion products and systemic disease. Systemic silicone toxicity has been documented after the injection of large volumes of liquid silicone for breast augmentation. Systemic toxicity has also been reported for the polymer, methylmethacrylate, during insertion of hip prostheses. No systemic toxicity has been reported with its use in craniofacial surgery. Cell-mediated hypersensitivity is an uncommon patient reaction, which can result in pain, bone nonunion, and dermatitis. Sensitivity can be confirmed by patch testing. Removal of the implant results in symptom resolution. Although hypersensitivity reactions to prefabricated polymer implants are extremely rare, the free monomer of methylmethacrylate can cause asthmatic reactions in operating room staff during procedures. The implant site itself affects morbidity. The chin and malar regions have the lowest complication rate, whereas the nose and ear have the highest complication rate. Surgical technique can also play a role in morbidity.

*Conclusions.*—Implantable biomaterials, such as metals, polymers, and ceramics, have become an important part of plastic surgery of the face. These materials are associated with a very low incidence of cancer, systemic disease, and hypersensitivity. Although all these implantable materials are successful in some applications, there is not one material that is ideal for all applications. Both implant site and surgical technique play a role in implant morbidity. Implantable device design must take into account the specifications and limitations of materials for specific sites of implantation to optimize results.

▶ The field of biomaterials and implants is expansive and complicated, even for one with an engineering background. Also, the technology advances very quickly. This article should be a basic reference for all those interested in biomaterials and facial implants (245 references!) and could be an introduction on the subject to medical students and residents. It is basic, but simple, with respect to materials theory at the molecular level, but good with clinical applications.

**G.R. Holt, M.D., M.S.E., M.P.H.**

**Clinical and Histologic Response of Subcutaneous Expanded Polytetrafluoroethylene (Gore-Tex) and Porous High-density Polyethylene (Medpor) Implants to Acute and Early Infection**
Sclafani AP, Thomas JR, Cox AJ, et al (St Louis Univ)
*Arch Otolaryngol Head Neck Surg* 123:328–336, 1997                    10–13

*Introduction.*—Several new synthetic materials are available for use in facial surgery. Host tissue response to the new implants is of particular interest. Porous implants, such as expanded polytetrafluoroethylene (e-PTFE, Gore-Tex), porous high-density polyethylene (PHDPE, Medpor), and calcium hydroxyapatite have recently been introduced. These implants allow soft tissue and bone ingrowth into the implant to varying degrees and provide stability to the implant, thus allowing the implant to act more like host tissue. The response of subcutaneously implanted e-PTFE and PHDPE to experimental infection in rats was examined in the acute and early postimplantation periods. Clinical and histologic findings are described.

*Methods.*—An 8-mm diameter, 1-mm-thick implant of either e-PTFE or PHDPE was placed in a subcutaneous pocket over the dorsum of 28 adult male Sprague-Dawley rats weighing 200–250 g. An inoculum of $10^9$ colony-forming units of *Staphylococcus aureus* was injected transcutaneously directly over each implant at either the time of implantation or 14 days later. Animals were observed for 7 days before being killed. The implants were harvested and analyzed with conventional light and scanning electron microscopy. The degree of capsule reaction, infection, inflammation, and implant degradation was assessed.

*Results.*—Clinical infection was more likely in implants inoculated at the time of implantation in both e-PTFE and PHDPE implants (5 of 5 for each group). Among implants inoculated 14 days after implantation, PHDPE implants were less likely to become infected than e-PTFE implants were (1 of 4 vs. 3 of 4). The e-PTFE implants inoculated at 14 days were significantly less likely to become infected than were PHDPE implants inoculated immediately after implantation (25% vs. 100%). There was a histologic correlation between resistance to infection and increasing fibrovascular ingrowth into the PHDPE implants. The inoculated PHDPE implant had little to no ingrowth, compared with PHDPE control implants. Early fibrovascular ingrowth into the peripheral pores of the implant was observed in the uninfected e-PTFE implant.

*Conclusion.*—The PHDPE implant promoted faster fibrovascular ingrowth than the e-PTFE implant because of its greater pore size. Vascularized host tissue in and around the implant allows stability and resistance to experimentally induced infection. Conservative management of clinical implant infections may be all that is needed if bacterial seeding occurs after adequate fibrovascular ingrowth occurs. e-PTFE and future alloplast designs should provide pore sizes that will promote invasion of the implant by the host tissue.

▶ The authors present excellent photomicrographs of their experimental findings. It has previously been shown that increased pore size facilitates ingrowth of fibrovascular tissue, which is important for stabilization of the implant and long-term bioacceptance. The authors highlight an additional benefit of the enhanced vascular-implant interface, namely, an enhanced resistance to infection. The e-PTFE soft tissue implants have rather small diameter pore size currently, and perhaps this needs to be revisited by their materials engineers. It's still an excellent implant, however.

**G.R. Holt, M.D., M.S.E., M.P.H.**

**Histologic Effects of the High-energy Pulsed $CO_2$ Laser on Photoaged Facial Skin**
Stuzin JM, Baker TJ, Baker TM, et al (Univ of Miami, Fla; Univ of Pennsylvania)
*Plast Reconstr Surg* 99:2036–2050, 1997                                    10–14

*Introduction.*—With an aging population that increasingly seeks interventions to improve the appearance of photoaged skin, physicians are pursuing resurfacing techniques that improve skin surface texture and roughness and are observing the histologic changes that accompany these improvements. The gold standard for long-standing amelioration of photodamaged facial skin continues to be the deep phenol peel, but its limitations and hazards make it a less popular choice than laser resurfacing among physicians. The appeal of the laser approach is that striking histologic changes occur only in the epidermis and dermis. A comprehensive histologic analysis of the structural changes induced by $CO_2$ laser resurfacing was conducted in patients with photodamaged skin.

*Findings.*—Laser test sites were biopsied in photodamaged skin in conjunction with performing a face lift. Five patients with severe photodamaged skin underwent bilateral resurfacing of the preauricular region using varying pulse energies and number of passes. Histologic examination of these biopsy specimens indicated a dose-dependent depth of laser injury. Increasing pulse injury resulted in a deeper wound, and increasing the number of passes similarly caused a larger band of necrosis.

Ten patients with photodamaged skin underwent resurfacing of the preauricular region at 15 days to 6 months before rhytidectomy. When the laser-resurfaced spot was compared with adjacent untreated photodamaged skin, epidermal atrophy and atypia were eliminated in laser-treated skin and regeneration of epithelium was seen. Melanocytic hypertrophy and hyperplasia were corrected after treatment, and density and function of epidermal melanocytes seemed normal. Treated specimens showed substantial new collagen formation that involved both the superficial and middermis. All treated specimens had advanced dermal damage; glycosaminoglycans were greatly increased and filled spaces where collagen had been destroyed. Collagenolysis was observed to be proportional to the degree of elastosis and glycosaminoglycans. Solar elastosis produced masses of thickened, curled, and hypertrophied abnormal elastic tissue occupying the deep and superficial dermis.

Laser resurfacing in 3 black patients produced aesthetically satisfactory results. All 3 patients had reepithelialization within 7 to 10 days that was pinkish and lighter than untreated skin. The resurfaced area returned to its normal color within 4 months. Biopsy of test sites showed histologic effects similar to those observed in white patients who underwent laser resurfacing. Complete repopulation of epidermal melanocytes was observed in biopsy specimens of black patients obtained 3 months after laser treatment.

*Conclusion.*—The histologic effects of laser resurfacing correspond to those observed for phenol peel in regard to the amelioration of photodamaged skin. Where these two approaches differ is in their effect on epidermal melanocytes, which seem to function normally after laser resurfacing.

▶ It is important to have well-planned and well-executed scientific studies to determine the true histologic effects and safety parameters with laser resurfacing. Although this study size is small, their data indicates safety to photodamaged skin treated with laser without apparent deleterious effects. However, it clearly is possible to injure the skin with the laser if inappropriate settings are used or the number of passes is excessive. Concomitantly, phenol peels can be dangerous as well. At least the laser has not been shown to cause cardiovascular irritability and liver damage, like phenol, when used excessively over a large region in a short period of time.

**G.R. Holt, M.D., M.S.E., M.P.H.**

---

**A Critical Appraisal of High-energy Pulsed Carbon Dioxide Laser Facial Resurfacing for Acne Scars**
Apfelberg DB (Atherton Plastic Surgery Ctr, Calif)
*Ann Plast Surg* 38:95–100, 1997                                                10–15

---

*Introduction.*—Laser resurfacing has yielded excellent results in treatment of rhytids and photoaging in several patient series. Few reports describe the use of laser for acne treatment. Reported are treatment outcomes in 13 patients with residual acne scars of the face.

*Methods.*—The average age of 11 female and 2 male patients was 38.5 years, and average follow-up was 7.18 months. Of 13 patients, 5 had severe acne with marked irregularity, soft-tissue defects and atrophy, and "cobblestoning," and 8 patients had more minor acne with more superficial irregularity, blotchy pigmentation, and occasional or scattered deeper pits or pocks. Nine patients underwent full-face laser resurfacing, and 4 patients received regional treatment only. All patients were pretreated with Retin-A.

*Results.*—Healing averaged 7.3 days. Erythema disappeared at an average of 7.6 weeks (2–11 weeks). Of 8 patients with mild acne, 1 had good results and 7 had excellent results. In the 5 patients with severe acne, 2 patients had fair results and 2 had good results; 1 was lost to follow-up.

*Conclusion.*—Laser resurfacing produced only moderate results in patients with severe atrophic acne and excellent results in patients with mild acne.

▶ Several modalities of skin treatment can improve mild acne scars, including chemical peel and dermabrasion, at a fraction of the cost of laser resurfacing. The real heartbreak for the practitioner, however, is seen in those patients with severe acne, where the scars are so deep, and the skin so atrophic, that one has a desire to totally excise the affected facial area and recover it with expanded skin. The pulsed $CO_2$ laser as utilized in this project may give some satisfactory results for a bad problem. If further testing reveals the optimal parameters and intervals between treatments, it may afford some improvement for that unfortunate patient with severe acne.

**G.R. Holt, M.D., M.S.E., M.P.H.**

## Secondary Healing of Mohs Defects of the Forehead, Temple, and Lower Eyelid

Deutsch BD, Becker FF (Eastern Virginia School of Medicine, Norfolk; Facial Plastic Surgery Ctr, Vero Beach, Fla; Univ of Florida, Gainesville)
*Arch Otolaryngol Head Neck Surg* 123:529–534, 1997                    10–16

*Objective.*—Healing by secondary intention of Mohs defects is an option rarely chosen by facial plastic surgeons. An analysis of Mohs defects of the forehead, temple, and lower eyelid that were allowed to heal by secondary intention over a 4-year period are presented.

*Methods.*—Mohs resections between January 1, 1989, and December 31, 1993, allowed to heal by secondary intention in 1 practice included 15 of 22 forehead, 13 of 17 temple, and 10 of 28 lower eyelid resections. Ten forehead, 6 temple, and 10 lower eyelid wounds were available for follow-up. Wound color, contour, distortion of surrounding structures, presence of telangiectasia or paresthesias, pain or infection during healing, and overall cosmetic result were rated as poor (0), fair (1), good (2), or excellent (3).

*Results.*—Patients with forehead wounds rated color match with surrounding skin as 2.2, texture and contour 2.2, overall cosmetic effect 2.4. One of 8 patients reported paresthesia, and 1 wanted scar revision. Physicians rated color, contour, and cosmetic effect as 1, 1.3, and 1.4, respectively. Nine patients had telangiectasis, and 1 had distortion of an adjacent structure. Patients with temple wounds rated scar color, texture, and contour, and cosmetic effect as 2.5, 2.7, and 2.7. Physicians rated color, contour, and cosmetic effect as 1, 1.4, and 1.4. Four of 6 patients had telangiectasis, and 2 of 6 had distortion of the temporal hairline. Patients with lower eyelid wounds rated scar color, texture, and cosmetic effect as 2.7, 3, and 3, respectively. One patient reported pain. Physicians rated color, contour, and cosmetic effect as 2.6, 2.5, and 2.4, respectively. One patient had telangiectasis, and 5 had mild notching.

*Conclusion.*—Secondary healing produced satisfactory results. Patients not wanting another procedure, who are poor surgical candidates, or who do not wish to incur added hospitalization costs are candidates for this technique.

▶ The authors provide evidence, based on objective analyses of actual cases, that secondary healing of Mohs defects can be quite acceptable in certain regions of the face. The main problem is telangiectasia, which is probably due to neoangiogenesis, induced by the healing wound. Revision of unacceptable scars can be carried out in time, if needed. Patients do need to understand the prolonged wound care requirements and must be patient while they wait for the final resort. This report notwithstanding, I am personally indebted to the senior author for his expert excision and primary closure of a forehead skin malignancy which looks quite good in its early healing!

**G.R. Holt, M.D., M.S.E., M.P.H.**

---

**The Liposhaver in Facial Plastic Surgery**
Becker DG, Weinberger MS, Miller PJ, et al (Tardy Facial Plastic Surgery Inst, Chicago; Oregon Health Sciences Univ, Portland; Univ of Virginia, Charlottesville)
*Arch Otolaryngol Head Neck Surg* 122:1161–1167, 1996                    10–17

---

*Introduction.*—The various modifications of the original blunt liposuction cannulas have all retained the basic avulsion principle as the method of fat extraction. With soft-tissue shaving cannulas, fat removal is more precise and less traumatic. The results of use of the liposhaver in cosmetic facial surgery were reported for 19 patients who participated in a multicenter clinical trial of the device.

*Methods.*—A nonrandomized, nonblinded evaluation of the liposhaver was undertaken in patients having submental lipectomy, facelift with need for defatting beneath the facelift flap, and/or correction of deep nasolabial folds. The liposhaver was designed to cut fat preferentially but to be less efficient at cutting adjacent muscle and other soft tissue. Within the blunt, outer cannula of this instrument lies a recessed oscillating blade that precisely cuts and extracts tissue as it is gently suctioned through the side port of the cannula. Surgeons at 3 centers reported details of each procedure and evaluated outcome. Preoperative and postoperative photographs were obtained.

*Results.*—The procedures were performed between August 1994 and April 1996. In all cases, the liposhaver was used successfully, and patients achieved the desired contour and profile results without any dimpling or asymmetry. There were no facial nerve injuries, and no hematomas developed in the immediate postoperative period. All surgeons believed that the liposhaver was a precise, minimally traumatic, and efficient method of lipectomy. Some surgeons were able to rely on direct visualization to avoid cutting soft tissue other than fat, whereas others initially used precise surgical technique and knowledge of anatomy without direct visualization.

*Discussion.*—The liposhaver offers several advantages compared with conventional liposuction. Fat is removed precisely in a minimally traumatic manner, without potentially bruising back-and-forth motion. There is the potential, however, for injury to vital nerves or vessels in the head and neck area when the device is used in the power mode without direct visualization.

▶ The authors are a team of excellent teachers and surgeons who have given us advice relative to the use of the liposhaver. Their experience has demonstrated its efficacy in debulking fatty regions of the face. They recommend using the power liposhaving mode only under direct visualization so that nonadipose tissues are not damaged. Their very low complication rate underscores the strength of their findings.

**G.R. Holt, M.D., M.S.E., M.P.H.**

# 11 Larynx and Airway

**Pediatric Flexible Fiberoptic Bronchoscopy Through the Laryngeal Mask Airway**
Tunkel DE, Fisher QA (Johns Hopkins Univ, Baltimore, Md)
*Arch Otolaryngol Head Neck Surg* 122:1364–1367, 1996                    11–1

*Introduction.*—In the evaluation of pediatric laryngeal and tracheobronchial disorders, fiberoptic bronchoscopy has been used more frequently. An alternative to the face mask and the endotracheal tube for airway support during general anesthesia is the laryngeal mask airway. To facilitate fiberoptic bronchoscopy in children, the laryngeal mask airway has been used. The usefulness and safety of the laryngeal mask airway as an adjunct to pediatric flexible fiberoptic bronchoscopy were determined.

*Methods.*—The charts of 17 patients, aged 3 months to 18 years, who had fiberoptic bronchoscopy with the use of laryngeal mask airway were retrospectively reviewed. The patients had general anesthesia for the fiberoptic bronchoscopy, with the laryngeal mask airway used to support the airway. The analysis included the number and type of complications, and the ability to perform airway evaluation with fiberoptic bronchoscopy and the laryngeal mask airway.

*Results.*—The use of the laryngeal mask airway failed in 2 patients—1 who could not have the laryngeal mask airway appropriately placed, and another who had airway obstruction with the laryngeal mask airway in place, which required intubation. Uncomplicated fiberoptic bronchoscopy through the laryngeal mask airway was performed in 15 patients, none of whom required unplanned endotracheal intubation. When the glottis could not be visualized at direct laryngoscopy, 2 patients with mandibular hypoplasia required laryngeal mask airway use for airway evaluation.

*Conclusions.*—As an adjunct to pediatric flexible fiberoptic bronchoscopy, the laryngeal mask airway can be used safely and effectively. Use of the laryngeal mask airway for flexible fiberoptic bronchoscopy allows the airway to be evaluated during spontaneous ventilation without an endotracheal tube or a face mask. Compared with pediatric flexible fiberoptic bronchoscopy performed through the nose or through an endotracheal tube, larger fiberoptic scopes can be used through the laryngeal mask airway.

▶ The authors report their comfort with using the laryngeal mask airway for diagnostic fiberoptic pediatric bronchoscopy. The decision to use the mask should be made between the otolaryngologist and the anesthesiologist— both should feel comfortable with the decision. Practice using the mask and scope is highly recommended (even on a mannequin) before trying the first patient. Intubation equipment and a rigid scope should be at the table, if needed. I don't believe this is the preferred method for approaching a known airway foreign body, however.

**G.R. Holt, M.D., M.S.E., M.P.H.**

**Laryngeal Biomechanics of the Singing Voice**
Koufman JA, Radomski TA, Joharji GM, et al (Wake Forest Univ, Winston-Salem, NC)
*Otolaryngol Head Neck Surg* 115:527–537, 1996                    11–2

*Introduction.*—Biomechanical analysis of athletic performance is accomplished by linking a videosystem to a computer system to evaluate movement critically. This technology allows patterns to be identified that are optimally efficient or maladaptive. Laryngeal biomechanics were studied to determine normal laryngeal biomechanics of healthy singers and to analyze sex, vocal training, and singing style that may influence laryngeal biomechanics.

*Methods.*—A total of 100 healthy singers were studied by transnasal fiberoptic laryngoscopy to assess patterns of laryngeal tension during normal singing and to determine whether sex, style of singing, or occupation influence laryngeal muscle tension. There were 61 female singers and 39 male singers, of whom 52 were amateurs and 48 were professional singers. A "blinded" otolaryngologist analyzed the study of volunteers performing standardized and nonstandardized singing tasks, which were recorded on a laser disk and then analyzed in a frame-by-frame fashion. Grades for muscle tension were assigned to each vocal task, and computations were made of objective muscle tension scores.

*Results.*—In female professional singers, the lowest muscle tension scores were seen, while amateur female singers had the highest muscle tension scores. Intermediate muscle tension scores were seen in professional and amateur male singers. Lower muscle tension scores were seen in classical singers when compared with nonclassical singers. Choral music produces the lowest muscle tension scores (41%), followed by art songs (47%) and opera (57%). Rock/gospel produced the highest muscle tension scores (94%), followed by bluegrass/country and western (86%), musical theater (74%), and jazz/pop (65%).

*Conclusions.*—Muscle tension scores were not influenced by alcohol use, tobacco use, prior vocal problems, and regular exercise. Significantly higher muscle tension scores were seen among black singers than white singers. Significantly higher muscle tension scores were seen in singers with vocal nodules compared with those who did not.

▶ I found this study both enlightening and educational. Although we know it really isn't true, it is commonly held that professional singers are supposed to utilize the best vocal habits possible. However, as the performer strays further away from classical singing (and training), it appears that the muscle tension dysfunctions increase. Even classical singers are not immune from misuse, but it may not affect them as much, or they are careful to misuse only occasionally. I wonder where all of those little girls who sang the role of "Annie" on Broadway would fall?

**G.R. Holt, M.D., M.S.E., M.P.H.**

---

**Analysis of Voice Outcomes in Pediatric Patients Following Surgical Procedures for Laryngotracheal Stenosis**
Clary RA, Pengilly A, Bailey M, et al (Great Ormond Street Hosp for Children, London; Royal Free Hosp, London; Charing Cross Hosp, London)
*Arch Otolaryngol Head Neck Surg* 122:1189–1194, 1996          11–3

---

*Introduction.*—The routine use of a tracheostomy has been replaced by various open procedures that augment the existing airway for pediatric subglottic stenosis. Even after these procedures, however, many studies show that a substantial proportion of children still have significantly impaired voice function. The long-term voice function was assessed in children at least 2 years after an airway augmentation procedure. Preoperative risk factors that identify children most likely to have voice problems were also assessed.

*Methods.*—Families of 33 patients who had augmentation procedures for laryngotracheal stenosis were contacted by mail and completed home questionnaires. A comprehensive hospital-based voice assessment was conducted on the 33 patients, and 28 had fiberoptic endoscopy performed. The Vocal Profile Analysis protocol was used by 3 speech and language therapists to assess perceptual voice from taped samples. Three otolaryngologists performed fiberoptic laryngeal endoscopy. Patients were assessed for the degree of stenosis, coexisting laryngeal lesions, and type of surgical procedure performed.

*Results.*—Normal voices were found in 8 of 33 children, as assessed by the Vocal Profile Analysis scheme. Abnormalities were found in the remaining 25 children, including harshness (52%), whisper (36%), ventricular band phonation (21%), continuity (27%), mean pitch (27%), and falsetto voice (12%). Three of 25 larynges were judged to be anatomically normal by endoscopy. The other patients had the following abnormalities: altered vocal fold mobility (42%), abnormal subglottis (38%), supraglottic vibration (31%), and anterior commissure blunting (31%). Ventricular band phonation type corresponded with supraglottic vibration, which was seen in children with glottic insufficiency. After surgical procedures were performed, 12% of parents indicated that deterioration of voice and dissatisfaction with voice function occurred.

*Conclusions.*—Chronic voice and endoscopic abnormalities have been demonstrated in a substantial proportion of children who had laryngotracheal surgical procedures for stenosis. In the pediatric population, the effects of pre-existing laryngeal abnormalities and these surgical procedures on the voice continue to be difficult to establish. For optimal voice function, speech and language therapists must carefully manage these children. Voice outcome may be predicted by the etiology and severity of the stenosis, as well as the history of surgical procedures. Poorer voice function was associated with stenoses that were acquired rather than those that were congenital. Stenosis that required more than 1 operation had a lower success rate in providing acceptable voices.

▶ I am sure that the surgeons who perform laryngotracheoplasty for stenosis are concerned about the voice quality and capability of these young patients, although the airway is of primary concern. We all know how vocal malfunctions can occur in individuals even after a case of laryngitis, so it is not hard to see that these children who undergo long-term cannulation and perhaps multiple airway procedures, will have a high likelihood of vocal dysfunction. I don't see how it could be otherwise. A team approach to these children is important, as they will require not only long-term speech therapy, but, also, educational guidance and psychosocial support as they grow.

**G.R. Holt, M.D., M.S.E., M.P.H.**

## Botulinum Neurotoxin Injection After Total Laryngectomy

Hoffman HT, Fischer H, VanDenmark D, et al (Univ of Iowa, Iowa City)
*Head Neck* 19:92–97, 1997                                                                11–4

*Background.*—Disturbance in the relaxation of the pharyngoesophageal (PE) segment is one cause of tracheoesophageal puncture (TEP) speech failure after total laryngectomy. The use of chemical denervation of the PE segment by botulinum neurotoxin injection to improve TEP speech was described.

*Methods.*—Eight patients received botulinum neurotoxin injections for TEP speech problems after total laryngectomy at 1 center between 1991 and 1994. Outcomes were analyzed prospectively by 1 speech pathologist. Outcomes were determined subjectively in all patients. In 6, pressure readings at the tracheostoma site during speech were recorded.

*Findings.*—Botulinum neurotoxin injection improved TEP speech in 7 of the 8 patients. Five of these 7 patients had substantial improvement in their speech, including 3 patients who had been completely unable to speak before the injection (Figs 2 and 4).

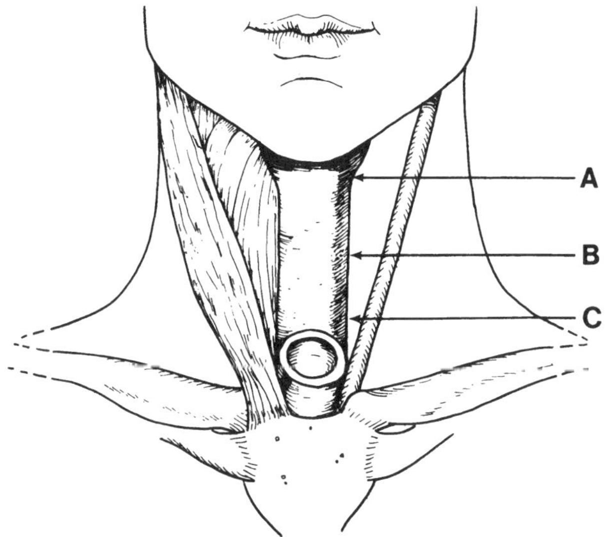


**FIGURE 2.**—Injection sites located: **A,** junction between the middle constrictor and the base of the tongue. **B,** mid-portion of the pharyngoesophageal segment midway between **A** and **C. C,** lower pharyngoesophageal segment adjacent to the tracheostome. (Courtesy of Hoffman HT, Fischer H, VanDenmark D, et al: Botulinum neurotoxin injection after total laryngectomy. *Head Neck* 19:92–97, 1997. Reprinted by permission of John Wiley & Sons, Inc.)

*Conclusion.*—Botulinum neurotoxin injection is a safe, effective technique for improving TEP speech in selected patients with disturbed relaxation of the PE. The positive responses to chemical denervation of the PE segment observed in this study support the notion that increased PE tone

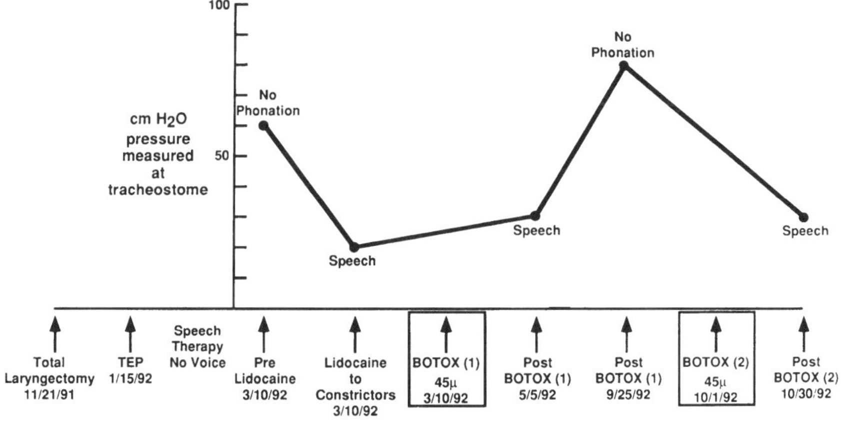


**FIGURE 4.**—Clinical course of patient 6 demonstrating the results of pressure generated at the tracheostome following interventions to improve tracheoesophageal puncture *(TEP)* speech. Botox is a brand name for botulinum toxin type A. (Courtesy of Hoffman HT, Fischer H, VanDenmark D, et al: Botulinum neurotoxin injection after total laryngectomy. *Head Neck* 19:92–97, 1997. Reprinted by permission of John Wiley & Sons, Inc.)

or a disorder in the relaxation of this segment can interfere with TEP speech.

▶ As more otolaryngologists become familiar with the use of botulinum toxin type A (Botox) and their comfort index rises, we will see more widespread use in clinical applications such as described in this Iowa study. Botox is not a "magical" medication, and when its appropriate use and dosage are identified, along with the capability to inject with or without electromyographic control, it can be used like other medications at our disposal. Obviously, care must be taken, as shown by the authors' gradual increase in initial dosage over time, but its application for improving tracheoesophageal speech is commendable.

**G.R. Holt, M.D., M.S.E., M.P.H.**

---

**Navigational Aids for Real-time Virtual Bronchoscopy**
Summers RM (NIH, Bethesda, Md)
*AJR* 168:1165–1170, 1997                                              11–5

---

*Introduction.*—Volume acquisition technology (CT and MRI), combined with computer graphics hardware and software, have made virtual endoscopy (VE) possible. This noninvasive medical imaging technique provides a three-dimensional (3D) data set of a part of the body that can be visualized from an internal perspective to simulate an endoscopic procedure. Virtual endoscopy has resolution of ≤1 mm; thus fine detail can be detected. It is easy to lose anatomic orientation with this approach with the lack of visual cues. A number of software navigational aids have been designed to help the endoscopist who wants to use VE images for medical diagnosis.

*Methods.*—Seven software tools were used to create virtual bronchoscopy (VB) images in 21 patients with suspected endobronchial or cavitary lung disease: co-ordinate axes, global maps, trail markers, cross-references to standard two-dimensional projections, rearview windows, collision avoidance, and stereoscopic displays. The computer program produced a 3D surface-rendered model of the desired anatomic structure; then an isosurface algorithm was used to produce a surface at a set threshold at the boundary between the detected lumen and the adjacent undetected border voxels ("wall" of the structure).

*Results.*—The navigational aids provided satisfactory views for VB in the 21 patients evaluated. It was possible to attain a frame rate of 1 to 7 frames per second, depending on the complexity of the bronchial model. Several of the navigational aids worked best when used selectively or when updated frequently, but not continuously. It was helpful to have several navigational aids, because no one method worked well for all circumstances.

*Conclusion.*—Navigational aids are potentially useful in VB studies. With the development of more robust software to create the VE model, navigational aids may make it possible for VE to become more user friendly and a more widely applicable tool for clinical radiologists.

▶ I found this article very fascinating. To have the capability of virtual imaging of the lower airway from CT data is mind-boggling. With further refinements in the future, it may well be possible to diagnose a foreign body (without the need for a flexible bronchoscopy) and plan the correct forceps for extraction preoperatively. Or the presence of an obstructive mucous plug vs. an intrabronchial tumor might be confirmed. While it clearly lacks therapeutic capabilities, it could provide the endoscopist with valuable information in a spatial orientation with which we are all familiar.

**G.R. Holt, M.D., M.S.E., M.P.H.**

## Laryngeal Adjustment in Whispering: Magnetic Resonance Imaging Study

Tsunoda K, Ohta Y, Soda Y, et al (Nissan Tamagawa Hosp, Japan; Hitachi Gen Hosp, Ibaragi, Japan; Univ of Tokyo; et al)
*Ann Otol Rhinol Laryngol* 106:41–43, 1997                    11–6

*Background.*—During whispering, the glottis is kept open to prevent vocal fold vibration, and the supraglottal structures are constricted. The exact contour of the laryngeal lumen in the frontal dimension during the production of whispering is not known. The nature of the laryngeal adjustment of the contour of the laryngeal lumen during whispering, especially the role of supraglottal contriction, was further investigated.

*Methods and Findings.*—Magnetic resonance imaging was used to examine laryngeal adjustment during whispering. During normal whispering and stage whispering, the laryngeal ventricle appeared to be narrowed, and the supraglottal structures (in particular, the false vocal folds) were shifted downward, impinging on the vocal folds. In both modes of whispering, the glottal closure appeared incomplete, and a clear glottal chink was evident at the level of the vocal folds.

*Conclusion.*—During whispering, the supraglottal structures are not only constricted but are shifted downward, attaching to the vocal fold to prevent vocal fold vibration completely. Suppression of vocal fold vibration therefore appears to be the underlying mechanism during whispering.

▶ Although this was a small study, it introduced some interesting clinical concepts for consideration. Whereas prolonged whispering is likely a maladaption for the larynx because of the high constrictive forces involved, can short-term whispering (say, after microlaryngeal surgery) be beneficial in resting the true vocal cords? This is an interesting concept because of the "braking" effect whispering has on true vocal fold vibration, which might be helpful to healing mucosa. Additionally, it seems to me that prolonged whispering is a close cousin to plicae dysphonia ventricularis, and further study of the former might lead to new treatment options for the latter.

**G.R. Holt, M.D., M.S.E., M.P.H.**

---

**MRI Evaluation of Vocal Fold Paralysis Before and After Type I Thyroplasty**
Bryant NJ, Gracco C, Sasaki CT, et al (Yale Univ, New Haven, Conn; Haskins Labs, New Haven, Conn)
*Laryngoscope* 106:1386–1392, 1996                                     11–7

---

*Background.*—Magnetic resonance imaging is useful in the 3-dimensional assessment of laryngeal anatomy. The findings of MRI in patients with vocal fold paralysis before and after type I thyroplasty are presented.

*Methods.*—Three men and 1 woman with vocal fold paralysis underwent MRI before and after thyroplasty. Videoendoscopic and acoustic measurements were also documented. Implant location was assessed by 3-dimensional descriptive parameters, and the success of the procedure was established by vocal and endoscopic assessment. The MR images of 2 patients with satisfactory outcomes were compared with the images and vocal analysis of the other 2 patients, whose results were unsatisfactory.

*Findings.*—Magnetic resonance imaging was useful for determining implant location after type I thyroplasty. It provided additional information to that provided by standard videoendoscopic and acoustic measures. In 2 patients, preoperative MR images were affected by severe artifact, which made 3-dimensional description impossible. Vocal fold height, length, and medial/lateral displacement could not be assessed on phonation or during resting. However, the implant was clearly seen on MR images in all patients. In the 2 patients with satisfactory outcomes, MR images showed an implant position somewhat superior, suggesting that such placement may affect vocal outcome less adversely than placement that is excessively anterior or medial. In 1 patient, anterior implant placement was observed to dampen anterior vocal cord vibration, increasing the mass and stiffness of the segment.

*Conclusion.*—Magnetic resonance imaging can provide useful information on implant location in patients with unsatisfactory outcomes after type I thyroplasty. However, MRI does not replace videostroboscopy. The latter demonstrates closure patterns and mucosal vibration not shown on MRI and can correlate with acoustic analysis. Thus, MRI should be seen as a valuable adjunct to endoscopic and acoustic assessment in planning for revision surgery.

▶ In the past, it seemed reasonable to me that any study of implant placement in the larynx should utilize MRI as a research component. The authors show us that the MRI can also be a good tool for the clinical evaluation of results in either a dissatisfied patient or one in which the vocal results are not optimal or as expected by the physician. What I do not yet see in the literature are studies that detail the results of repositioning of the implant or secondary implantation in an attempt to improve the results. We revise ("fine tune") other implants, so why not laryngeal implants?

**G.R. Holt, M.D., M.S.E., M.P.H.**

### Ideal Timing of Pediatric Laryngotracheal Reconstruction

Zalzal GH, Choi SS, Patel KM (Georgetown Washington Univ, Washington, DC)

*Arch Otolaryngol Head Neck Surg* 123:206–208, 1997                    11–8

*Background.*—The initial treatment of laryngotracheal stenosis and airway compromise not amenable to cricoid split in infants and young children is the placement of a tracheotomy tube. A definitive laryngotracheal reconstruction (LTR) is planned for when the child is older and the laryngotracheal stenosis is mature. The timing of pediatric LTR is important, because high morbidity and mortality are still associated with tracheotomy in children and because the speech and language development of children with tracheotomy tubes is greatly debated. The best age for performing LTR was investigated.

*Methods.*—Forty-eight infants and children, aged 48 months or younger, with laryngeal stenosis were included in the study. The children underwent a total of 50 LTRs. Twenty-two patients (group 1) were 8 to 24 months of age at the time of LTR, and 26 patients (group 2) were 25 to 48 months of age at LTR.

*Findings.*—The degree of laryngotracheal stenosis was more severe in the children in group 2, as determined by the duration of stenting. There was no difference in multiple sites of stenosis or type of repair needed to correct the laryngotracheal stenosis. Decannulation was more likely to be successful in the children in group 2.

*Conclusion.*—Performing LTR before the patient is 25 months of age is important for speech and language development and for eliminating the morbidity and mortality associated with tracheotomy. However, the risk of failure is higher in children undergoing LTR at a younger age, despite a lesser degree of abnormality.

▶ The authors warn us that there is a price to be paid for early LTR to enable speech development: a higher failure rate and more revision surgeries. Obviously, each patient's care must be individualized, and there must be full and open discussion with the parents regarding both sides of the issue. As there is no "right" answer to the timing, the parents must share in the dilemma and the decision.

**G.R. Holt, M.D., M.S.E., M.P.H.**

## Association of Esophageal Reflux and Globus Symptom: Comparison of Laryngoscopy and 24-Hour pH Manometry

Woo P, Noordzij P, Ross J-A (New England Med Ctr, Boston; Tufts Univ, Boston)

*Otolaryngol Head Neck Surg* 115:502–507, 1996　　　　　　　　　　11–9

*Background.*—Globus symptom, a lumplike sensation in the throat, is a common throat disorder that prompts otolaryngologist consultation. Recent studies have suggested that gastroesophageal reflux disease (GERD) is a cause of globus. The laryngoscopic findings of GERD in patients with globus sensation and the role of acid reflux in globus symptoms were investigated.

*Methods and Findings.*—Thirty-one patients with globus sensation underwent dual probe pH manometry and videolaryngoscopy. Seventeen patients had abnormal laryngeal findings, including grossly abnormal as well as subtle changes. Pharyngeal erythema was present in 12 patients, interarytenoid pachydermia in 11, laryngeal edema in 11, arytenoid erythema in 9, and thick mucus in 3. Gastroesophageal reflux disease was found in 21 of the 31 pH probe studies, with Johnson and DeMeester composite scores for the distal probe. There was no correlation between the upright and supine positions, nor was there correlation between positive laryngeal findings and a positive pH probe study.

*Conclusion.*—In many patients, globus sensation appears to be a nonspecific symptom of laryngopharyngeal irritation in which gastroesophageal reflux disease has an important role. Careful laryngoscopic assessment combined with pH probe studies can help clinicians differentiate between patients with organic abnormalities resulting from GERD and those with other nonspecific laryngopharyngeal disorders.

▶ It has been my understanding that the symptom of globus has a number of causes. First, because lymphoid tissue is present in the hypopharynx down to the upper esophageal inlet, inflammation of this tissue could produce a sensation of swelling and discomfort. Second, edema of the endolarynx could cause a "lump" in the throat, although most of the symptoms would likely be vocal in nature. Finally, inflammation of the mucosa inside the esophagus at the level of the upper esophageal sphincter, as well as a reflex spasm of the underlying sphincter muscle, could give rise to the globus sensation as well as the dysphagia that commonly accompanies it.

**G.R. Holt, M.D., M.S.E., M.P.H.**

## Endoscopic Laser Medial Arytenoidectomy Versus Total Arytenoidectomy in the Management of Bilateral Vocal Fold Paralysis

Wani MK, Yarber R, Hengesteg A, et al (Univ of Tennessee, Memphis)
*Ann Otol Rhinol Laryngol* 105:857–862, 1996                    11–10

*Background.*—Severe airway compromise is associated with bilateral laryngeal paralysis. Endoscopic laser total arytenoidectomy (TA) is a widely accepted treatment for bilateral laryngeal paralysis. Unfortunately, the vocal results of this procedure are usually poor. Resection of only the medial part of the arytenoid (MA) may result in less vocal impairment but may not provide a sufficient airway. Endoscopic laser MA and TA are compared in the treatment of bilateral vocal fold paralysis in an animal model.

*Methods and Results.*—Twelve dogs were subjected to bilateral laryngeal paralysis. Laryngeal resistance was measured in vivo and ex vivo after TA, MA, and no surgery. Laryngeal resistance was found to be significantly lower in the control group than in the dogs undergoing TA and MA. However, it did not differ significantly between the TA and MA groups. The glottic area was also significantly greater in dogs treated by MA and TA compared with the control group but did not differ significantly between the TA and MA groups. Phonation could be elicited in all the control group animals, in 2 of the 4 dogs in the MA group, and in none of the dogs in the TA group.

*Conclusion.*—In this canine model, MA and TA produced similar glottic airway resistance at physiologic flow rates, even though a greater amount of cartilage was removed with TA. In addition, MA and TA resulted in essentially the same cross-sectional area of the glottis. Thus, MA appears to be a promising alternative to TA for restoring the airway while preserving vocal function in patients with bilateral laryngeal paralysis.

▶ Based on previous work pioneered by Ossoff and Crumley, the authors work has used an animal model to study laser MA vs. surgical TA. As there was little difference in the objective findings between the 2, it would appear that the laser procedure, being less invasive, should be considered first. There may also be a role for MA in the management of these patients with a contralateral reinnervation procedure.

**G.R. Holt, M.D., M.S.E., M.P.H.**

## Muscle Tension Dysphonia and Spasmodic Dysphonia: The Role of Manual Laryngeal Tension Reduction in Diagnosis and Management

Roy N, Ford CN, Bless DM (Univ of Wisconsin, Madison)
*Ann Otol Rhinol Laryngol* 105:851–856, 1996                    11–11

*Background.*—Excessive activity of the extralaryngeal muscles affects laryngeal function, contributing to a spectrum of symptoms and syndromes, such as muscle tension dysphonia and spasmodic dysphonia.

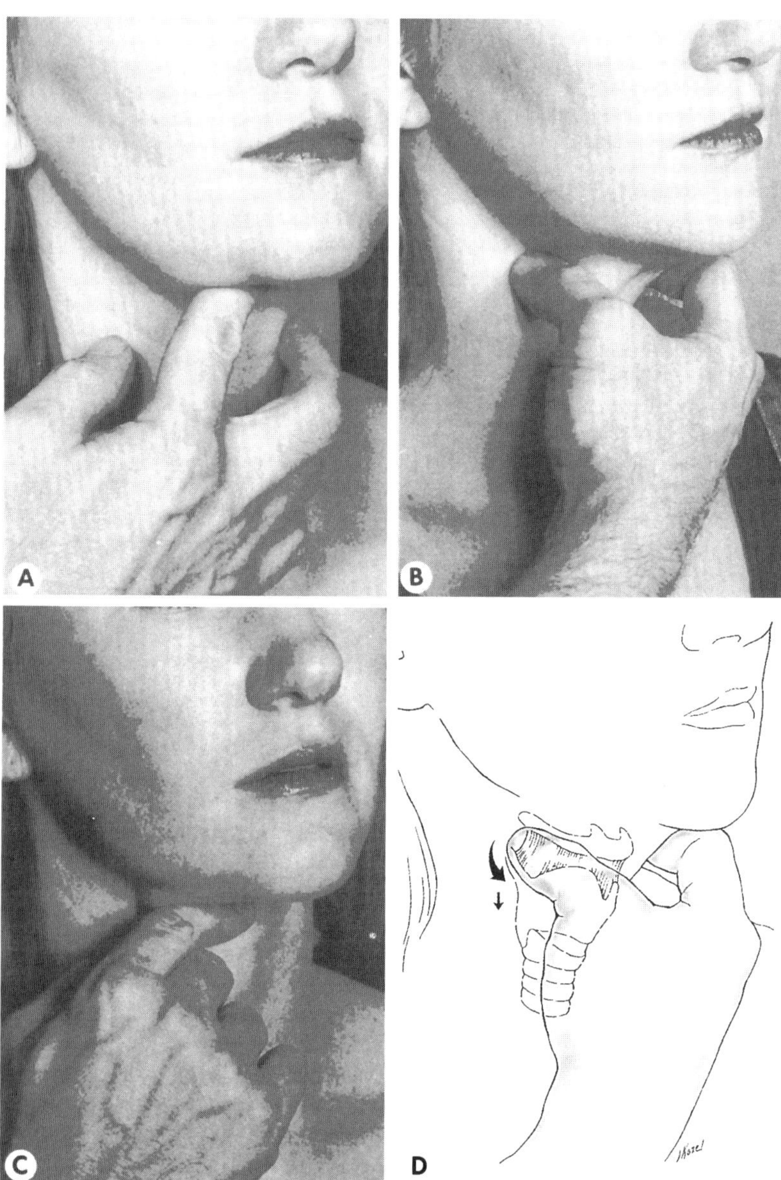

**FIGURE.**—Manual laryngeal tension reduction. **A,** medial suprahyoid musculature is palpated at rest and during upward pitch glide maneuvers. Focal sites of tenderness and taut bands signal excessive muscle activity. **B,** signs of excess laryngeal tension are assayed by (1) evaluating presence of focal sites of pain or nodularity, (2) determining size of thyrohyoid space, and (3) observing voice effect of downward traction over superior border of thyroid lamina and during circumlaryngeal massage. **C,** larynx is compressed by exerting anterior-to-posterior pressure over inferior border of hyoid bone. **D,** manual tension reduction procedure (circumlaryngeal massage) with hand configuration and placement. Pressure is applied in circular motion over tips of hyoid bone and within thyrohyoid space. Procedure is repeated over posterior borders of thyroid cartilage and larynx is gently pulled downward. (Courtesy of Roy N, Ford CN, Bless DM: Muscle tension dysphonia and spasmodic dysphonia: The role of manual laryngeal tension reduction in diagnosis and management. *Ann Otol Rhinol Laryngol* 105:851–856, 1996.)

Recognizing the role of extralaryngeal tension is useful for correct diagnosis and treatment decision making. The use of manual laryngeal musculoskeletal tension reduction methods in the diagnosis and treatment of laryngeal hyperfunction syndromes was discussed.

*Discussion.*—The technique involves focal palpation to determine the degree of laryngeal elevation, focal tenderness, the effect of downward pressure over the superior border of the thyroid lamina on the voice, and the extent of sustained voice improvement after circumlaryngeal massage (Figure). During palpation, the finding of laryngeal pain and tenderness, stiffness, and elevation suggests the presence of excessive musculoskeletal tension. The clinician can confirm the role of abnormal muscular tensions by eliciting a positive response to diagnostic treatment with laryngeal reposturing methods such as circumlaryngeal massage. The identification of patients with neurologic spasmodic dysphonia and generalized laryngeal hypertonicity will help clinicians to interpret suboptimal responses to botulinum therapy. Thus, clinicians can prospectively advise a treatment regimen that combines manual laryngeal tension reduction and botulinum injections.

*Conclusion.*—Regardless of cause, all patients with voice disorders should be evaluated for the presence of excess laryngeal musculoskeletal tension as a primary or secondary cause of the dysphonia. The use of manual laryngeal methods can ensure correct diagnosis and proper treatment for patients with muscle tension dysphonia and spasmodic dysphonia.

▶ Athletes, both amateur and professional, understand the benefits of muscle massage to their performance. By analogy, vocal performers also utilize a specific set of muscles in their specialty. Hyerpfunctioning of the larynx can be as debilitating for a vocal performer as muscle spasms can be in a basketball player. Self-massage techniques should be easy to teach the patient, and perhaps there will develop a whole new subset of massage therapy—for the neck and larynx.

**G.R. Holt, M.D., M.S.E., M.P.H.**

---

**Reinke's Edema: Phonatory Mechanisms and Management Strategies**
Zeitels SM, Bunting GW, Hillman RE, et al (Harvard Med School, Boston; Massachusetts Eye and Ear Infirmary, Boston)
*Ann Otol Rhinol Laryngol* 106:533–543, 1997                    11–12

---

*Objective.*—Reinke's edema, chronic inflammation of the vocal cords, is generally associated with smoking, vocal abuse, or reflux. Whereas previous tests of vocal function have used only perceptual and acoustic analysis, this study employed stroboscopic, acoustic, and aerodynamic measures before and after phonomicrosurgical resection to provide insights into underlying vocal mechanisms that could potentially be associated with the development of this disorder.

*Methods.*—Twenty patients (1 male) underwent reflux management for 1 month prior to surgery. Pre- and postoperative vocal assessments using videolaryngoscopy with stroboscopy, voice assessments by speech-language pathologists, acoustic assessment to determine maximum phonation time, and aerodynamic testing to determine glottal airflow rate and subglottal air pressure were performed.

*Results.*—Five patients (POST-2) who resumed smoking had recurrent Reinke's edema, but 4 had an improved glottal appearance. Vestibular fold compression decreased in 7 of 14 patients with nonrecurrence (POST-1); 11 had normal mucosal waves, and 10 had decreased anteroposterior compression. Supraglottal strain problems persisted in the 4 POST-2 patients. Women with abnormally low (123 Hz) speaking voices before surgery, had even lower voices after surgery. Abnormally low speaking voices create abnormally high average subglottal pressures (9.7 cm $H_2O$). Voice quality improved after surgery in 18 patients.

*Conclusion.*—Reinke's edema appears to be caused by an abnormally low speaking voice that increases subglottal pressure to the point of hyperfunction. Smoking cessation programs and voice therapy may be helpful for these patients.

▶ This treatise nicely summarizes what is known about Reinke's edema and postulates that vocal hyperfunction may be commonly associated. If the hyperfunction is not addressed (preferably pre-operatively), then the edema is likely to return. Additionally, it is helpful to begin anti-reflux therapy well before the microsurgical therapy to debulk the edema, so that control may be gained pre-operatively. Adequate vocal rest is required ( 2 to 3 days) for resealing of the vocal fold flap, with voice conservation utilized for perhaps another week. I am likely to resume speech therapy 1 week following a microlaryngeal procedure.

**G.R. Holt, M.D., M.S.E., M.P.H.**

---

**Indications for Flexible versus Rigid Bronchoscopy in Children With Suspected Foreign-Body Aspiration**
Martinot A, Closset M, Marquette CH, et al (Centre Hospitalier et Universitaire, Lille, France)
*Am J Respir Crit Care Med* 155:1676–1679, 1997                                11–13

---

*Objective.*—Early diagnosis and removal of foreign bodies (FBs) from the airways of children is necessary to prevent life-threatening airway obstruction, chronic wheezing, or recurrent pneumonia. Diagnosis and extraction is usually accomplished with a rigid bronchoscope. Diagnostic indications for flexible fiberoptic bronchoscopy have not been investigated. Results are reported of a prospective study to determine the positive predictive value of history, signs, and symptoms of FB aspiration at prebronchoscopic examinations; to examine the complications of flexible and

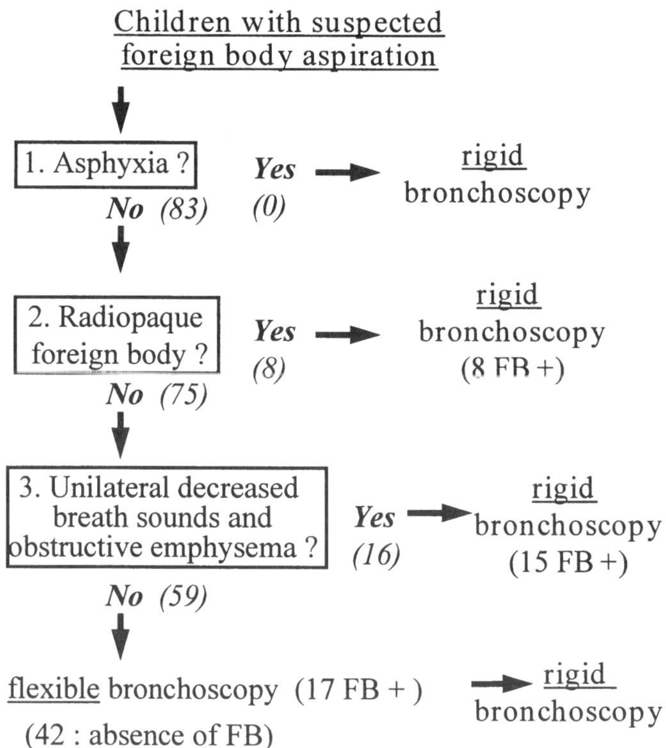



FIGURE 2.—Proposed management algorithm for children with suspected FB aspiration, and simulated results when applied retrospectively to the study population. Simulated results are based on pediatricians' chest x-ray interpretations. *Abbreviations:* ( ), number of patients; *FB+*, presence of an FB. (Courtesy of Martinot A, Closset M, Marquette CH, et al: Indications for flexible versus rigid bronchoscopy in children with suspected foreign-body aspiration. *Am J Respir Crit Care Med* 155:1676–1679, 1997.)

rigid bronchoscopy; and to evaluate the value of a management algorithm combining flexible and rigid bronchoscopy.

*Methods.*—Histories and chest radiographs were obtained for 83 children, average age 24 months, with suspected FB aspiration. Rigid bronchoscopy was performed on all children with asphyxiating FB aspiration or clear evidence of an FB. Flexible bronchoscopy was performed on all others. If an FB was found, it was removed using a rigid bronchoscope.

*Results.*—There were 68 children with a history of choking. Of 28 children undergoing rigid bronchoscopy, 23 had an FB. Of 55 children undergoing flexible bronchoscopy, 17 had an FB and rigid bronchoscopy (Fig 2). One patient had laryngospasm and 6 patients had laryngeal edema after rigid bronchoscopy; 1 child had dyspnea after flexible bronchoscopy. A radiopaque FB and unilaterally decreased breath sounds and obstructive emphysema had a positive predictive value of 94%.

*Conclusion.*—The algorithm is a useful tool for managing children with suspected FB aspiration. A radiopaque FB and unilaterally decreased breath sounds and obstructive emphysema had a positive predictive value of 94%.

▶ The discussion about flexible vs. rigid bronchoscopy for suspected foreign bodies in children continues. As I understand it, if there is absolutely no objective evidence for a foreign body being present, then the authors recommend flexible bronchoscopy for diagnosis. While I realize I'm not a pediatric otolaryngologist, I have performed my share of rigid pediatric bronchoscopies during the past 25 years. I can count on less than 5 fingers the times I have come up lacking a foreign body—I just don't think it is very common, when one takes a careful history, conducts a complete physical examination and performs appropriate radiological testing. I think flexible is okay, but I'd want a rigid scope right there in the endoscopy suite to get the foreign body out if/when it was found.

**G.R. Holt, M.D., M.S.E., M.P.H.**

---

**Arytenoidopexy for Bilateral Vocal Fold Paralysis in Young Children**
Triglia J-M, Belus J-F, Nicollas R (Univ of Marseille, France)
*J Laryngol Otol* 110:1027–1030, 1996                                    11–14

---

*Background.*—Bilateral vocal fold paralysis is uncommon but can be disabling in young children. In severe cases, with little chance for spontaneous recovery, intervention is indicated. This retrospective report assesses arytenoidopexy in children with life-threatening bilateral vocal fold paralysis.

*Methods.*—Between October 1988 and January 1995, 34 children were seen at La Timone Children's Hospital in Marseille, France, with evidence of vocal fold paralysis. Of these 34 children, 15 underwent arytenoidopexy. The average age at operation of these children was 20 months. All underwent direct endoscopic larynx examination and were found to have life-threatening airway obstruction. Arytenoidopexy was performed by the external laterocervical approach. The files of all 15 cases were retrospectively examined.

*Findings.*—After arytenoidopexy, 14 of the 15 patients were successfully decannulated within 42 days. The final patient remained tracheotomy dependent and aryenoidectomy was performed 10 months later. All decannulated patients remained in good health, with an average follow-up of 3.5 years. The patients' parents were generally satisfied with the quality of breathing, feeding, and voice.

*Conclusions.*—These results suggest that arytenoidopexy is a safe and effective surgical treatment for life-threatening bilateral vocal fold paralysis in young children.

▶ I was impressed that 14 of 15 children were able to be decannulated after unilateral arytenoidopexy for bilateral vocal cord paralysis. Also interesting was the information that 12 of the original 34 children did not require a procedure because of partial or complete recovery. I do not know how long they waited for recovery before operating, however. Although their results are quite encouraging, we do not have information on their exercise tolerance and whether the children are able to do the things that children like to do—run, skip, play, bike, skate, swim, and so on. Finally, is there a role for neuromuscular pedicle reinnervation attempts in children?

**G.R. Holt, M.D., M.S.E., M.P.H.**

## Vocal Fold Vibration Viewed From the Tracheal Side in Living Human Beings

Yumoto E, Kadota Y, Mori T (Ehime Univ, Japan)
*Otolaryngol Head Neck Surg* 115:329–334, 1996                    11–15

*Background.*—Vocal fold vibration, the propagation of a mucosal wave that travels upward from the lower surface of the vocal fold, has been studied in canine models. The vibratory behavior of the in vivo human vocal fold, viewed from the tracheal side, was assessed.

*Methods.*—Fourteen men and 6 women, aged 22 to 70 years, who had had tracheostomy for various head and neck diseases participated in the study. A rigid oblique-view endoscope was inserted through a tracheostoma to visualize the inferior apsect of the vocal fold during phonation. Each participant enunciated the vowel /a/ at a comfortable pitch and volume (easy phonation) and again at a higher pitch.

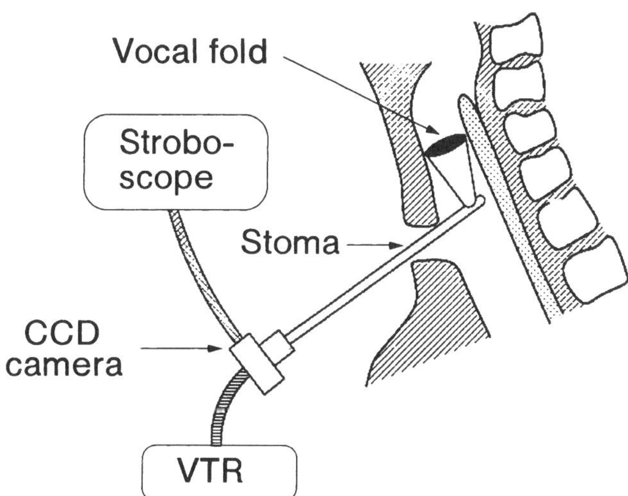


FIGURE 1.—Observation of vocal fold vibration from the tracheal side. A rigid oblique-view endoscope was inserted into the subglottic space through a tracheostoma. Cotton gauze was used to prevent air leak around the rigid endoscope. *Abbreviations: CCD,* charge-coupled device; *VTR,* videotape recorder. (Courtesy of Yumoto E, Kadota Y, Mori T: Vocal fold vibration viewed from the tracheal side in living human beings. *Otolaryngol Head Neck Surg* 115:329–334, 1996.)

*Findings.*—During easy phonation, the mucosal upheaval appeared on the lower surface of the vocal fold between the anterior commissure and the vocal process in all 19 subjects in whom inferior glottoscopy could be performed. During high-pitched phonation—studied successfully in 10 subjects—the vocal folds elongated, and the subglottic vault surrounded by the bilateral mucosal upheavals narrowed, compared with those during easy phonation. In 1 subject, the use of a dilated blood vessel as a landmark showed the location of the mucosal upheaval on the vocal fold mucosa to actually shift medially toward the oral side during high-pitched phonation (Fig 1).

*Conclusion.*—In these subjects, the mucosal wave was observed to begin at the mucosal upheaval and propagate upward. Although there were structural differences between the human and canine vocal folds, the infraglottic aspect of the vocal fold vibration in the living human larynx was found to be quite similar to that in the excised canine larynx.

▶ The notion of development of the mucosal wave in the superior subglottic region, with migration of that wave to the free margin of the vocal fold, is intriguing and easy to accept. Although I question the inclusion in this study of patients who had vocal cord fixation or whose larynx had been irradiated, other patients provided an observation platform for the better understanding of this physiologic activity involved in sound behavior. The study also helps explain the vocal difficulties in patients with idiopathic subglottic stenosis.

**G.R. Holt, M.D., M.S.E., M.P.H.**

---

**Supraglottic Stenosis in Infants and Children: A Preliminary Report**
Walner DL, Holinger LD (Children's Hosp, Cincinnatti, Ohio; Children's Mem Hosp, Chicago)
*Arch Otolaryngol Head Neck Surg* 123:337–341, 1997          11–16

---

*Objective.*—Supraglottic stenosis/collapse (SS/C) has been observed in a small number of pediatric patients. The condition involves a thickening of soft tissues of the supraglottic larynx, posterior displacement of the epiglottis, and anterior displacement of the posterior supraglottis. SS/C is primarily acquired and can be a major cause of upper airway obstruction. The factors present and the potential causes of this condition are discussed.

*Methods.*—Records of 17 children (7 females), aged 7 months to 14 years, evaluated between October 1985 and June 1993 at Children's Memorial Hospital in Chicago were reviewed retrospectively.

*Results.*—All patients had undergone laryngoscopy, bronchoscopy, and tracheostomy primarily for respiratory failure. Only 1 patient had supraglottic edema at the time of tracheostomy. SS/C was found from 4 months to 14 years after tracheostomy. Ten patients had laryngotracheal (LTR) reconstruction. SS/C was found 1 to 36 months after LTR. All 17 patients were diagnosed with SS/C, 10 with posterior displacement of the epiglottis and 10 with anterior arytenoid displacement. Sixteen patients were also found to have subglottic stenosis varying from 40% to 75% obstruction. Nine patients had gastroesophageal reflux disease.

*Conclusion.*—SS/C is a new form of supraglottic narrowing that appears to be primarily acquired as a result of laryngeal or tracheal surgery.

▶ The authors present us with the possibility of a new and distinct clinical entity—SS/C. They postulate the etiologies and comment that the otolaryngic community should be observant about this condition for future definition. It occurred to me that since this was found overwhelmingly in children who had been instrumented or had undergone a tracheotomy, that it could also result from perichondritis or chondritis secondary to the procedure. Healing of the inflammation might well lead to softening of the cartilage and loss of integral support. At any rate, keep your eyes open for this new observation.

**G.R. Holt, M.D., M.S.E., M.P.H.**

## p53 Protein Expression in Benign Lesions of the Upper Respiratory Tract

Ingle RR, Setzen G, Koltai PJ, et al (Albany Med College, NY)
*Arch Otolaryngol Head Neck Surg* 123:297–300, 1997                    11–17

*Objective.*—Inactivation of p53 suppressor genes results in functional loss and unrestrained cell growth. Whereas the literature is replete with p53 overexpression studies in cancers of various organs, there is little information about p53 expression in normal tissue or benign lesions. p53 immunoreactivity was evaluated in a variety of common epithelial proliferations of the upper respiratory tract.

*Methods.*—p53 expression was demonstrated by immunohistochemical studies in 16 cases of juvenile laryngeal papillomatosis, 36 cases of adult laryngeal papillomatosis, 10 cases of laryngeal nodules, 10 cases of laryngeal polyps, 17 cases of inverted papilloma, and 20 cases of nasal polyps. Staining for p53 positivity was scored from 0 to 4+.

*Results.*—p53 reactivity was demonstrated in 14 (88%) of 16 cases of juvenile laryngeal papillomatosis, 33 (92%) of 36 cases of adult laryngeal papillomatosis, 4 (40%) of 10 cases of laryngeal nodules, 8 (80%) of 10 cases of laryngeal polyps, 7 (41%) of 17 cases of inverted papilloma, and 2 (10%) of 20 cases of nasal polyps. Most of the staining in the papilloma and papillomatosis cases appeared in the basal ad intermediate layers. The presence of significant overexpression of p53 protein in the papillomatosis cases is suggestive of a possible pathogenic role for p53.

*Conclusion.*—p53 overexpression in benign epithelial lesions of the upper respiratory tract, particularly in the basal cell layer, shows that p53 accumulation can occur without mutation of the gene, may correlate with epithelial proliferative activity, and does not indicate the presence of malignancy.

▶ The p53 protein seems to play a role, albeit incompletely defined, in the growth of malignancies of the head and neck. Further work may lead to the mass screening of patients for p53 gene (as with the prostate specific antigen test), which could identify high risk patients who need to be closely followed and who may need to alter their risk factors. The same approach might well be prescribed in the future for patients with a risk for benign lesions of the upper aerodigestive tract. Certainly screening of groups exposed to mucosal irritants would be helpful, and of course, if gene therapy becomes available, who knows how much help that could be for us and our patients.

**G.R. Holt, M.D., M.S.E., M.P.H.**

---

**Instability of Voice in Adolescence: Pathologic Condition or Normal Development Variation?**
Boltežar IH, Burger ZR, Žargi M (Univ Dept of Otorhinolaryngology, Ljubljana, Slovenia)
*J Pediatr* 130:185–190, 1997                                      11–18

---

*Introduction.*—As a result of growth of the phonatory, resonatory, and respiratory organs, the voices of boys and girls start to change in puberty and adolescence. There is a high prevalence of dysphonia, and these adolescents often need professional help. For successful treatment, the most critical disordered system in voice production must be found. To distinguish normal variation of voice development from pathologic disorders, the main characteristics of adolescent voice were identified and the characteristics to distinguish the variations were determined.

*Methods.*—There were 51 adolescents, 22 boys and 29 girls between the ages of 10 and 17 years, who were divided into 4 groups: candidates for singing lessons without voice problems; those with mutation voice disorders; those with functional dysphonia; and those with vocal cord nodules. They were divided into the groups by using indirect laryngoscopy and stroboscopy. Each adolescent had the fundamental frequency evaluated, along with the variability of pitch and amplitude, and the presence of noise. Voice analysis was done by using the Multi-Dimensional Voice Program.

*Results.*—In boys and girls, all mean values of variables that describe variability of pitch and amplitude were abnormal, with boys having greater abnormalities. In most adolescents, the variability of loudness and pitch were abnormal. Only boys had a significant negative correlation between age and fundamental frequency. Only girls had a significant negative correlation between age and variability of amplitude. There were positive correlations between variables that express variability of pitch and amplitude. No significant differences were found between the candidates for singing lessons or those with mutational disorders, vocal cord nodules, or functional dysphonia. Also, no differences were found between those without voice problems, those with functional voice disorders, and those with vocal cord nodules.

*Conclusions.*—The instability of amplitude and pitch are the main characteristics of adolescent voice. There is more stability with female voices than with male voices. The more gradual adaptation of the afferent and efferent nervous control to the rapid growth of the respiratory, phonatory, and resonatory organs seems to be the reason for this instability. Optimal phonatory patterns can be created in the growing speech apparatus. For treatment of functional voice disorders, adolescence is an ideal period for treatment.

▶ This article was of personal interest to me because I now have a 13-year-old son with a changing voice. Only shortly ago he could sing so purely, and now he seemingly has little control over volume and pitch. This study addresses the worse instability of the male adolescent voice, yet states that this same period of instability is also a great window of opportunity for speech therapy. At least in my experience, I have not seen many vocal abnormalities present at adolescence that do not straighten out with time. However, for cheerleaders, that does not seem to hold true. So, physicians and parents, be patient and that voice, like a squawky saxophone, may develop into a rich baritone with time.

**G.R. Holt, M.D., M.S.E., M.P.H.**

---

**Tenuous Airway in Children With Trisomy 21**
de Jong AL, Sulek M, Nihill M, et al (Baylor College of Medicine, Houston; Texas Children's Hosp, Houston)
*Laryngoscope* 107:345–350, 1997                                              11–19

---

*Introduction.*—One of the most frequent congenital syndromes recognized at birth is trisomy 21 or Down syndrome, with an estimated incidence of 1 in 600 live births. Anatomical features include typical facies, brachycephaly, flat nasal bridge, and anterior-posterior flattening of the skull. Heart defects are found in up to 40% of these patients, and many require general anesthesia at an early age, which places them at increased risk for upper airway compromise. The frequency of postoperative upper airway obstruction and the cause of this obstruction were retrospectively studied in patients with Down syndrome who had major cardiovascular surgery.

*Methods.*—A total of 99 patients with trisomy 21 who had cardiovascular surgery were studied. They were evaluated for race, age at the time of the procedure, growth percentile for weight, initial diameter of the endotracheal tube used, predicted endotracheal tube diameter for age, number of required reintubations, total time the patient was intubated, presence of stridor, and presence or development of subglottic stenosis. Follow-up ranged from 1 month to 5 years.

*Results.*—Younger age, lower growth percentile for weight, and increased frequency for reintubation were significant factors for the development of stridor. There were 69 patients (69.7%) who did not have stridor and 24 (24.2%) who had stridor. In 6 other patients (6.1%), subglottic stenosis was found, and all 6 of these patients were less than the 10th percentile for weight. An endotracheal tube of larger diameter than predicted for age was used in 4 of these patients.

*Conclusions.*—Postextubation stridor is more common in patients with Down syndrome who have cardiovascular surgery. If the 6 patients with subglottic stenosis are included, the overall frequency of postextubation stridor among patients studied was 33.3%. For successful airway management, patients with Down syndrome deserve special considerations and modifications of standard intubation techniques. The use of an oversized endotracheal tube may be a key factor in the development of subglottic stenosis in trisomy 21 patients.

▶ The authors present sound management advice for handling the airway in children with Down syndrome. In addition to the high incidence of unsuspected subglottic stenosis, there is the daunting challenge of the enlarged tongue. It is wise to inform our colleagues in anesthesia and surgery (perhaps by offering to speak at their department meetings) of the pitfalls in intubating and extubating these patients. In this study, the anesthesiologists were not always aware of the potential problems before treatment. Remember, too, that subluxation of the cervical spine is also prevalent during hyperextension of the neck. Obviously, adult patients with Down syndrome also pose problems. The recovery room nurses should also be in-serviced (trained) in recognizing the problems associated with the airway in Down syndrome patients.

**G.R. Holt, M.D., M.S.E., M.P.H.**

# 12 Head and Neck Oncology

**Changes in Quality-of-Life Scores in a Population of Patients Treated for Squamous Cell Carcinoma of the Head and Neck**
McDonough EM, Varvares MA, Dunphy FR, et al (Saint Louis Univ)
*Head Neck* 18:487–493, 1996                                                12–1

*Introduction.*—The successful rehabilitation of patients with head and neck cancer requires careful consideration of quality of life (QOL) or satisfaction with physical, emotional, and social functioning. Global functional measures, such as those of Karnofsky or Zubrod, make use of nurse or physician ratings and may not reflect QOL as perceived by the patient. A prospective study of patients with head and neck cancer used self-evaluations to assess QOL before, during, and after treatment.

*Methods.*—Study participants were 24 patients (21 men and 3 women) with an average age of 54 years. All had advanced stage III or IV head and neck cancer and were enrolled in an experimental organ-preservation protocol. One group was treated with chemotherapy (paclitaxel and carboplatin) followed by radiation therapy, and the other group received the same chemotherapeutic agents followed by surgery and radiation. Patients completed the University of Washington Quality of Life Questionnaire and the Social Avoidance and Distress Scale at various time points.

*Results.*—Social avoidance was significantly negatively correlated with QOL; thus QOL scores decreased as social avoidance scores increased. As there was also a significant correlation between social avoidance and social distress, high levels of social distress were associated with high levels of social avoidance. At the last treatment point reported, QOL was significantly higher in the nonsurgical group than in the surgical group. The nonsurgical group also had lower social distress/avoidance scores.

*Discussion.*—Preliminary findings in this small series of patients with head and neck surgery suggest that the treatment protocol followed is associated with differences in QOL and social distress/avoidance. Patients who fail chemotherapy and undergo surgery followed by radiation have compromised QOL compared with patients successfully treated with chemotherapy and radiation. Thus, treatment that is less invasive and disfiguring and has fewer adverse effects on eating and communication abilities helps to preserve QOL.

▶ I readily admit that I have selected a number of articles for the YEARBOOK OF OTOLARYNGOLOGY/HEAD NECK SURGERY on "quality of life" issues because I believe we, as surgeons, must make every effort to consider this factor and to have the patient consider it, as well, when making therapeutic decisions on head and neck tumors. Although we have been trained primarily as surgical specialists, there are times when we are *capable* of performing resections, but perhaps we should not do them.

This article strongly suggests that QOL in non–surgically treated patients is self-perceived to be better. But there is always the issue of QOL vs. actual longevity (albeit of a poorer quality). The patient has to understand these trade-offs when making a decision. I often ask myself, when weighing the choices for a patient in my own mind, what I would want to happen to (for) my own father or late mother. Although we are supposed to remain "objective" when dealing with the patient, we can still be human, and this is my way of seeking that "human factor" in these cases.

**G.R. Holt, M.D., M.S.E., M.P.H.**

---

**Critical Pathways for Head and Neck Surgery: Development and Implementation**
Cohen J, Stock M, Andersen P, et al (Oregon Health Sciences Univ, Portland)
*Arch Otolaryngol Head Neck Surg* 123:11–14, 1997                    12–2

---

*Background.*—Application of the concept of the "critical pathway" in medicine allows each discipline involved in a patient's care to determine the critical elements of care and their expected time course, cost, and outcome, and to define methods of coordination. Because of its complicated surgical procedures, lengthy hospitalizations, and need for many ancillary services, head and neck oncologic care is an ideal area for the development and implementation of critical pathways. The 4 critical pathways for head and neck surgery reported here were developed at Oregon Health Sciences University (OHSU).

*Methods.*—The critical pathways identified were chemotherapy, clean head and neck surgery, clean contaminated head and neck surgery, and clean contaminated head and neck surgery with reconstructive flap. A generic critical pathway set up as a grid had already been developed at OHSU. The grid was completed for head and neck surgery using data obtained by polling all departments involved in the care of these patients. When possible, standing orders already formulated were incorporated into the grid. Copies of the critical pathways were posted on doors to patients' room and served as a guide to everyday care. The outcomes of critical pathways were assessed in patients admitted for head and neck oncologic surgery or chemotherapy.

*Results.*—Sixty-eight patients were admitted from December 1, 1995 through May 31, 1996, when clinical pathways were used. Outcome (length of stay, cost of hospitalization, and variance tracking) in this group was compared with that of 30 historical controls who had similar diagnoses and underwent surgical procedures during the year before critical pathways were implemented. With critical pathways, length of stay for the clean contaminated group without flap reconstruction decreased by 1.5 days; costs were reduced by $7,407 per patient. Length of stay decreased 1.6 days and costs decreased $9,845 per patient in the clean contaminated group with flap reconstruction. Nine patients (13%) had a prolonged period of hospitalization while on a critical pathway.

*Conclusion.*—Patients admitted for treatment of head and neck cancer are a diverse group and various procedures are required, but their care can be organized into 4 critical pathways. The implementation of these critical pathways at OHSU has reduced length of stay and hospitalization costs and has allowed for better coordination and documentation of patient care.

▶ I believe this is, perhaps, the best overall article on health care delivery that I reviewed for this issue, because it is a key element in the management of resources through proactive steps taken by *the health care team*—not some "for-profit" entity. As physicians and leaders of the health care team, it is our responsibility to initiate such critical pathways and to monitor their use for constant improvement. Not only were length of stay and costs reduced, but I believe that patient care was enhanced because of attention focused on the main items of care for these patients.

**G.R. Holt, M.D., M.S.E., M.P.H.**

---

**Informed Consent in Head and Neck Surgery: How Much Do Patients Actually Remember?**
Hekkenberg RJ, Irish JC, Rotstein LE, et al (Univ of Toronto)
*J Otolaryngol* 26:155–159, 1997                                         12–3

---

*Introduction.*—To comply with the requirements of informed consent, physicians in Canada must inform the patient of the risk that a reasonable or prudent person would want to know about concerning a particular procedure or treatment. Signing of the consent form is a portion of the consent process, but the key element lies in the specific communication between physician and patient. A prospective study of 54 patients scheduled for head and neck surgery evaluates how much recall they had of the information communicated by the physician.

*Methods.*—The patients were undergoing routine thyroidectomy, parathyroidectomy, or parotidectomy. Four participating surgeons were given a checklist of risks to outline to the patient at the preoperative visit. Patients were to have their questions answered and then to sign a standard surgical consent form. One to 8 weeks later, they were interviewed and asked to recall the specific risks of the operation. Patient data collected included sex, age, educational level, and type of surgical procedure.

*Results.*—Patients were 40 women and 14 men with an average age of 46.9 years. The average follow-up was 33 days. For all procedures, the overall recall of all complications was 48%. Patients who underwent parotidectomy were most likely to recall the risk for a facial nerve injury (93%) and for a greater auricular nerve injury (60%). The best recall for thyroidectomy or parathyroidectomy—procedures with similar risks— were for recurrent laryngeal nerve injury (77%); 44% in these groups recalled a risk for hypocalcemia. Patient gender did not appear to influence recall success, but those who were younger and better educated had higher recall rates (more than 50% of risks).

*Discussion.*—Even at a relatively short period after the surgical procedure, these patients recalled only 48.5% of the risks described to them before operation. Both patient age and educational level were significant determinants of recall. Some patients might retain more if they were given written information sheets regarding the material presented orally by the physician.

▶ How many times have you had a patient say, "I don't remember you telling me about that"? Or, more commonly, when the nurse obtains the consent after physician counseling, the patient does not recognize the possible complications listed? This study found that younger, more educated patients had a better recall for 6 specific complications. Although this is a very helpful study, I think 2 additional factors need to be considered. First, if really concerned about the surgery, the patient may be preoccupied and may not pay attention well. Second, the way the surgeon states the complications may make a difference—for instance, just reading out the complications on a list is not as conducive to understanding as is presenting a practical explanation on a level understandable by *that* particular patient and the family. For that reason, I usually state the complications *3* times, in some manner or fashion, to emphasize by repetition.

**G.R. Holt, M.D., M.S.E., M.P.H.**

---

**Management of the Orbit During Anterior Fossa Craniofacial Resection**
Andersen PE, Kraus DH, Arbit E, et al (Mem Sloan-Kettering Cancer Ctr, New York; Staten Island Univ, NY)
*Arch Otolaryngol Head Neck Surg* 122:1305–1307, 1996        12–4

---

*Background.*—Paranasal sinus tumors may invade the orbital contents. The need for orbital exenteration in such cases is debated. Research has shown that effective tumor control and preservation of the orbit can be achieved even when the bony limits of the orbit have been breached and periosteal invasion has occurred. However, surgery and radiation therapy may result in the loss of ocular function. Postoperative ocular function in patients undergoing anterior fossa craniofacial resection with orbital preservation was studied.

*Methods.*—The medical records of 58 consecutive patients undergoing anterior fossa craniofacial resection with orbital preservation for tumors involving the anterior skull base between 1973 and 1994 were reviewed. Patients were followed for a median of 38 months.

*Findings.*—Forty-three percent of the patients had some ocular complications related to treatment. Twenty-one patients had epiphora, 8 had diplopia, 6 had visual loss, and 2 had pain and enophthalmos. Twelve patients needed surgery: dacryocystorhinostomy in 8, ectropion repair in 3, drainage of orbital mucocele in 1, and corneal transplant in 1. Ocular complications were more common in patients treated with postoperative radiation therapy. Visual loss occurred only in this group. Fifty of the 58 patients had functional vision in the ipsilateral eye.

*Conclusion.*—Ocular sequelae are common in patients undergoing anterior fossa craniofacial resection with orbital preservation. Revision surgery may be needed. In most patients, functional vision can be preserved.

▶ Among those conditions for which retaining the globe after anterior cranial fossa resection would lead to a terminal ocular disorder are optic nerve injury/disruption and a painful, nonseeing eye. The others—including diplopia, enophthalmos, and epiphora—can be dealt with by reconstructive procedures. The key is to preserve ocular function without compromising the oncologic extirpation.

**G.R. Holt, M.D., M.S.E., M.P.H.**

## Secondary Squamous Cell Carcinoma of the Orbit

Johnson TE, Tabbara KF, Weatherhead RG, et al (King Saud Univ, Riyadh, Saudi Arabia; Univ of Cincinnati, Ohio; Univ of Arkansas, Little Rock)
*Arch Ophthalmol* 115:75–78, 1997                    12–5

*Introduction.*—Squamous cell carcinoma (SCC) of the orbit is often a slow-growing tumor affecting older patients, but in some areas this type of cancer tends to affect younger individuals and acts in an aggressive manner. Conjunctival SCC is common in Saudi Arabia, and secondary orbital invasion occurs frequently. A retrospective review of 30 consecutive patients aged 19 years or older was conducted to examine factors that may contribute to the aggressive behavior of SCC in this geographic region.

*Methods.*—Patients were admitted to a large ophthalmic hospital in Saudi Arabia from 1983 through 1991. Data recorded were patient age, sex, laterality of the tumor, duration of symptoms, clinical findings, histopathologic features, and outcome. Of 51 patients with secondary orbital tumors, 30 were found to have SCC and 28 of these had tumors of conjunctival origin. These patients, 16 men and 14 women, ranged in age from 38 to 80 years (mean age, 65 years). Nineteen patients were available for follow-up (mean, 21 months).

*Results.*—The right orbit was involved in 15 of 28 cases and the left orbit in 13. Although the mean duration of symptoms was 6 months, 75% of patients had a duration of more than 6 months. In 22 cases, the tumor was localized inside the orbit only; 4 patients had both intraocular extension and orbital invasion at the initial visit. Twenty-two patients had orbital exenteration, with or without radiation therapy, and 6 were referred for more extensive surgery because of regional lymph node involvement. Three patients had another primary neoplasm elsewhere in the body (a primary carcinoma of the lung, a primary hepatoma, and a basal cell carcinoma of the contralateral lower eyelid). Seven patients (23%) died of their disease.

*Discussion.*—Most cases of orbital SCC are secondary tumors resulting from direct tumor extension from adjacent structures. In contrast to reports from the United States, where most secondary SCC extends to the orbit from the paranasal sinuses or eyelid skin, the most common cause of secondary orbital tumor invasion in Saudi patients was conjunctival SCC. Because of prolonged exposure to ultraviolet radiation, chronic irritation from sandstorms, and the high prevalence of trachoma, conjunctival SCC is a common disease in Saudi Arabia. Genetic factors may also be involved.

▶ Most of the orbital tumors found in this Saudi Arabian study were the result of direct extension from SCCs of the eyelids. Having spent some "quality" time in the Arabian desert during the Gulf War, I know that the conditions there are very similar to those of the Southwestern United States (including south Texas). Those of us who practice in these environments need to provide patient education as to the risks to vision from untreated eyelid cancers, and we need to be prepared to develop screening clinics, if appropriate. Primary care physicians need to be reminded by us—the ophthalmologists, the dermatologists, and the plastic surgeons—on the importance of identifying suspicious lesions.

**G.R. Holt, M.D., M.S.E., M.P.H.**

---

**Cancer of the Tongue in Patients Younger Than 40 Years: A Distinct Entity?**

Atula S, Grénman R, Laippala P, et al (Turku Univ, Finland; Univ of Tampere, Finland)

*Arch Otolaryngol Head Neck Surg* 122:1313–1319, 1996          12–6

---

*Introduction.*—Oral cancer has been primarily a disease of older men who have been smokers, but the incidence is increasing among individuals younger than 40 years who have never smoked or consumed alcohol excessively. Some reports suggest that oral cancer behaves more aggressively in younger patients. Records of 34 patients aged under 40 years were reviewed to assess the clinical and biological behavior of tongue cancer in this age group.

*Methods.*—The study group included all patients younger than 40 years who had a squamous cell carcinoma of the tongue diagnosed in Finland from 1980 through 1989. All but 1 of the original paraffin-embedded specimens obtained before therapy were available for analysis. Smoking habits were reported for 24 patients, 11 of whom were heavy smokers. Alcohol consumption was known in 18 patients: 16 were social drinkers and 2 were heavy consumers. Eighteen patients had neck dissection, 24 underwent radiotherapy, and 5 received chemotherapy. Immunocytochemical staining was used to assess the expression of p53 and bcl-2 proteins; *p53* mutation analysis was performed by means of the nonradioactive single-strand conformation polymorphism technique.

*Results.*—The number of cases of tongue cancer in young adults increased from 302 cases between 1953 and 1962 to 585 cases between 1983 and 1992. During the period of this study (1980–1989) the number of younger patients fluctuated from 1 to 6 per year. Overall 5-year survival in the study population was 70.6%, indicating that tongue cancer was not more aggressive in patients younger than 40 years compared with those older than 60 years. Seventeen tumors (51.5%) were found to have *p53* mutations, and approximately one third of samples had strong or moderate p53 and bcl-2 protein expression. An association between intense p53 protein expression and larger tumor size was noted. Patients whose tumors exceeded 4 cm in diameter and those with moderately or poorly differentiated cancer had the poorest prognosis. There was a tendency toward shorter survival for an interaction between tumor grade and *p53* mutations.

*Conclusion.*—Patients younger than 40 years did not differ substantially from older patients with cancer of the tongue in clinical course, prognosis, and function of *p53*. Mutations of *p53* may be a molecular prognostic marker for identification of high-risk patients.

▶ The more I hear about the prognostication capability of the *p53* marker, the more it seems to provide important information. This article surprised me, because I have previously believed that those young people who have oral cancer have a real defect in their immune surveillance systems and a worse prognosis than older adults. At least in Finland, this did not hold to be true. I hope these investigators and others will continue to pursue the *p53* mutation, not only in high-risk groups but also in those lower-risk groups (nonsmokers, nondrinkers) who seem to have aggressive tumors in spite of their otherwise good health.

**G.R. Holt, M.D., M.S.E., M.P.H.**

## Preoperative Parathyroid Localization With Sestamibi

Malhotra A, Silver CE, Deshpande V, et al (Albert Einstein College of Medicine, Bronx, NY)
*Am J Surg* 172:637–640, 1996                    12–7

*Introduction.*—Initial parathyroid surgery, when performed by an experienced surgeon, achieves a high rate of success (95%) without preoperative localization studies. But before reoperation in cases of failed initial exploration or recurrent disease, a sensitive noninvasive method of localization would be invaluable. Patients in this study underwent preoperative parathyroid localization with $^{99m}$Tc-labeled sestamibi.

*Methods.*—Between November 1993 and September 1995, 51 patients underwent surgery for hyperparathyroidism at the study institution. Forty-four were surgically treated for the first time and 7 underwent re-exploration for recurrent or persistent disease. Preoperative scintigraphy with sestamibi was performed in all cases before surgical exploration. Double radionuclide studies were used when the single study failed to localize a parathyroid lesion. In several cases single photon emission CT (SPECT) provided a useful adjunct to the sestamibi technique. The results of radionuclide studies were compared with surgical and pathologic findings.

*Results.*—Solitary adenomas were present in 26 patients, and all 26 lesions were localized preoperatively with sestamibi scanning. Sixty-nine pathologic glands were found at surgery in the 18 patients with multiglandular pathology. The scans localized 36 of these glands in 15 patients; there were no false positives. Six of 7 pathologic glands found at surgery in patients undergoing re-exploration were correctly localized by the scan. Sestamibi scanning also accurately localized ectopic lesions in 2 patients.

*Conclusion.*—Sestamibi scanning offers a reliable, noninvasive test for localizing hyperfunctioning parathyroid glands. Sensitivity was 100% and positive predictive value was 92.8% in the group of patients with solitary adenomas. Among those with multiglandular pathology, sensitivity for individual enlarged glands was 52% and positive predictive value was 100%. Both the sensitivity and positive predictive value of sestamibi scanning were 71% in patients undergoing re-exploration. Overall, the sensitivity of sestamibi scanning was superior to that of other noninvasive means of localization.

▶ Although many otolaryngologists do not perform parathyroid surgery, those who do will appreciate this study and the suggestion that the task is made easier by preoperative identification of the adenomas with sestamibi. The authors' best returns were in those patients with solitary adenomas and those who had failed an earlier exploration. This type of scan may take much of the "educated" and expensive "guesswork" out of identifying these adenomas. The risks for the nuclear scan appear to be minimal.

**G.R. Holt, M.D., M.S.E., M.P.H.**

## Growth Patterns of Piriform Sinus Carcinomas

Zbären P, Egger C (Univ of Bern, Switzerland)
*Laryngoscope* 107:511–518, 1997
                                                                12–8

*Introduction.*—Many surgeons now treat piriform sinus carcinomas by classic conservation surgery or endoscopic laser surgery rather than by more radical techniques. This trend has been influenced by advances in functional surgery and the knowledge that these tumors have a poor prognosis independent of local control. To define criteria for appropriate application of voice preservation surgery, investigators analyzed patterns of tumor spread to laryngeal and parapharyngeal structures.

*Methods.*—Forty-two surgical specimens were obtained from patients who had undergone primary surgical resection for piriform sinus or post-cricoid carcinoma. The hypopharyngeal carcinomas were divided into 3 groups: tumors occupying mainly the lateral wall (group A, 6 cases); tumors occupying the medial wall with or without postcricoid involve-ment (group B, 16 cases); and extensive tumors occupying both lateral and medial walls (group C, 20 cases).

*Results.*—Because group A tumors tended to extend laterally beyond the thyroid ala, rarely infiltrating the intrinsic laryngeal muscles, conservation surgery was possible in many cases (even in T4 carcinomas). In contrast, carcinomas confined to the medial wall or occupying the whole piriform sinus tended to infiltrate laryngeal structures early. In these groups, 61% of tumors exhibited hemilaryngeal fixation and 64% had tumor spread to the contralateral side. Invasion of the intrinsic laryngeal muscle was the cause of hemilarynx fixation. There were no instances of isolated perineural or cricoarytenoid joint involvement. Tumor spread in group B indicated that conservation surgery is inadequate in most cases, even T2 carcinomas. Similarly, group C tumors had histologic extension patterns of both groups A and B and were rarely candidates for conservation surgery.

*Conclusion.*—Despite the potential benefits of functional surgery, most piriform sinus carcinomas exhibit a growth pattern that makes conserva-tion techniques inadequate. Conservation surgery may be possible in cases in which tumors are confined to the lateral wall.

▶ The findings presented in this article coincide with the common sense and experiential understanding that the location of the piriform sinus carcin-omas will affect their invasion course and subsequent areas of surgical resection. In my own experience, the lateral cancers tend to metastasize sooner or grow directly into the lateral neck; the larynx can often be pre-served, but the hypopharynx and/or esophagus may need reconstruction. Those that directly infiltrate the larynx are, in my opinion, best treated with a total laryngectomy with partial pharyngectomy. If the tumor extends to involvement of the cricopharyngeus and inferior constrictor muscles, a gas-tric pullup or colon interposition is usually required.

**G.R. Holt, M.D., M.S.E., M.P.H.**

## CT Surveillance of the Thorax in Patients With Squamous Cell Carcinoma of the Head and Neck: A Preliminary Experience

Mercader VP, Gatenby RA, Mohr RM, et al (Temple Univ, Philadelphia; MetroHealth Med Ctr, Cleveland, Ohio)
*J Comput Assist Tomogr* 21:412–417, 1997                    12–9

*Introduction.*—Patients with squamous cell carcinoma (SCC) of the head and neck have an increased incidence of second primary malignancies and should undergo careful examination of the chest. Because there is no consensus concerning the method of surveillance after diagnosis and treatment of head and neck SCC, investigators sought to determine the number of malignancies detected by chest CT at various stages in the disease process.

*Methods.*—The retrospective analysis included 168 CT scans of the thorax performed in 93 patients with biopsy-proven SCC of the neck. Most had stage III or IV disease. All patients were under the care of a single otorhinolaryngologist who obtained the scans in 3 specific clinical settings: at the time of diagnosis of the primary neck tumor (57 patients), at yearly intervals after treatment of the primary cancer (93 examinations in 43 patients), and when there was clinical evidence of local or regional recurrence (18 patients). The CT scans were reviewed by an examiner blinded to the results of the CT examinations, chest radiographs, endoscopic findings, and pathologic determinations.

*Results.*—The CT scans obtained at diagnosis identified additional malignancies in 9 of 46 patients with stage III or IV primary neck SCC; none were detected in the 11 patients with stage I or II disease. During routine follow-up, 9 malignancies were found on thoracic CT scans of 39 patients, all with initial stage III or IV disease. Four of these malignancies were detected within the first year and 3 in the second year after diagnosis. Examination of the 18 patients with local or regional neck recurrence yielded 6 chest tumors, 4 in the 12 patients with initial stage III or IV SCCA of the head and neck and 2 in the 6 patients with initial stage I or II disease.

*Discussion.*—Chest CT, performed at diagnosis and during follow-up, identifies a large number of additional chest malignancies in patients with advanced SCC of the head and neck. Early detection offers an opportunity for cure of both the neck and thoracic cancers and may spare some patients extensive, mutilating surgery when an incurable thoracic malignancy is found. Regardless of the initial stage, patients with locally recurrent tumor have a very high number of intrathoracic malignancies.

▶ The number of positive identifications of metastases or second primaries through CT chest screening in patients with SCC of the head and neck appears to justify its use. It seems that chest radiographs (posteroanterior and lateral) will demonstrate fairly macroscopic lesions, whereas the fine-cut CT imaging is getting better and better through improved technology and software. Although we do not, in general, subscribe to the routine use of bronchoscopy in staging, CT surveillance could direct us to do so when a suspicious lesion is shown. Cost effectiveness needs to be looked at here.

**G.R. Holt, M.D., M.S.E., M.P.H.**

**Markers for Assessment of Nodal Metastasis in Laryngeal Carcinoma**
Takes RP, Baatenburg de Jong RJ, Schuuring E, et al (Univ Hosp Leiden, The Netherlands)
*Arch Otolaryngol Head Neck Surg* 123:412–419, 1997        12–10

*Introduction.*—Regional metastasis determines treatment and prognosis in patients with head and neck squamous cell carcinoma. Current imaging techniques are not adequate and US-guided fine-needle aspiration biopsy has a sensitivity of only 76%. Results of histologic, immunohistochemical, and molecular biological analysis were correlated with clinical and histopathologic data to determine whether biological markers could be identified that could predict the presence of metastases, based on features of the primary tumor, in 31 patients with laryngeal carcinoma.

*Methods.*—Several histologic features and biological markers were analyzed. These markers were used because of their putative role in the process of metastasis and were analyzed by immunohistochemical and/or Southern blot techniques: proliferating cell nuclear antigen, *p53*, retinoblastoma tumor-suppressor gene (*Rb*), *myc*, *bcl-2* (inhibitor of apoptosis), epidermal growth factor (*EGF*), *EGF*-receptor, *neu*, *nm23* (also known as *NME1*, putative metastasis suppressor), *desmoplakin*, neuron cell-adhesion molecule (*N-CAM*), epithelial cell-adhesion molecule (*Ep-CAM*), E-*cadherin*, cyclin D1 (*CCND1*), and *EMS1*.

*Results.*—Nodal metastasis was correlated with the presence of an inflammatory reaction surrounding the tumor, eosinophilic infiltration, positive immunostaining for *Rb*, negative immunostaining for *Ep-CAM*, and amplification of *CCND1* and *EMS1*. There were no correlations between differentiation and growth pattern and lymph node metastasis. No correlation was determined between *p53*, *E-cadherin*, *EGF*, *nm23*, *desmoplakin*, or *N-CAM* staining and the presence of lymph node metastasis.

*Conclusion.*—It is feasible to predict and exclude lymph node metastasis by evaluating the features of the primary tumor only. Use of immunohistochemical staining was easy, quick, and cost-effective in evaluating the markers analyzed in this trial.

▶ The authors report their preliminary data in identifying a series of biological or chemical markers found on the primary tumor that may indicate the risk or possibility for nodal metastases. I do feel that fine imaging sections of the neck can identify all but the smallest of nodal metastases, and this may improve in the future. However, identifying histologic markers on primary tumor biopsy specimens would be a major step forward in assisting our developing a therapeutic plan for each individual patient—much like estrogen receptors in breast tumors do for the oncologist.

**G.R. Holt, M.D., M.S.E., M.P.H.**

---

**Surgical Salvage After Radiotherapy for Advanced Laryngopharyngeal Carcinoma**
Davidson J, Keane T, Brown D, et al (Univ of Toronto; Princess Margaret Hosp, Toronto)
*Arch Otolaryngol Head Neck Surg* 123:420–424, 1997                    12–11

---

*Objective.*—Patients with advanced laryngopharyngeal carcinoma are generally treated with primary radiotherapy to preserve the function of the laryngopharyngeal complex. Surgery is used only if needed for salvage. The results of patients undergoing surgery after failure of radiotherapy for advanced laryngopharyngeal carcinoma were evaluated.

*Methods.*—Three hundred thirty-six patients with T3 or T4 or N+ laryngopharyngeal carcinoma were entered into a randomized clinical trial. One group received standard fractional radiotherapy, 51 Gy in 20 fractions, while the other group received hyperfractionation radiotherapy, 58 Gy twice daily in 40 fractions. Salvage surgery was performed as required for recurrent disease. The patients were followed up prospectively for complications, tumor recurrences, and survival.

*Results.*—Of 191 patients in whom primary radiotherapy failed, 163 had local or regional tumor recurrence. Salvage surgery was performed in 108 of these patients. The remaining 55 patients did not have surgery because of unresectable disease, patient refusal, medical contraindications, or death from other causes. Sixty-one patients underwent total laryngectomy and 1 had partial laryngectomy. The surgical complication rate was 27%, with considerable variation by site. The complication rate was 6% for patients having neck dissection only, 15% for those having surgery at the primary site only, and 40% for those having surgery at both sites. Actuarial survival for patients undergoing surgical salvage was 37% at 3 years and 18% at 5 years. Of 25 patients with positive resection margins, none were alive at 3 years.

*Summary.*—As in previous reports, the surgical complication rate of surgical salvage after failure of primary radiotherapy for advanced laryngopharyngeal carcinoma was high, especially in patients undergoing more complex procedures. Positive resection margins were observed in one fourth of patients undergoing surgery for recurrence at the primary tumor site.

▶ The topic of surgical salvage after radiation failures for advanced head and neck disease has been debated for a long time. The corollary question is—should patients be selected for radiation therapy only on the basis of data such as is presented here, which suggests that surgical salvage is feasible? As more clinicians write about laryngeal preservation protocols, we must look not only at survival rates but also quality-of-life issues ("Is having an intact larynx in the face of recurrent disease better or worse than no larynx and recurrent disease?"). The patient *must* understand the goals, risks, and uncertainties in laryngeal preservation protocols.

**G.R. Holt, M.D., M.S.E., M.P.H.**

---

**Concomitant Pilocarpine During Head and Neck Irradiation Is Associated With Decreased Posttreatment Xerostomia**

Zimmerman RP, Mark RJ, Tran LM, et al (Univ of California, Los Angeles)
*Int J Radiat Oncol Biol Phys* 37:571–575, 1997                    12–12

---

*Background.*—Patients who have undergone radiation therapy for head and neck cancer may experience xerostomia. In addition to oral dryness and discomfort, patients report problems with mastication, speech, and sleep and are at high risk for the development of dental caries and periodontal disease. Two recent trials showed pilocarpine hydrochloride to be effective in reducing the symptoms of radiation-induced xerostomia when administered beginning at least 4 months after the conclusion of radiotherapy. This retrospective study compared patients who received pilocarpine from the first day of radiotherapy until 3 months after the completion of radiotherapy with patients not given pilocarpine.

*Methods.*—Twenty-two consecutive patients, each of whom had both parotid glands treated to a dose of at least 45 Gy, were treated with pilocarpine (5 mg 4 times a day). The 18 patients who did not receive pilocarpine also had parotid glands treated to a dose 45 Gy or more. Patient charts were reviewed for primary tumor site, radiotherapy ports, and prescribed tumor dose, and patients completed a xerostomia questionnaire using a visual analogue scale.

*Results.*—Seventeen patients treated with concomitant pilocarpine and 18 who did not receive the treatment were available for follow-up. The mean interval between completion of radiation and evaluation of xerostomia was 17 months for the pilocarpine group and 16 months for the no pilocarpine group. The 2 groups were also similar in mean total prescribed tumor dose, tumor site, and other noted variables. Patients treated with concomitant pilocarpine had significantly less subjective complaints of oral dryness; discomfort; and difficulty with speech, sleep, and eating. The overall xerostomia score was also significantly less in the pilocarpine-treated group than in the other group.

*Conclusion.*—Pilocarpine taken after head and neck radiotherapy reduces xerostomia by stimulating the major salivary glands through its cholinergic parasympathomimetic action. Oral pilocarpine should be taken during and for 3 months after radiotherapy; longer-term administration was required in only 1 patient in this series.

▶ Although this is a preliminary report on a retrospective study, I was heartened by the improvement in salivation in patients treated with pilocarpine. Why it works, I don't know, but I do know that dry mouth is one of the most bothersome side effects of radiation therapy according to patients. I am hopeful that the authors' double-blind study is underway and will soon be reported.

**G.R. Holt, M.D., M.S.E., M.P.H.**

**Detailed Quality of Life Assessment in Patients Treated With Primary Radiotherapy for Squamous Cell Cancer of the Base of the Tongue**
Harrison LB, Zelefsky MJ, Pfister DG, et al (Mem Sloan-Kettering Cancer Ctr, New York)
*Head Neck* 19:169–175, 1997                                    12–13

*Purpose.*—There is a new emphasis on measuring the quality-of-life (QOL) effects of alternative treatments for head and neck cancer. In patients with cancer of the base of the tongue, primary radiotherapy and surgery both offer a high cure rate. Because it preserves the tongue, radiotherapy would be expected to have functional as well as QOL advantages; however, there is some morbidity associated with radiotherapy. A detailed QOL analysis of patients undergoing primary radiotherapy for cancer of the base of the tongue was done.

*Patients.*—The study included 36 patients with primary squamous cell carcinoma of the base of the tongue. Disease stage was T1 in 11 patients, T2 in 14, T3 in 10, and T4 in 1. Eighty-six percent of the patients had palpable cervical lymph node metastases at presentation. All received primary radiotherapy, consisting of external beam radiotherapy to the primary tumor site and neck and a brachytherapy boost to the tongue. Neck dissection was performed in those with positive lymph nodes. At a median follow-up of 5 years, actuarial 5-year local control was 85%, regional control was 96%, survival with freedom from distant metastases was 87.5%, and overall survival was 85%.

*Methods.*—A detailed QOL assessment was performed in 29 of 30 long-term survivors. This assessment included the Memorial Symptom Assessment Scale (MSAS), Functional Assessment of Cancer Therapy, Performance Status Scale for Head and Neck Cancer, and sociodemographic and economic assessment. When their cancer was diagnosed, 62% of patients were employed full time, 21% were employed part time, 83% had annual incomes of more than $20,000, and 59% had incomes of more than $60,000.

*Results.*—There were few differences in annual income at follow-up. Seventy-two percent of the patients who had been working full-time and 83% of those who had been working part-time were still doing so. Performance scores were high for eating in public and understandability in speech, and reasonably good for normalcy of diet. Sixty-nine percent of patients had a Karnofsky Performance Scale score of 100, indicating no impairment (Table 2). Frequent symptoms on the MSAS included xerostomia, difficulty in swallowing, decreased energy, pain, worrying, insom-

**TABLE 2.**—Performance Status Scale for Patients With Head and Neck Cancer

| | |
|---|---|
| **Eating in public** | |
| 100 | No restriction of place, food, or companion (eats out at any opportunity) |
| 75 | No restriction of place, but restricts diet when in public (eats anywhere, but may limit intake to less "messy" foods, eg, liquids) |
| 50 | Eats only in presence of selected persons in selected places |
| 25 | Eats only at home in presence of selected persons |
| 0 | Always eats alone |
| **Understandability of speech** | |
| 100 | Always understandable |
| 75 | Understandable most of the time; occasional repetition necessary |
| 50 | Usually understandable, face-to-face contact necessary |
| 25 | Difficult to understand |
| 0 | Never understandable; may use written communication |
| **Normalcy of diet** | |
| 100 | Full diet (no restrictions) |
| 90 | Peanuts |
| 80 | All meats |
| 70 | Carrots, celery |
| 60 | Dry bread and crackers |
| 50 | Soft, chewable foods (eg, macaroni, canned/soft fruits, cooked vegetables, fish, hamburger, small pieces of meat) |
| 40 | Soft foods requiring no chewing (eg, mashed potato, applesauce, pudding) |
| 30 | Pureed foods (in blender) |
| 20 | Warm liquids |
| 10 | Cold liquids |

(From Harrison LB, Zelefsky MJ, Pfister DG, et al: Detailed quality of life assessment in patients treated with primary radiotherapy for squamous cell cancer of the base of the tongue. *Head Neck* 19:169–175, 1997. Courtesy of List M, Ritter-Sterr C, Lansky S: A performance scale for head and neck cancer patients. *Cancer* 66:564–569, copyright © 1990 American Cancer Society. Reprinted by permission of Wiley-Liss Inc., a subsidiary of John Wiley & Sons, Inc.)

nia, cough, drowsiness, alterations of taste, and irritability (Table 3). Scores of the functional assessment were better than those reported in a cancer population with mixed tumor types.

*Conclusion.*—Patients treated with primary radiotherapy for squamous cell cancer of the base of the tongue have excellent functional status and quality of life at follow-up. Outcome includes preservation of their preillness earning potential and employment status. The findings demonstrate the importance of performing QOL analyses of treatments for head and neck cancer.

▶ Although the authors report excellent 5-year data, they referred to the study patients as having "advanced" disease of the base of the tongue—I could not find a breakout of the lower stages vs. higher stages as far as those 29 long-term survivors are concerned. Did most of them have lower stage cancers? At any rate, I was impressed with the functional status of their patients according to their QOL test battery. Preservation of the

**TABLE 3.**—Memorial Symptom Assessment Scale (MSAS): Prevalent
Symptoms and Degree of Distress

| Symptom | Percentage of patients who report symptom prevalent in their life (%) | Percentage with symptom who report moderate to severe distress from symptom (%) |
|---|---|---|
| Xerostomia | 100 | 89 |
| Difficulty swallowing | 76 | 90 |
| Decreased energy | 48 | 64 |
| Pain | 43 | 89 |
| Worrying | 38 | 63 |
| Insomnia | 41 | 78 |
| Cough | 36 | 38 |
| Drowsiness | 34 | 25 |
| Change in Taste | 34 | 70 |
| Irritability | 31 | 57 |

(From Harrison LB, Zelefsky MJ, Pfister DG, et al: Detailed quality of life assessment in patients treated with primary radiotherapy for squamous cell cancer of the base of the tongue. *Head Neck* 19:169–175, copyright © 1997 John Wiley & Sons, Inc. Reprinted by permission of John Wiley & Sons, Inc.)

larynx and base of tongue is a godsend for these patients, and protocols such as this are clearly headed in the right direction. We all *must* pay attention to QOL as a strong decision parameter for the patient's selection of therapy.

**G.R. Holt, M.D., M.S.E., M.P.H.**

## Postoperative Radiation of Open Head and Neck Wounds: Updated
Isaacs JH Jr, Stiles WA, Cassisi NJ, et al (Univ of Florida, Jacksonville; Univ of Florida, Gainesville)
*Head Neck* 19:194–199, 1997                                    12–14

*Introduction.*—When postoperative radiation rather than preoperative radiation is used, surgical complication rates are lower or less serious when operating for head and neck cancer. If a problem develops with postoperative wound healing, a major concern is the delay in irradiation. It is recommended that irradiation begin within as short a period as possible after surgery. The authors' study in 1987 is the only study that reviewed the use of radiotherapy on an open postoperative wound in humans. This retrospective study updates their prior series.

*Methods.*—A total of 462 patients had postoperative radiotherapy within a 13-year period; of these, 33 had unhealed wounds when irradiation began. Their average age at time of surgery was 57 years. Twenty-eight were men and 5 were women, and they were followed up at least 24 months. Histopathologic findings were used to base the decision to begin irradiation therapy with an open wound. The analysis included the type of postoperative wound and the use of surgical closure. An average of 67 Gy was given to each patient.

*Results.*—The wounds healed spontaneously in 22 of 33 patients (67%) within a mean of 98 days. After surgical closure, 5 more patients achieved successful wound healing within a mean of 281 days. Four patients died before healing was complete, and 2 were lost to follow-up before wound healing occurred. No evidence of disease was found in 9 patients who are alive. Five patients died of other causes and 19 died of cancer.

*Conclusion.*—It is desirable to initiate treatment within 6 weeks of the date of surgery when there are indications to deliver irradiation in the postoperative setting. When it is anticipated that healing time will be prolonged, some consideration must be given to initiating irradiation in the face of incompletely closed wounds, although it is preferable to have completely closed operative wounds before irradiation. The wounds will stabilize or will continue to heal during the course of irradiation in some patients. After irradiation is completed, the wound can be surgically managed or it may spontaneously heal after treatment. Excessive delays in beginning appropriate cancer therapy may lead to recurrence before irradiation. These recurrences are rarely successfully treated.

▶ The authors address a difficult topic—namely, balancing the need for timely radiation therapy to reduce the risk of recurrence, and the desire to have a surgical wound close for the convenience of patient care and to avoid having to reoperate on irradiated tissue. Although this is a reasonably sized series, 6 patients died before healing was complete, so we do not know what their outcome might have been. I guess it boils down to individualizing the decision for each patient, *with* the patient's *full* understanding of the issues and choices.

**G.R. Holt, M.D., M.S.E., M.P.H.**

---

**Role of Interstitial Brachytherapy in Oral and Oropharyngeal Carcinoma: Reflection of a Series of 1344 Patients Treated at the Time of Initial Presentation**
Pernot M, Hoffstetter S, Peiffert D, et al (Centre Alexis Vautrin, Vandoeuvre Les Nancy, France)
*Otolaryngol Head Neck Surg* 115:519–526, 1996                    12–15

---

*Introduction.*—Brachytherapy has often been used in the treatment of oral and oropharyngeal carcinoma, but advances in plastic surgery, anesthesia, and external-beam irradiation have expanded treatment options for the disease. Current applications of brachytherapy using low-dose $^{192}$Ir were reported.

*Methods.*—Between 1973 and 1992, 1,344 cases of carcinoma of the oral cavity and oropharynx were treated with brachytherapy at the study institution. Methods for treatment of primary lesions included external radiotherapy, complementary brachytherapy after external irradiation, complementary brachytherapy after surgery, and brachytherapy alone. Techniques reported for treatment of the oral cavity varied according to site: mobile tongue, floor of mouth, postoperative brachytherapy for patients with positive or narrow margins after surgery (using the modified bridge technique for lesions located in the mandible), and buccal mucosa. Techniques for treatment of the oropharynx were directed to the base of the tongue and to the faucial arch, soft palate, and tonsillar area. Neck dissection had been used since 1980 for tumors of the oral cavity of more than 1.5 cm when the primary lesion was treated by brachytherapy only.

*Results.*—Local control rates and overall survival rates for 565 cases of mobile tongue at 5 years were, respectively, 92% and 70% for T1 disease, 62% and 42% for T2, and 50% and 29% for T3. For the 207 cases of floor-of-mouth carcinoma, local control and overall survival rates at 5 years were, respectively, 97% and 71% for T1 disease, 72% and 42% for T2, and 51% and 35% for T3. The T3T4 patients were not considered surgical candidates. There were only 42 cases of carcinomas of the buccal mucosa; the overall survival rate in this group was 48%. The overall survival rate in the group of 72 patients with epidermoid cancers of the base of the tongue was 44%.

The loop technique of brachytherapy combined with external-beam irradiation was used for 361 patients with carcinomas of the tonsil, soft palate, and pillars. Local control rates were 84% and 65%, respectively, for tonsil, soft palate, and posterior pillar carcinomas and for carcinomas of the anterior pillar and the pharyngoglossal sulcus. Overall survival rates in these groups were 57% and 38%, respectively. Minor complications occurred in approximately 20% of patients and severe complications in approximately 5%. The risk of complications was increased by tumor location near the mandible, a total irradiation dose of more than 80 Gy, a dose of more than 0.7 Gy/hr, a treated volume greater than 30 mL, and no leaded protection of the mandible.

*Conclusion.*—Brachytherapy still has many advantages in the treatment of head and neck cancers. High doses can be delivered to small volumes, the dose can be rapidly decreased at the periphery of the treatment volume, and leaded protection of the mandible is possible.

▶ The authors report on an extensive series of patients who have been treated with interstitial brachytherapy "boosts" to tumors present after external beam irradiation or positive margins after radiation and surgery. Not all radiation oncologists in the United States use these implants, so it is wise for you to discuss this with their own therapists. I wasn't sure what the authors meant when they stated that the T3T4 patients were not considered surgical candidates. Such floor-of-mouth tumors can be operated on, but many surgeons in the United States will look toward induction chemotherapy and radiation therapy before deciding upon a surgical procedure. A mandibulectomy of some sort with reconstruction is usually required.

**G.R. Holt, M.D., M.S.E., M.P.H.**

**Endovascular Management of Hemorrhage in Patients With Head and Neck Cancer**
Morrissey DD, Andersen PE, Nesbit GM, et al (Oregon Health Sciences Univ, Portland)
*Arch Otolaryngol Head Neck Surg* 123:15–19, 1997                    12–16

*Introduction.*—Hemorrhage in patients with head and neck squamous cell carcinoma has traditionally been managed with surgical exploration and ligation of the involved vessel. Endovascular embolization may provide selected patients with the advantages of decreased morbidity and reduced length of hospital stay, with equal or greater efficacy than open surgical ligation. A retrospective review of 12 patients with squamous cell carcinoma of the head and neck confirmed the benefits of endovascular management of hemorrhage.

*Methods.*—The patients, 9 men and 3 women, were treated with angiography and selective embolization for 13 episodes of hemorrhage. Eleven had previously undergone surgery and 7 were treated with preoperative irradiation. Charts were reviewed for diagnosis, stage, factors contributing to hemorrhage, bleeding site, treatment, and outcome.

*Results.*—Causes of hemorrhage included recurrent tumor in 5 patients, pharyngocutaneous fistula in 4, radiation necrosis in 3, and postoperative complication in 1. Vessels involved were the external carotid artery or its branches in 8 cases, the common carotid artery in 4, and the internal jugular vein in 1. Endovascular embolization successfully controlled hemorrhage in all patients, and there were no recurrences of bleeding. In 1 patient, a permanent left-sided hemiplegia and facial weakness developed after emergent occlusion of the right common, internal, and external carotid arteries. The hospital stay from embolization averaged 7.6 days. At follow-ups ranging from 6 months to 4.5 years, 4 patients had died of disease and 2 had died of unrelated or unknown causes; 2 patients are alive with disease and 4 are alive without evidence of disease.

*Conclusion.*—Angiography followed by embolization successfully stopped hemorrhage in all 13 cases reported here, and no patient experienced recurrent bleeding. This technique offers an effective, safe, and fast alternative to surgical ligation.

▶ Interventional radiology for hemorrhage works if there is time to get the radiologist into the hospital, get the angiography team ready, and get the patient to the embolization suite. Unfortunately, some bleeds will be so precipitous that there isn't time for an embolization—the patient must go to the operating room *right then*. However, this embolization technology is quite helpful for the right patient and should be used when indicated. Having an agreed-to protocol with the radiologist/technical team will reduce the response time and allow for the management of more time-sensitive cases.

**G.R. Holt, M.D., M.S.E., M.P.H.**

## Selective Neck Dissection and the Management of the Node-positive Neck

Traynor SJ, Cohen JI, Gray J, et al (Oregon Health Sciences Univ, Portland)
*Am J Surg* 172:654–657, 1996                                    12–17

*Introduction.*—With an increased emphasis on improved postoperative function and cosmesis in the treatment of head and neck cancer, surgeons have investigated means of modifying the radical neck dissection (RND). The use of selective neck dissection (SND) is controversial, however, in patients with clinical and histologic evidence of metastatic neck disease. The cases of 29 patients who underwent 36 SNDs were reviewed to determine the oncologic effectiveness of this technique.

*Methods.*—Patients in the study group had undergone an SND at a single tertiary care referral center. All had newly diagnosed upper aerodigestive tract squamous cell carcinoma and both clinically and pathologically proven regional metastases. Site of the primary tumor determined the type of SND performed. Mobile nodes were required for study entry; thus, most patients were staged N2 and nodes were less than 3 cm. Minimum follow-up was 2 years (median 3 years).

*Results.*—Patients were 23 men and 6 women with an average age of 59 years. Primary site locations were the oral cavity in 9 cases, the oropharynx in 8, the larynx in 8, and the hypopharynx in 4. Primary site staging was T3 or T4 in 24 of 29 patients. Nodal staging was N1 in 11 patients, N2A in 1, N2B in 8, and N2C in 9. Unilateral SND was performed in 22 patients and bilateral SND in 7. Postoperative radiation to the neck was administered to 20 patients. Overall actuarial disease-specific survival at 4 years was 47%: 67% in N1 cases and 42% in N2 cases. The 4-year actuarial local recurrence and distant failure rates were 36% each; there was only 1 case of neck recurrence (4%).

*Discussion.*—In patients with head and neck cancer and a clinically negative neck, SND offers treatment results and staging information comparable with those obtained with RND. The patients reviewed here would traditionally be managed surgically with RND. Increased knowledge of the cervical drainage pattern allows selected patients with clinically and histologically apparent regional metastases to be managed successfully with less extensive neck dissection.

► The efficacy of SND in the positive neck depends a great deal on the precise identification of nodal disease on fine-cut CT imaging. The patient should be counseled that the decision to perform an RND may be made at the time of surgery and that the patient must consent preoperatively.

**G.R. Holt, M.D., M.S.E., M.P.H.**

## Supraomohyoid Neck Dissection

Spiro RH, Morgan GJ, Strong EW, et al (Mem Sloan-Kettering Cancer Ctr, New York)
*Am J Surg* 172:650–653, 1996

12–18

*Introduction.*—In a previous report, the authors present their experience with supraomohyoid neck dissection (SOHND) in patients treated for squamous cell carcinoma (SCC). This technique has grown in importance as a staging lymphadenectomy in patients with $N_0$ oral and oropharyngeal SCC, and it is also used as a potentially curative procedure in selected patients with limited metastatic disease in the neck. In this retrospective study, the charts of 287 patients who underwent SOHND are reviewed.

*Methods.*—The patients, 161 men and 126 women, underwent 320 SOHNDs from 1986 through 1993. Their primary tumor site (in 82%) was the oral cavity. Procedures were performed electively in 268 necks judged clinically to be $N_0$ on initial assessment. Fifty-two patients had SOHND as a therapeutic procedure for clinically positive nodes. Twelve patients underwent simultaneous bilateral SOHND. Patients were followed for control of disease in the neck after SOHND; the median follow-up was 38 months.

*Results.*—Occult metastases were confirmed pathologically in 67 (25%) of the 268 necks judged clinically negative. In 18 cases (35%), enlarged nodes in 52 necks considered metastatic were found to be pathologically negative. Neck recurrence was documented in 10 patients (5%) among the 205 proved pathologically negative at dissection. Six of these failures occurred in the 152 patients who did not receive postoperative radiation therapy. Four of 53 dissected necks had tumor recurrence despite radiation therapy. The incidence of neck failure was similar in the subgroup of patients with occult metastases (7%); 3 of 4 patients with neck failure had received postoperative radiation therapy. There were 2 recurrences within the dissected field among the 31 SOHNDs performed for resection of palpable metastases. Overall, 9 of 16 patients with neck recurrence had received postoperative radiation therapy, and 9 recurrences were within the field of SOHND.

*Conclusion.*—A modification of radical neck dissection, SOHND provides a reliable staging procedure in patients with $N_0$ oral or oropharyngeal SCC. In conjunction with postoperative radiation therapy, therapeutic SOHND can effectively control neck metastases in selected patients with limited disease in the upper neck while avoiding the cosmetic deformity and functional disability of conventional radical neck dissection.

▶ I have come to use the SOHND in $N_0$ necks with anterior oral cavity and lip lesions. It helps me stage the disease, as I find it difficult to palpate small nodes in levels I and II under the mandible. This study looked at patients through 1993; since then some advances in CT imaging of the neck have occurred that increase the sensitivity for identifying suspicious nodes. However, I still believe that SOHND adds little morbidity to the surgical procedure on the primary tumor and gives valuable information.

**G.R. Holt, M.D., M.S.E., M.P.H.**

### Spindle Cell Carcinoma of the Larynx and Hypopharynx

Olsen KD, Lewis JE, Suman VJ (Mayo Clinic and Found, Rochester, Minn)
*Otolaryngol Head Neck Surg* 116:47–52, 1997                    12–19

*Introduction.*—Spindle cell carcinomas, rare and unusual neoplasms of the upper aerodigestive tract, are thought to be epithelial in origin. A recent review of 26 cases confirms this view and supports the neoplastic nature of the spindle cell tumor population. Clinical records of 34 patients with laryngeal (25 patients) or hypopharyngeal (9 patients) spindle cell carcinomas are examined for tumor behavior, treatment results, and prognostic factors.

*Methods.*—The patients were all treated at the Mayo Clinic between 1960 and 1990. Three who were seen for recurrent tumors after an initial operation elsewhere were excluded from the study group. The remaining patients, 25 men and 6 women, had an average age of 64.6 years. Most (96%) were current or past smokers, and 8 had received radiation therapy to the larynx or overlying neck skin in the past. Hoarseness was the most common symptom, affecting 24 patients; 5 had dysphagia and 3 reported pain. A T1 glottic tumor was identified in 16 cases. Two patients had no additional treatment after undergoing biopsy; the remaining patients had various surgical procedures. All spindle cell carcinomas were studied using paraffin section immunostains. Ploidy analysis of the sarcomatoid component was performed in 31 patients.

*Results.*—Patients treated for recurrent tumors were followed for less than 2 years; 1 had died of recurrent tumor. Median follow-up for the 31 patients treated at the Mayo Clinic was 3.7 years. Twelve patients were alive without disease, 8 died of their tumors, 9 died of other causes, and 2 died of unknown causes. Ten of 31 patients had tumor progression or recurrence after the initial therapy. The Kaplan-Meier estimate of survival at least 3 years after the initial treatment was 56.8%. Spindle cells were nondiploid in 86% of carcinomas, and 74% had positive keratin immunostains. Keratin had an adverse effect on the overall survival rate. Patients with laryngeal lesions had better survival rates than patients with hypopharyngeal tumors.

*Conclusion.*—Findings from this study and previous reports support the epithelial origin of spindle cell carcinoma. As is the case with squamous cell carcinoma, the main cause of spindle cell carcinoma appears to be tobacco use. The most important prognostic factors appear to be location, tumor size, and the presence of cervical metastasis.

▶ This article caught my eye because I recently saw my first patient with spindle cell carcinoma of the glottis. After an extensive review of the literature, a colleague and I both recommended conservation laryngeal surgery. The patient refused and, instead, selected radiation therapy. To date he is free of disease, and I hope he has as good an outcome as the 1 patient in this series who was treated with primary radiotherapy. Although this is an unusual tumor, it appears to act more like an epithelial malignancy than a supporting tissue sarcoma.

**G.R. Holt, M.D., M.S.E., M.P.H.**

---

**Familial Papillary Carcinoma of the Thyroid**
Kraimps J-L, Bouin-Pineau M-H, Amati P, et al (Jean Bernard Hosp, Poitiers, France)
*Surgery* 121:715–718, 1997                                                12–20

---

*Introduction.*—Epidemiologic and familial studies suggest that a subset of nonmedullary forms of thyroid cancer may have a genetic basis. The 7 families reported here had at least 2 members with papillary thyroid carcinoma (PTC), supporting the idea of the involvement of a genetic susceptibility.

*Methods.*—Eleven patients from 7 families were among the 105 consecutive patients operated on for PTC at the study institution between 1991 and 1996. An additional 4 relatives with PTC were identified from the same 7 families. A complete pedigree was obtained to at least the second-degree relatives. One family underwent DNA analysis, and linkage analysis was performed to test the *RET* proto-oncogene as a candidate gene for PTC.

*Results.*—The rate of familial PTC (FPTC) was 10.5% in the series of patients operated on during the study period. There were 26 nodular goiters in the 7 families. Twenty-four patients, (mean age 33 years) had undergone operation; 15 had PTC and 9 had multinodular goiters. The PTC group included 10 women and 5 men. Multifocal carcinoma occurred at a higher rate in the 15 patients with FPTC (47%) than in the 94 patients with sporadic PTC (22%) operated on during the same period. None of the patients had a history of cervical irradiation, familial polyposis, or multiple endocrine neoplasia. The DNA analysis of family 1 yielded negative lod scores value and haplotype analysis, excluding *RET* prot-oncogene as a candidate gene for the disease.

*Discussion.*—The familial incidence of PTC in this series of patients was 10.5%, supporting the view that FPTC is a new familial cancer syndrome. Because there may be a relationship between PTC and colon cancer, patients older than 40 years with a family history of PTC should have annual fecal occult blood testing. Case studies in the literature and findings in 4 of these 7 families are consistent with an autosomal dominant trait. The relatives of patients with PTC should be examined to rule out the disease, and total thyroidectomy is recommended because of the frequency of multifocality.

▶ Although the disease is uncommon, the authors present us with convincing evidence that PTC *can* be familial. We should be sensitive to this possibility when treating a patient with PTC and take the time to look into the family history, even if it takes time and phone calls to track down Uncle Henry and Cousin Bob to determine what kind of thyroid tumor they had. Why do this? Because it might allow for an earlier diagnosis of an unsuspected tumor in an at-risk family member.

**G.R. Holt, M.D., M.S.E., M.P.H.**

**Ultrasound-guided 1.2-mm Cutting-needle Biopsies of Head and Neck Tumours**
Elvin A, Sundström C, Larsson SG, et al (Univ Hosp, Uppsala, Sweden)
*Acta Radiol* 38:376–380, 1997                                    12–21

*Background.*—Fine-needle aspiration biopsy has been used for a long time in thyroid nodules, lymph nodes, and tumors in the cervical region. Some lesions in the head and neck are not easily palpable and, therefore, are often unsuitable for unguided needle biopsy techniques. Image-guided techniques can provide high tissue yields without significant complications. Ultrasound is the most common image-guided technique in the head and neck. A biopsy gun provides safe and accurate biopsies for diagnosing tumors in other regions of the body. The safety and efficacy of mid-sized needle biopsy in head and neck tumors were examined.

*Methods.*—During a 5-year period, 74 biopsies were performed in 72 patients with tumors of the head and neck. There were 42 men, 29 women, and 1 girl aged 5 years. A biopsy gun with a 1.2-mm biopsy needle (mid-sized needle biopsy) was used. There were 24 biopsies from the salivary glands, 29 from the lymph nodes, and 21 from various other locations. Thyroid tumors were not included. Mid-sized needle biopsy with US guidance was used in 33 patients after a blinded fine-needle aspiration biopsy did not provide accurate diagnostic material.

*Results.*—In 91% of cases, the mid-sized needle biopsy result and the final diagnosis were identical, and in 9% of cases, mid-sized needle biopsy results were false negative or nonrepresentative. In 17 of 33 patients, mid-sized needle biopsy provided more diagnostic information than fine-needle aspiration biopsy. In 12 of these 17 patients, both methods were equally accurate, and in 4 patients, the information from fine-needle aspiration biopsy was superior to the information from mid-sized needle biopsy. The nondiagnostic sampling rate was 25% for fine-needle aspiration biopsy and 3% for mid-sized needle biopsy. The results of mid-sized needle biopsy were diagnostically correct in 24 of 26 patients with lymphoma, and the results of fine-needle aspiration biopsy were diagnostically correct in 2 of 9 patients with lymphoma. There were no complications related to biopsy.

*Discussion.*—In these patients, mid-sized needle biopsy was safe and had high diagnostic accuracy. When results of fine-needle aspiration biopsy are negative, mid-sized needle biopsy may offer additional diagnostic information. Mid-sized needle biopsy is recommended as the primary diagnostic method in patients with lymphoma.

▶ I recently wanted to perform a fine-needle aspiration of a mass that was located behind the carotid artery. I stewed and fretted over the potential mishap of introducing tumor cells into the carotid circulation by skewering both the tumor and the artery. Perhaps ultrasound (US) could have guided me right to the mass without injury to the artery, vein, or sympathetic plexus. Certainly, when lymphoma is suspected, a larger core-sampling needle can provide more specimen for flow cytometry and alleviate the need for an open biopsy. Perhaps this technique could be considered when the result of fine-needle aspiration is suggestive of, but not diagnostic for lymphoma, before going to an open procedure.

**G.R. Holt, M.D., M.S.E., M.P.H.**

---

**Human Papillomavirus in Head and Neck: Squamous Cell Carcinomas in Nonsmokers**
Fouret P, Monceaux G, Temam S, et al (Hôpital Tenon, Paris)
*Arch Otolaryngol Head Neck Surg* 123:513–516, 1997                    12–22

---

*Background.*—Smoking and alcohol consumption are the most important risk factors for head and neck squamous cell carcinomas (SCCs). Whether infection with oncogenic types of human papillomavirus (HPV) have an independent effect in the head and neck is unknown. The current study determined relationships between smoking and HPV in patients with head and neck SCCs.

*Methods and Findings.*—One hundred eighty-seven consecutive patients with head and neck SCCs were included in the study. Human papillomavirus infection was detected in 10.7%. Such infection was found in 18.6% of patients with oropharyngeal SCCs, compared with only 6.1% in patients with SCCs in other locations. Only 5% of the patients were nonsmokers. These 10 patients had an HPV incidence of 50%, which was significantly greater than the 8.5% incidence among smokers. Nonsmokers appeared to have no occupational risk factors. No *p53* gene mutations were noted in cancer cells.

*Conclusion.*—Human papillomavirus infection may play a role in head and neck SCCs in nonsmoking patients. Though inactivation of the *p53* gene seems to be a common step in the development of HPV-positive and

-negative head and neck SCC, it is not known whether the outcomes between these 2 groups differ.

► This article is not directed toward those cases of viral respiratory papillomatosis that undergo malignant transformation. Rather, the issue is whether HPVs exert an influence in the development of cancers in nonsmokers or whether they are merely "coincidental inhabitants" of the neoplastic tissue, much like a saprophytic fungus on external ear canal debris. I have previously addressed the issue of environmental toxicant exposure causing cancers in nonsmokers, but such exposure was ruled out by history in this study group. If Epstein-Barr virus can be a player in nasopharyngeal carcinoma, so perhaps can the papilloma virus.

**G.R. Holt, M.D., M.S.E., M.P.H.**

## Patterns of Care for Cancer of the Larynx in the United States

Shah JP, Karnell LH, Hoffman HT, et al (Mem Sloan-Kettering Cancer Ctr, New York; Univ of Iowa, Iowa City; Connecticut Ctr of Plastic Surgery, New Haven; et al)
*Arch Otolaryngol Head Neck Surg* 123:475–483, 1997                    12–23

*Background.*—The annual Patient Care Evaluation studies, sponsored by the Commission on Cancer of the American College of Surgeons and the American Cancer Society, have provided valuable data on case-mix characteristics, patterns of diagnosis and treatment, and outcomes. Patterns of care for U.S. patients with laryngeal cancer were reported.

*Methods.*—Data for 16,936 patients with laryngeal cancer seen at 769 U.S. hospitals from 1980 through 1985 and from 1990 through 1992 were analyzed. Most patients had squamous cell carcinomas (SCCs).

*Findings.*—The incidences of stage IV disease and of radiation therapy, with or without surgery and/or chemotherapy, increased slightly between these periods. Overall, management approaches, by site and stage, were diverse. Analysis of 5-year survival rates showed a large difference between modified groupings of the T and N classifications, with stages III and IV separated into localized disease (87.5% for T1–T2 and 76% for T3–T4) and regional metastasis (46.2%).

*Conclusion.*—These findings suggest that efforts to detect laryngeal cancer early have not been successful. More rigorous standards are needed for entering data in hospital records. The increased use of radiation may reflect an increase in nonsurgical treatments for early-stage disease and organ-sparing radiochemotherapy protocols for advanced disease. Predicting survival appears to be more accurate when stages III and IV cases are regrouped as localized disease vs. regional metastasis.

► This study has some important implications for us. One, it actually was performed on retrospectively collated records at multiple hospital sites—not an easy task. Its purpose was clearly a desirable one, namely, the evaluation of patterns of care across the U.S. Two, valuable insight was gained regarding the deficiencies in our reporting and staging systems, which can lead to improvements. The patients want such information, and the physicians need it in order to make rational decisions about treatment options. What we don't have, however, is data on the patterns of care in non-tertiary, community hospitals.

**G.R. Holt, M.D., M.S.E., M.P.H.**

---

**Communication After Laryngectomy: An Assessment of Patient Satisfaction**
Clements KS, Rassekh CH, Seikaly S, et al (Univ of Texas, Galveston)
*Arch Otolaryngol Head Neck Surg* 123:493–496, 1997                    12–24

---

*Background.*—Various methods of alaryngeal communication have been described, but few studies have reported patient satisfaction with these different methods. Patient satisfaction with their current method of alaryngeal communication, with a focus on patients' perception of their own speech, was investigated.

*Methods.*—Forty-seven patients who had undergone total laryngectomy because of cancer were mailed a questionnaire. Thirty-one patients returned the survey. Methods of communication included the use of tablet writing, esophageal speech, electrolarynx, and tracheoesophageal speech.

*Findings.*—Compared with patients in the other 3 groups, the patients using tracheoesophageal speech were significantly more satisfied with their speech. These patients believed their speech was of better quality and that they had greater ability to talk on the telephone and had fewer limitations in their interactions with others. Patients using tracheoesophageal speech also rated their overall quality of life as higher.

*Conclusion.*—After laryngectomy, patients who use tracheoesophageal speech judge their own speech as being significantly better than do patients who use other methods. The former group most likely has a better overall quality of life.

▶ It's been awhile since I have had a patient of mine learn esophageal speech. Perhaps it's a thing of the past. Tablet writing is also uncommon, for those who are functionally illiterate must find another method, and those who are literate and educated tend to pursue the best form of communication available to them. Using all practical parameters, tracheoesophageal speech is undoubtedly the best, as the Galveston group has shown in their survey. However, in some patients in whom for some reason tracheoesophageal puncture failed or could not be accomplished, the Cooper-Rand oral device can enable good speech in a motivated patient.

**G.R. Holt, M.D., M.S.E., M.P.H.**

## Why Has Induction Chemotherapy for Advanced Head and Neck Cancer Become a United States Community Standard of Practice?

Harari PM (Univ of Wisconsin, Madison)
*J Clin Oncol* 15:2050–2055, 1997

12–25

*Background.*—The use of induction chemotherapy for advanced head and neck cancer has become common in the United States, despite the failure of clinical trials for 2 decades to demonstrate a clear benefit in locoregional tumor control or overall survival. Some of the factors that may have contributed to this were studied.

*Methods.*—Three hundred community cancer specialists were mailed a questionnaire to elicit data on their treatment approaches for patients with locoregionally advanced, nonmetastatic head and neck cancer. The response rate was 73%.

*Findings.*—The most common treatment approach, used by 61% of the respondents, was sequential chemoradiation. Specifically, these physicians used induction chemotherapy with fluorouracil/cisplatin followed by radiation therapy. Only 4% of respondents gave induction chemotherapy in controlled clinical trials. The main reasons cited for using induction chemotherapy were the desire to improve locoregional tumor control (reported by 67%), to improve overall survival (56%), to maintain a spirit of multidisciplinary care (34%), to improve quality of life (29%), and to reduce distant metastases (26%).

*Conclusion.*—Despite the lack of clear evidence that induction chemotherapy improves locoregional control or overall survival in patients with advanced head and neck cancer, this treatment strategy has become common among US community cancer specialists. Furthermore, more than half the physicians responding to the current survey specifically identified improved locoregional control and overall survival as primary objectives for using induction chemotherapy in such patients.

▶ Everyone who performs head and neck surgery should discuss this article with radiation and medical oncologists. In fact, it should be the topic for discussion at every head and neck tumor board. Are the data sufficiently strong to warrant the continued (and apparently widespread) use of induction chemotherapy, or is it taking a "shot in the dark" and hoping for a bull's eye? On the other hand, the efficacy of induction chemotherapy followed by radiation therapy may be an evolving clinical science, and we haven't yet reached the point to give it up considering the occasional encouraging report. For myself, I believe it must be a treatment option for the patient.

**G.R. Holt, M.D., M.S.E., M.P.H.**

## Videoendoscopic Biofeedback: A Simple Method to Improve the Efficacy of Swallowing Rehabiliation of Patients After Head and Neck Surgery

Denk D-M, Kaider A (Univ of Vienna)
*ORL J Otorhinolaryngol Relat Spec* 59:100–105, 1997                12–26

*Introduction.*—The flexible videoendoscope can be left in place during swallowing to provide noninvasive direct visualization and analysis before and after swallowing. The use of this technology in swallowing rehabilitation has not been tested. Videoendoscopic biofeedback during swallowing rehabilitation was compared with conventional swallowing therapy to determine whether videoendoscopic biofeedback could improve the efficacy of swallowing rehabilitation.

*Methods.*—Thirty-three patients who underwent radical resection of malignant tumors of the oropharyngolaryngeal swallowing structures underwent swallowing therapy after the healing process was completed. All patients had prolonged postoperative aspiration that persisted more than 1 week after surgery. There were 14 patients in the conventional therapy group and 19 patients in the biofeedback therapy group.

*Results.*—Videoendoscopic biofeedback significantly enhanced the chance of therapeutic success and shortened the period of functional rehabilitation, compared with conventional swallowing therapy. After the first 40 days, there was no difference in chance of success in either group. The effect of biofeedback therapy was still present 80 days after treatment. Only 2 patients indicated that videoendoscopy was uncomfortable. One patient with poor cognitive skills had to discontinue treatment.

*Conclusion.*—The efficacy of swallowing therapy was enhanced with videoendoscopic biofeedback. This method should be used in the first 40 days of swallowing therapy as an adjunct to conventional treatment of aspiration in patients who have undergone head and neck surgery.

▶ This is an interesting concept: let the patient visualize the response of the hypopharyngeal/laryngeal structures to swallowing therapy as part of a positive biofeedback loop. It is certainly easier to do than repeated modified barium swallows. There is always the risk, however, that *no* improvement will be seen on the video examination, which then could serve as negative feedback. The wise physician, then, chooses when to re-scope the patient, based on history and symptoms, to pick the best reinforcement opportunities. If the insurance company rejects all of these endoscopies, send them this article.

**G.R. Holt, M.D., M.S.E., M.P.H.**

## Metastasis to the Thyroid Gland: A Report of 43 Cases

Nakhjavani MK, Gharib H, Goellner JR, et al (Mayo Clinic and Mayo Found, Rochester, Minn)
*Cancer* 79:574–578, 1997                                                      12–27


*Purpose.*—Autopsy reports vary as to the incidence of thyroid metastasis, (from 1.25% to 24%). Clinical thyroid metastasis may be rarer still. A 10-year experience with metastasis to the thyroid gland was reviewed, focusing on current diagnosis and treatment.

*Methods.*—The experience included 43 patients with metastasis to the thyroid gland. There were 23 women and 20 men (mean age, 66 years). The primary tumor site was known in all patients but 2. In each case, the thyroid metastasis was confirmed by fine-needle aspiration cytology or histologic examination. The analysis included the frequency and types of malignancies, the clinical course, and the patients' prognosis after diagnosis of thyroid metastasis.

*Results.*—Thirty-three percent of patients had primary renal tumors. Other primary sites included the lung and breast (16% of patients each), the esophagus (9%), and the uterus (7%). The mean time from diagnosis of the primary tumor to thyroid gland metastasis was 106 months for patients with renal cell adenocarcinoma, 131 months for those with breast cancer, and 132 months for those with uterine cancer. For 28% of patients, the interval was longer than 120 months. In 29 of 30 patients studied, the metastasis was diagnosed by fine-needle aspiration cytology. Thyroidectomy was performed in 23 patients, lobectomy in 14, and subtotal or total thyroidectomy in 9. The mean survival was 34 months for patients treated by thyroidectomy, alone or with adjuvant therapy, vs. 25 months for those treated nonsurgically. Disease regression—with no signs of tumor recurrence—occurred in 3 patients: 2 with uterine adenocarcinoma and 1 with breast adenocarcinoma.

*Conclusion.*—A thyroid mass occurring in a patient with a history of malignancy should be considered a recurrent cancer, until proven otherwise. This is so regardless of how long ago the primary cancer was diagnosed and treated. The prognosis is generally poor for patients with metastasis to the thyroid. However, with aggressive surgical and medical therapy, survival is possible for some.


▶ It is noteworthy that of this substantive group of patients with metastatic cancer to the thyroid gland, the upper aerodigestive tract was not a site of origin in any patients. Why is that? Is the thyroid gland "protected" from metastasis from a primary tumor superior to the vascular supply to the thyroid? Is the thyroid better dealt with in the surgical procedure? Does radiation therapy to the neck atrophy the gland and/or alter its blood supply? These are all worth considering.

**G.R. Holt, M.D., M.S.E., M.P.H.**

## Combined Pectoralis Flap and Gastric Pull-Up for Pharyngeal Reconstruction

Marks SC, Steiger Z (Wayne State Univ, Detroit)
*Head Neck* 19:134–136, 1997

12–28

*Introduction.*—For patients undergoing total laryngopharyngectomy, the gastric transposition flap—or "gastric pull-up"—is a standard reconstructive technique. However, this flap does not always provide enough tissue for tension-free closure. In a new approach to dealing with this problem, the gastric pull-up was combined with the pectoralis major myocutaneous flap.

*Technique.*—The procedure starts after the definitive resection and gastric transposition have been performed and the stomach has been positioned in the pharyngeal defect. Using the anterior surface of the stomach, the surgeon creates a full-thickness, inferiorly

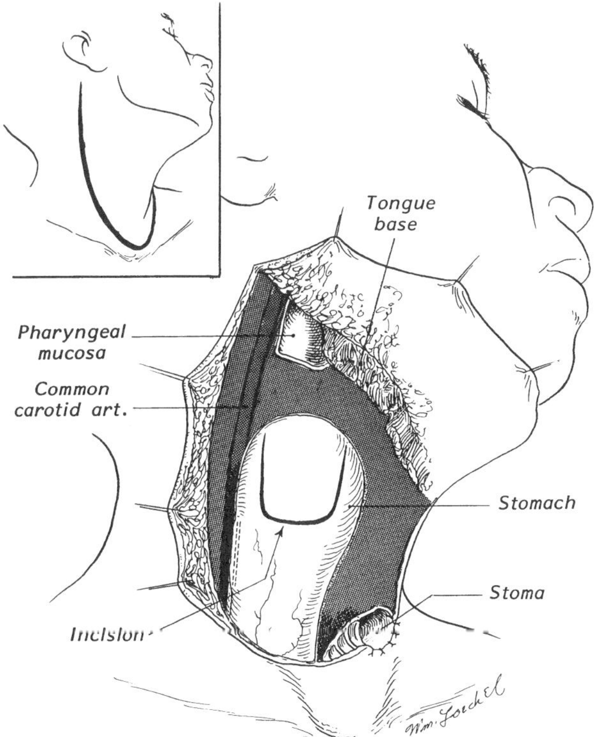


FIGURE 1.—Line drawing demonstrates the position of the gastric flap in the neck before anastomosis to the pharynx. An anterior wall inferiorly based rotation flap using full thickness of the stomach is outlined. The inset demonstrates a typical apron flap used for skin incision. (Courtesy of Marks SC, Steiger Z: Combined pectoralis flap and gastric pull-up for pharyngeal reconstruction. *Head Neck* 19:134–136, copyright 1997. Reprinted by permission of John Wiley & Sons, Inc.)

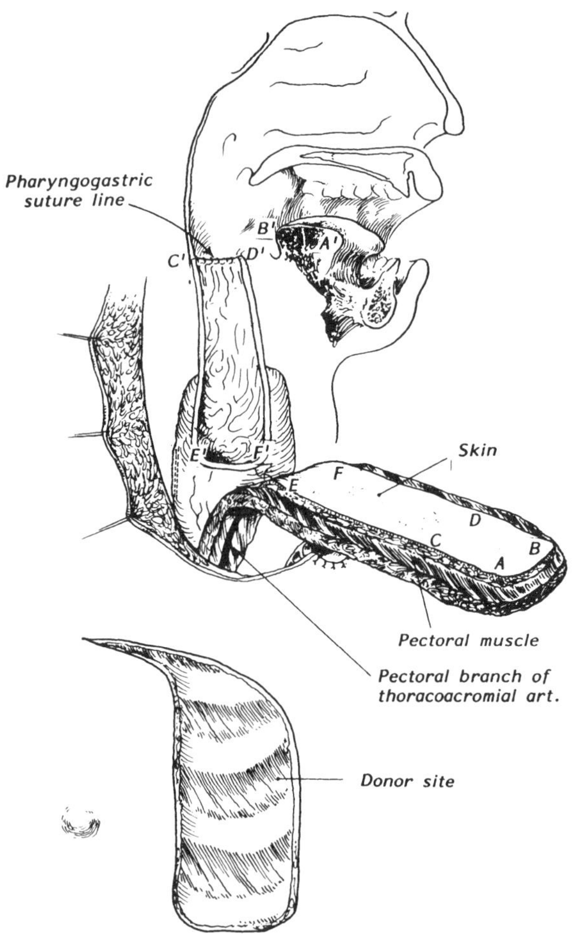


FIGURE 2.—Line drawing demonstrates the technique of combining the 2 flaps. The flap from the anterior wall of the stomach has been rotated and anastomosed to the pharyngeal wall (C' to D'). The pectoralis flap has been rotated into the neck. The pectoralis flap will be anastomosed to the stomach, pharynx, and tongue joining A to A', B to B', C to C', etc. (Courtesy of Marks SC, Steiger Z: Combined pectoralis flap and gastric pull-up for pharyngeal reconstruction. *Head Neck* 19:134–136, copyright 1997. Reprinted by permission of John Wiley & Sons, Inc.)

based flap (Fig 1). After being rotated superiorly, this flap is anastomosed to the posterior pharyngeal wall (Fig 2). The rotation flap is made long enough to fit without too much laxity or tension and with a wide base to ensure a good blood supply. A pectoralis major myocutaneous flap, designed to fit the remaining defect, is then rotated into the field. The distal end is usually the width of the tongue base and the proximal end the width of the anterior stomach wall defect. The pectoralis flap is then sutured into place, and the anastomosis is completed in an inferior to superior direction.

The anastomosis is completed from the distal surface of the pectoralis flap to the tongue base.

*Experience.*—The authors have used this combined technique in 3 patients over an 8-year period. At the start of each operation, the surgeon believed that the gastric pull-up would be sufficient for closure. In each case, however, the surgeons ran into the unexpected dilemma of the stomach not providing adequate tissue for complete closure. All patients healed without wound infection or fistula. Recovery was uncomplicated in 2 patients, who were able to swallow within 3 weeks. The other patients had a number of postoperative complications leading to death, but none were believed to be related to the reconstructive technique.

*Conclusion.*—For patients undergoing total laryngopharyngectomy in whom a gastric flap alone is insufficient, the gastric transposition may be combined with a pectoralis flap. This technique provides a tension-free closure without the need for patient repositioning or free-tissue transfer. The authors believe the combined pectoralis flap and gastric pull-up should be sufficient for reconstructing virtually any defect of the upper aerodigestive flap.

▶ This technique utilizes the best of both techniques—combining the gastric pull-up with the "workhorse" pectoralis myocutaneous flap. The muscle surrounding the anastomosis should also tend to help seal off salivary leakage. Perhaps the pectoralis flap could also be used when an anastomotic leak of the pharyngogastric neojunction occurs.

**G.R. Holt, M.D., M.S.E., M.P.H.**

---

## Re-irradiation With Concomitant Chemotherapy of Unresectable Recurrent Head and Neck Cancer: A Potentially Curable Disease

Haraf DJ, Weichselbaum RR, Vokes EE (Univ of Chicago)
*Ann Oncol* 7:913–918, 1996                                          12–29

---

*Background.*—Many patients with head and neck cancer are seen with advanced stage disease, for which cure rates are poor after traditional surgical and radiation treatment. Local and regional failure are the main causes of death after treatment. The results of concomitant chemotherapy and radiation therapy for previously irradiated patients with locally or regionally recurrent disease or persistent disease considered unresectable for cure were reported.

*Methods.*—Forty-five patients treated between 1986 and 1993 with unresectable locally or regionally recurrent disease were included in the study. The patients were treated with 1 of 4 concomitant chemotherapy phase I/II trials. All received hydroxyurea, 5-fluorouracil, and concomitant radiation therapy on an alternate week schedule (FHX); cisplatin was added to FHX in 3 trials.

*Findings.*—At 5 years, overall survival was 14.6%, progression-free survival was 13.5%, and local/regional control was 20%. This cohort would have been expected to have a fatality rate of nearly 100%. Eleven percent of the patients had fatal treatment-related complications. Two complications were associated with radiation therapy. Dose and protocol were significantly associated with survival, progression-free survival, and local/regional control in a stepwise Cox regression analysis. There was a direct association with radiation dose and an inverse correlation with initial FHX dose escalation. Patients given more than 58 Gy had a 2-year survival rate of 35%, compared with 8% for those given less than 58 Gy.

*Conclusion.*—Aggressive repeat radiation therapy with concomitant chemotherapy in patients with recurrent head and neck cancer can result in cure with acceptable toxicity when the dose used is tumoricidal. This treatment approach should be studied further as an alternative to chemotherapy alone.

► This article caught my eye because of the 13% to 20% local/regional control at 5 years of previously irradiated and unresectable disease. To have the opportunity to give even a 1 in 6 chance to a patient with an otherwise fatal disease seems to me to be worthy of further investigation.

**G.R. Holt, M.D., M.S.E., M.P.H.**

---

**Postoperative Radiotherapy for Malignant Tumors of the Parotid Gland**
Garden AS, El-Naggar AK, Morrison WH, et al (Univ of Texas, Houston)
*Int J Radiat Oncol Biol Phys* 37:79–85, 1997                    12–30

---

*Background.*—Postoperative radiation is a widely accepted treatment for patients thought to be at high risk for recurrence of malignant tumors of the parotid gland. Two commonly used radiation techniques are a pair of $^{60}$Co or high-energy photon beams oriented at oblique angles to encompass the parotid bed and an ipsilateral field treated primarily with electrons. A retrospective analysis was done to determine the outcomes of such treatment.

*Methods.*—One hundred sixty-six patients with parotid gland malignancies treated between 1965 and 1989 were included in the analysis. All received postoperative radiation therapy and were free of macroscopic disease at the time. Twenty-eight percent had mucoepidermoid carcinoma, and 27% had adenocarcinoma. Postoperative radiation was indicated by inadequate margins in 63% of the cases, extraglandular disease extension in 49%, perineural invasion in 34%, and nodal disease in 26%. In 142 patients, radiation was administered through an ipsilateral field of mainly high-energy electrons; in 19, wedged paired $^{60}$Co fields were used. The median dose was 60 Gy, usually given at 2 Gy per fraction. The median follow-up among survivors was 155 months.

*Findings.*—Disease recurred in 29% of the patients. Nine percent had local recurrences, and 6% had regional recurrences. Radiation dose was

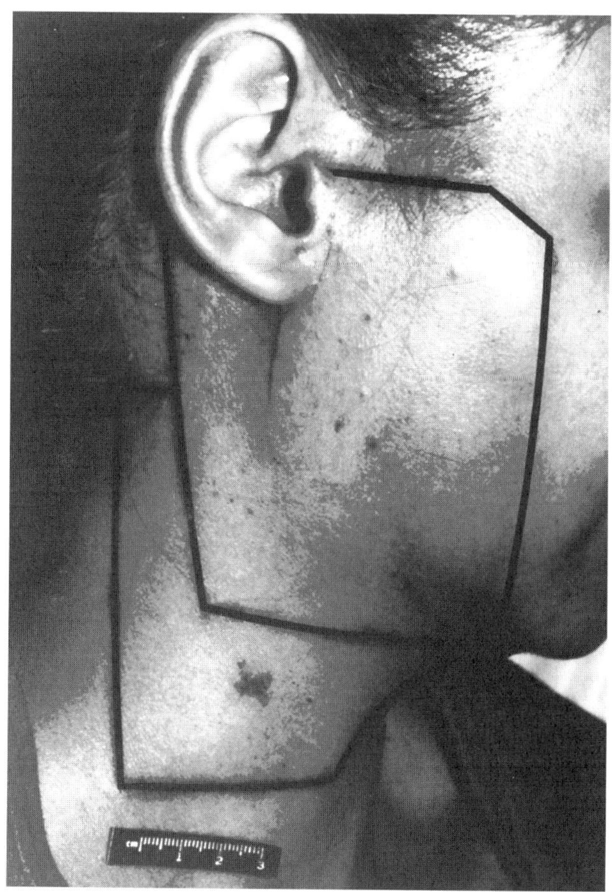

FIGURE 3.—This 39-year-old man underwent a superficial parotidectomy in 1982. An acinic cell carcinoma was dissected off the branches of the facial nerve. Postoperative radiation consisted of 50 Gy delivered through a mixed beam technique of 17 MeV electrons and 18 MV photons. A boost of 10 Gy was delivered with 13 MeV electrons. The total dose of 60 Gy was specified at a depth of 4 cm. Twelve years later he, the patient, is alive without evidence of disease. (Reprinted by permission of the publisher from Garden AS, El-Naggar AK, Morrison WH, et al: Postoperative radiotherapy for malignant tumors of the parotid gland. *Int J Radiat Oncol Biol Phys* 37:79–85, copyright 1997 by Elsevier Science Inc.)

unassociated with local failure, except for a trend toward improvement in local control after doses exceeding 60 Gy in patients with positive margins and/or named nerve involvement. Failure rates did not differ between patients treated with wedged pair methods or ipsilateral fields. However, the complication rate in the former was greater. Overall, chronic sequelae attributable to radiation occurred in 22% of the patients. Hearing decreased in 12 patients, and soft-tissue or bone necrosis or exposure occurred in 15 (Fig 3).

*Conclusion.*—Excellent local and regional control rates are achieved in high-risk patients with parotid gland carcinomas undergoing postoperative radiation therapy. The use of an ipsilateral field encompassing the parotid bed and treated with high-energy electrons often mixed with photons is effective and is associated with minimal severe late toxicity.

▶ Although we must remember that high-grade tumors of the parotid gland are potentially fatal, the authors have shown excellent *control* rates. Cure rates should not be the only major focus of this therapy, which should include concern for decreasing significant complications of irradiation (exposed bone), as well as quality of life. The patient should be well aware of the realities of the disease and the ramifications of the therapy to make an informed decision.

**G.R. Holt, M.D., M.S.E., M.P.H.**

## Does TANIS (T and N Integer Score) Help Predict Survival?

Hall SF, Groome PA, Dixon PF (Queen's Univ, Kingston, Ont, Canada)
*J Otolaryngol* 26:8–12, 1997                                    12–31

*Background.*—The use of the tumor/node/metastasis (TNM) staging system in patients with head and neck cancer has not been successful, as myriad factors affect outcomes in such patients. One team of researchers has proposed that the T and N integers be added arithmetically to create groups on a scale of 1 to 7. Three combinations of the 7 TANIS (T and N integer score) levels, created to maximize group size, resulted in significantly different survival curves. An increase in the TANIS appears to be associated with a poorer response to radiotherapy and reduced survival. The validity of the TANIS model as a predictor of survival was investigated.

*Methods and Findings.*—The Cox Proportional Hazards model was used to examine the subgroups of the TANIS score levels to determine whether they were homogeneous on survival. Data on 594 patients with cancer of the head and neck were obtained. Cancers were classified according to TNM and TANIS and analyzed for the outcome dead of disease, using relative risk estimates. The stages of TNM and levels of TANIS were found to contain patient subgroups with different survival rates.

*Conclusion.*—The major assumption of the TNM stages and TANIS when used to predict survival is that the groups are homogeneous on survival. In a Cox Proportional Hazards analysis of the relative risk of dying with disease, the levels of these classifications were found to contain TNM-defined patient groups with very different survival rates.

▶ This study raises the question, again, of the strength of staging systems in predicting survival. The problem seems to lie in the large number of possible categories of tumor sizes, sites, nodes, and treatment modalities. Although complicated regression analyses can be applied to these large categories, the powers still remain somewhat low. Attention continues to be focused on either simplification of the systems or the clumping of singular categories to achieve greater statistical significance.

**G.R. Holt, M.D., M.S.E., M.P.H.**

**Carcinoma of the Larynx in Patients With Gastroesophageal Reflux**
Freije JE, Beatty TW, Campbell BH, et al (Med College of Wisconsin, Milwaukee)
*Am J Otolaryngol* 17:386–390, 1996                                    12–32

*Background.*—Gastroesophageal reflux disease (GERD) is associated with chronic irritation of the larynx, and reports have long suggested that chronic laryngitis may be a precursor to laryngeal carcinoma in some patients. Series of nonsmoking patients with GERD in whom early laryngeal carcinoma developed suggest that GERD alone may have an etiologic role in this disease. The relationship between GERD and laryngeal cancer in patients with no other known risk factors for the development of squamous cell carcinoma of the larynx was investigated.

*Methods and Findings.*—Nine patients who had never smoked and who had stage 1 or 2 carcinoma of the larynx and GERD were identified. An additional 14 patients who had quit smoking more than 15 years before the development of laryngeal carcinoma and who had evidence of GERD were also studied. Men outnumbered women in both groups. One patient in each group had T2 lesions at diagnosis, the rest having T1 lesions. In the majority of the patients, alcohol consumption was variable but, at most, moderate. In several patients, recurrent leukoplakia and chronic erythema resolved when antireflux therapy was begun after laryngeal carcinoma treatment.

*Conclusion.*—These findings are consistent with previous suggestions that GERD likely plays an etiologic role in the development of squa-mous cell carcinoma of the larynx. Many of the patients in the series had chronic laryngeal abnormalities that only resolved with aggressive antireflux therapy.

▶ Although the authors want to raise our awareness of the association they found between laryngeal cancer and gastroesophageal reflux, I am certain they do not predict that untreated GERD will lead to laryngeal cancer. However, we do have a model in the lower esophagus in Barrett's disease, in which the risk of cancer is well documented. Finally, we must also give some consideration to the possibility of the patient's exposure to environmental carcinogens such as wood dust, pesticides, resins, and glues. Most physicians do not take a comprehensive environmental exposure history— but we definitely should.

**G.R. Holt, M.D., M.S.E., M.P.H.**

## Neck Surgery in Patients With Primary Oropharyngeal Cancer Treated by Radiotherapy

Peters LJ, Weber RS, Morrison WH, et al (Univ of Texas, Houston)
*Head Neck* 18:552–559, 1996

12–33

*Background.*—Authorities disagree regarding the value of neck surgery in node-positive patients with primary tumors treated by definitive radiotherapy. The risks associated with withholding planned neck dissection in patients with a complete nodal response to irradiation was assessed.

*Methods.*—The records of 100 patients with oropharyngeal cancers metastatic to the neck treated between 1984 and 1993 were reviewed. In all patients, the primary tumors were treated by radiotherapy, using the concomitant boost regimen. In 75 patients, nodal disease was treated definitively by radiotherapy. Sixty-two patients who had complete clinical resolution of all nodal disease had no planned surgery, and 13 had neck dissection for presumed residual disease. Of the remaining patients, 8 had node excision and 17 had neck dissection before radiotherapy.

*Findings.*—Isolated neck failure occurred in 8 patients, including 3 of the 62 having no planned surgery, none of the 13 having surgery for presumed residual disease, and 5 of the 25 patients having initial neck surgery. Among those responding completely to definitive radiotherapy, the risk of neck relapse was unassociated with pretreatment nodal size.

*Conclusion.*—Neck observation after complete nodal response to full-dose irradiation in patients with primary oropharyngeal cancer treated by radiotherapy is safe and cost-effective. Imaging should be performed to confirm resolution of nodal disease.

▶ This study addresses the long-debated issue of when to pursue an elective radical neck dissection when radiation therapy has (apparently) eradicated the neck disease. The authors reviewed their data and concluded that close observation was appropriate. They further advised that the current sophistication in soft-tissue imaging of the neck can provide valuable evidence (or lack thereof) of residual neck disease. I tend to hold with their recommendations but would be more likely to operate on a patient who continues to smoke and drink or on one who is a poor follow-up candidate as his risk for recurrence might be greater.

**G.R. Holt, M.D., M.S.E., M.P.H.**

## Morbidity of Combined Therapy for the Treatment of Supraglottic Carcinoma: Supraglottic Laryngectomy and Radiotherapy

Steiniger JR, Parnes SM, Gardner GM (Albany Med College, New York)
*Ann Otol Rhinol Laryngol* 106:151–158, 1997

12–34

*Background.*—Both supraglottic laryngectomy (SGL) and external beam radiotherapy (XRT) are common treatment modalities for patients with supraglottic carcinoma. Both procedures, however, are often associated with significant complications as a result of abnormal laryngeal and pharyngeal function. Many surgeons have noted that morbidity is greater in patients receiving SGL if XRT is performed as well; however, documentation of this interaction has been poor. The effect of subsequent XRT on morbidity after SGL was evaluated in this retrospective study.

*Methods.*—Mean follow-up for 29 patients who had been treated with SGL for supraglottic carcinoma was 64 months. XRT had been performed postoperatively in 17 of the 29 patients. The morbidity associated with SGL alone and SGL with subsequent XRT was evaluated, and a morbidity index score, an average of the total number of morbid events experienced by each patient, was created for both treatment groups.

*Results.*—Mortality during the 2- and 5-year period after treatment did not vary between the two groups. The most common cause of treatment failure was regional metastasis in the neck or the appearance of second primary tumors. The incidence of acute airway obstruction was significantly greater in patients treated with SGL and XRT (29%) than in those treated with SGL alone (0%), as was the incidence of permanent gastrostomy dependence (35% vs. 0%, respectively). Although not-significant, the time until independent swallowing was substantially greater in the SGL with XRT group (34.8 weeks) than in the SGL group (7.8 weeks), as was the incidence of aspiration pneumonia and tracheostomy dependence, at 35% and 24% in the SGL with XRT group, compared with 9% and 0% in the SGL group. The morbidity index score for the SGL with XRT group was 2.29 events per patient, compared with 0.83 events per patient for the SGL group ($P = 0.039$).

*Conclusion.*—The morbidity associated with SGL is significantly increased by subsequent radiotherapy. Although XRT is a beneficial adjunct to SGL in some patients with supraglottic carcinoma, its sequelae require that it be reserved for a strictly defined patient subset.

▶ This article pins down a commonly held clinical suspicion that XRT after supraglottic laryngectomy does not benefit the patient. The authors support a protocol of supraglottic laryngectomy with some form of bilateral neck dissections and only use XRT for very definitive criteria. One criterion, that of extracapsular spread of nodal disease, has been questioned recently as a nonsignificant prognosticator. However, their approach seems quite reasonable. These patients should probably have a percutaneous endoscopic gastrostomy placed before to definitive surgery.

**G.R. Holt, M.D., M.S.E., M.P.H.**

---

**One-Stage Reconstruction of Partial Laryngopharyngeal Defects**
Schuller DE, Mountain RE, Nicholson RE, et al (Ohio State Univ, Columbus)
*Laryngoscope* 107:247–253, 1997                                    12–35

---

*Background.*—Subtotal laryngopharyngectomy is frequently performed in the treatment of advanced-stage neoplasms involving the tongue base or hypopharynx and extending into the larynx. Reconstruction of the resulting laryngopharyngeal defects, however, may be problematic, potentially excluding this procedure in favor of a more disfiguring surgery. The outcome of patients receiving a 1-stage reconstruction of laryngopharyngeal defects using a pectoralis musculocutaneous flap is described in this article.

*Patients.*—Twenty one patients with oropharyngeal or hypopharyngeal squamous cell neoplasms were treated by partial laryngopharyngectomy, with reconstruction performed immediately with a pectoralis myocutaneous flap. Two patients had received prior radiotherapy, and 16 patients were treated with radiotherapy and 9 with chemotherapy postoperatively. The region of the pectoralis muscle from which the musculocutaneous flap was harvested was chosen based, in part, on the bulk of tissue required for the reconstruction. Mean patient follow-up was 28 months.

*Results.*—Pharyngocutaneous fistulae and minor wound infections each occurred in 2 patients (9.5%). Two patients had myocardial infarctions, and 1 patient had a perforated colon with septic shock culminating in fatal pulmonary embolism, yielding a 14.3% incidence of major complications. Twelve of the 21 patients had a patent airway immediately after the procedure, and their tracheotomy tubes were decannulated before discharge. The remainder had tracheotomy tubes in place for 62 to 262 days. Stenosis with occlusion of the airway did not occur in any of the reconstructed segments. Oral consumption of both solids and liquids was tolerated by 5 patients (23.8%) at the time of discharge, and by an additional 8 patients (38.1%) by the end of the follow-up period. A liquid diet alone was tolerated by 3 patients (14.3%), and the remaining 5 patients (23.8%) were unable to consume either liquids or solids. At the end of the observation period, 3 patients (14.3%) each had died as a result of their disease, had died of another cause, or were alive with their disease. The remaining 12 patients (57.1%) were alive and were apparently free of their initial disease.

*Conclusion.*—This is the first report of the use of a pectoralis musculocutaneous flap to reconstruct partial laryngopharyngeal defects. The failure rate for this treatment is consistent with that expected for the patient population involved in this study. In most patients undergoing this reconstructive technique, swallowing and speech functions are preserved. The use of a pectoralis major musculocutaneous flap is an effective method of immediate reconstruction of laryngopharyngeal defects in patients with tongue base or hypopharyngeal neoplasms.

▶ This experience again shows the versatility of the pectoralis flap when properly designed for specific use in reconstructing large defects of the base of tongue to hypopharynx. The proper positioning of the skin paddle, its appropriate bulk and thickness, and the need for reducing the tissue in the laryngeal area are all important considerations. I would submit that in some situations, it might be possible to use only the muscular component of the flap thus reducing unwanted bulk. Reepithelialization of the muscle occurs rather quickly.

**G.R. Holt, M.D., M.S.E., M.P.H.**

**Prognostic Value of Histologic Findings in Neck Dissections for Squamous Cell Carcinoma**

Pinsolle J, Pinsolle V, Majoufre C, et al (Centre Hospitalier Universitaire de Bordeaux, France)
*Arch Otolaryngol Head Neck Surg* 123:145–148, 1997                    12–36

*Background.*—The number of involved cervical nodes and the presence or absence of extracapsular spread are regarded as reliable prognostic indicators for squamous cell carcinoma of the head and neck. Recent studies, however, have found a connection between extracapsular spread and prognosis to be lacking. A confirmation of this observation was sought in this retrospective study.

*Methods.*—Records of 337 patients with histologically confirmed, previously untreated squamous cell carcinoma of the oral cavity, oropharynx, hypopharynx, and larynx were reviewed. Cancer was classified as stage III or IV in 270 patients (80.1%). Lymph node involvement was classified as N0 in 171 patients (50.7%). Distant metastases were absent in all patients at the beginning of the observation period. The patients were followed for a mean of 6 years.

*Results.*—Survival rates for the 2- and 5-year periods after neck dissection were 71.2% and 50.8%. The presence of neoplastic cervical nodes was strongly correlated with the incidence of distant metastasis, neck recurrences, and with survival probabilities ($P < 0.001$). The number of positive nodes was a strong indicator of subsequent survival probability ($P < 0.001$). The presence of extracapsular spread in positive nodes was a significant predictor of distant metastasis ($P < 0.05$); however, it was not predictive of survival probability ($P = 0.45$).

*Conclusion.*—The well-established utility of cervical node involvement as a prognostic indicator for head and neck cancer is again supported. Although previously asserted to be a useful prognostic tool, the presence of extracapsular spread appears to be unreliable as a predictor of survivorship, possibly because of the effectiveness and recent widespread use of combinations of chemotherapy and irradiation in the treatment of squamous cell carcinoma.

▶ Although the authors found that extracapsular spread of tumor in positive lymph nodes conveyed no more prognostic information than positive nodes without extracapsular spread, it still must be taken into consideration, especially in the preoperative planning, if identified on MR or CT scanning. Perhaps as a multifactorial consideration, when looking at the total number of nodes, their size, and the presence or absence of capsular spread the findings would be helpful.

**G.R. Holt, M.D., M.S.E., M.P.H.**

---

**Delphian Lymph Node in Laryngeal Carcinoma: A Whole Organ Study**
Thaler ER, Montone K, Tucker J, et al (Univ of Pennsylvania, Philadelphia; Albert Einstein Med Ctr, Philadelphia)
*Laryngoscope* 107:332–334, 1997                                    12–37

---

*Objective.*—Although it is known that laryngeal carcinoma metastasizes to the Delphian or cricothyroid (CT) lymph nodes, there have been no studies on the frequency of this event. In conservation laryngeal surgery, the CT node may not be resected. The frequency of CT node involvement in 92 whole organ sections of total laryngectomy specimens was investigated.

*Methods.*—A total of 92 total laryngectomy specimens were examined histologically. The pathologic site of the primary tumor and the presence or absence of CT node involvement was recorded. Fisher's exact test was used to compare results.

*Results.*—Eight patients had cricothyroid node involvement. In addition, the conus elasticus was involved in all 8 individuals, the anterior subglottis was in 7, and the crinoid cartilage was in 6. In specimens without CT node involvement, only one third had involvement of 1 of these sites. CT node positive patients were significantly more likely to have involvement of 1 of these sites. The rate of cervical lymph node involvement was 38% in patients with a CT node and 18% in patients without a CT node. Mortality rates were similar in both groups, although there was a significantly higher stomal recurrence rate in patients with CT node involvement than in patients without CT node involvement (38 vs. 6%). In patients with a similar primary site, significantly more patients with a positive CT node than a negative CT node had a stomal recurrence. Four patients died; 3 of them had stomal recurrence.

*Conclusion.*—Whereas the incidence of CT involvement is low, CT node positive patients were significantly more likely to have involvement of the conus elasticus, anterior subglottis, or crinoid cartilage and significantly more likely to have stomal recurrence.

▶ While most head and neck surgeons recall the importance of the Delphian (cricothyroid) node in thyroid gland cancer, some of us need to be reminded of its potential significance in the outcome of laryngeal cancer which has progressed beyond the endolarynx. The authors raise an important issue— attention should be paid to the paratracheal nodes when performing partial laryngeal resection surgery. This might include a node sampling in the crico-tracheal region or could involve a full paratracheal cleanout.

Enhanced CT scanning preop might identify abnormal paratracheal or crico-thyroid nodes.

**G.R. Holt, M.D., M.S.E., M.P.H.**

---

**Induction Chemotherapy Followed by Radiotherapy Versus Radiotherapy Alone in Patients With Advanced Nasopharyngeal Carcinoma: Results of a Matched Cohort Study**
Geara FB, Glisson BS, Sanguineti G, et al (Univ of Texas MD Anderson Cancer Ctr, Houston)
*Cancer* 79:1279–1286, 1997                                                     12–38

---

*Introduction.*—Definitive radiation therapy results in up to 35% long-term survival for patients with head and neck carcinomas; however up to 40% fail at distant sites. For many years, the role of adjunctive chemotherapy in advanced nasopharyngeal carcinoma has been explored, but findings have been inconsistent. A group of 61 patients who received cisplatin and 5-fluorouracil (5–FU) induction chemotherapy before definitive radiation therapy were matched by T classification, N classification, histologic type, and level of cervical lymph node metastases to another 61 patients who were treated by radiotherapy alone.

*Methods.*—During a 7-year period, 61 patients with advanced locoregional nasopharyngeal carcinoma in received induction chemotherapy consisting of cisplatin, 100 mg/m² on day 1, and 5-FU, 1,000 mg/m² on days 1–5, for 3 cycles before receiving definitive radiation therapy. They were compared with 61 patients who received radiation therapy alone. Both groups received radiation therapy of 66–72 gray in 6.5–7 weeks. In both groups, 59 patients (97%) had stage IV disease. Lower cervical lymph node metastasis was evident in 15 patients (25%) in both groups. In the cisplatin/radiation therapy group, the median follow-up time was 4.9 years.

*Results.*—For the cisplatin/radiation therapy group, the 5-year cumulative incidence of distant metastasis was 19%, and for the radiation therapy group it was 34%. In patients with intermediate or high risk of distant metastasis, this reduction in distant failure was more prominent. Improvement in disease-free survival and overall survival resulted from this reduction in distant metastasis. For the cisplatin/radiation therapy group, the 5-year actuarial disease-free survival rate was 64% and for the radiation therapy group it was 42%. For the cisplatin/radiation therapy group, the overall 5-year actuarial survival rate was 69%, and for the radiation therapy group it was 48%. There was no statistical significance in the difference of the incidence of locoregional failure between the 2 groups, in the incidence and severity of acute mucositis, or in the 5-year cumulative incidence of grade 3 or higher late complications.

*Conclusions.*—For patients with locoregional stage IV nasopharyngeal carcinoma, induction chemotherapy with cisplatin and 5-FU before definitive radiation improves freedom from distant metastasis, disease-free survival, and overall survival without increasing treatment-related morbidity.

▶ The therapy of nasopharyngeal carcinoma has, for a long time, resided in external beams and implants. Periodically, the notion of craniofacial surgical approaches for this cancer surfaces, but has not been widely accepted by patients and surgeons. This study raises the issue that if induction chemotherapy before radiation is helpful in advanced tumors, would it also be effective in early tumors? The authors could not answer that, but they intend to look further into it. However you look at it, nasopharyngeal carcinoma is not a very nice tumor, and I appreciate these efforts toward controlling it.

**G.R. Holt, M.D., M.S.E., M.P.H.**

---

**Tracheal Advancement Flap for Postlaryngectomy Stomal Stenosis**
Campbell BH, Rubach BW, McAuliffe TL, et al (Med College of Wisconsin, Milwaukee)
*Head Neck* 19:211–215, 1997                                                    12–39

---

*Introduction.*—Stomal stenosis after laryngectomy is a troublesome complication, with an incidence of 4% to 34%. The patient usually requires continuous use of a stent when stenosis occurs and may have shortness of breath as well as increased problems with bleeding, crusting, and retained secretions. One stomal revision technique involves the tracheal advancement flap, which allows construction of a widely patent, maintainable stoma without disrupting the posterior superior stomal wall. The technique was performed on patients requiring stoma revision, and its success rate was evaluated.

*Methods.*—The procedure was performed on 15 patients. The procedure involves advancing the trachea out of the stoma, dividing the anterior tracheal wall, and leaving the posterior tracheal wall undisturbed. The area to be excised is usually a 1.25-cm to 2-cm width of skin from each side of the stoma, which leaves an inverted V-shaped piece of skin inferiorly (Fig 1). Two to three rings of the trachea are dissected out of the stoma after the skin is excised, leaving the membranous trachea undisturbed. Then the anterior wall is divided and the trachea is splayed (Fig 3, B). The inverted V-shaped skin is secured to the depths of the tracheal cut after the mobilized trachea is sutured to the new tissue bed (Fig 4, B). A stable, trouble-free stoma requiring no stenting was the definition of success. An improved stoma requiring no stenting was the definition for partial success. No improvement and continuous stenting was the definition of failure. Patients were followed up for a median of 23 months.

*Results.*—Ten months was the median time from laryngectomy to revision. There was an increase in median stoma size from 63 mm² before surgery to 135 mm² after surgery. Seven patients had a successful procedure, 6 patients had a partially successful procedure, and 2 had a procedure that failed.

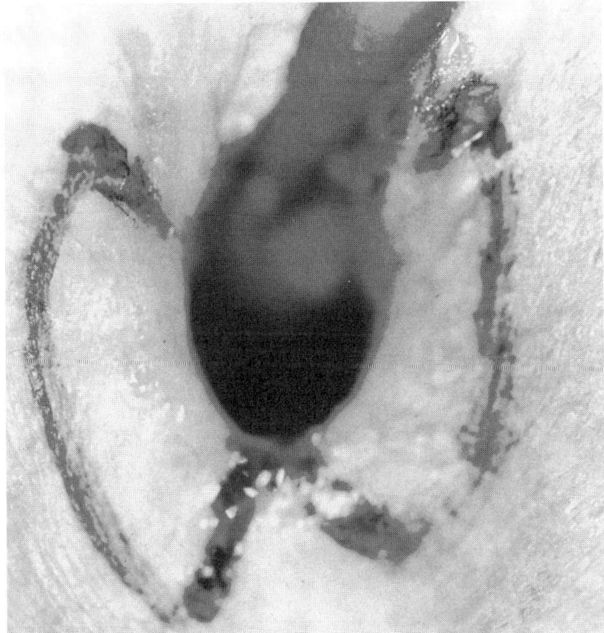

**FIGURE 1.**—A 66-year-old woman who had undergone tracheoesophageal puncture for voice restoration but was unable to tolerate the size of the prosthesis. She had been wearing a modified silastic laryngectomy tube prior to the revision. Areas of skin excision have been outlined. The rubber catheter is in the tracheoesophageal puncture tract. (Courtesy of Campbell BH, Rubach BW, McAuliffe TL, et al: Tracheal advancement flap for postlaryngectomy stomal stenosis. *Head Neck* 19:211–215. Copyright 1997, reprinted by permission of John Wiley & Sons, Inc.)

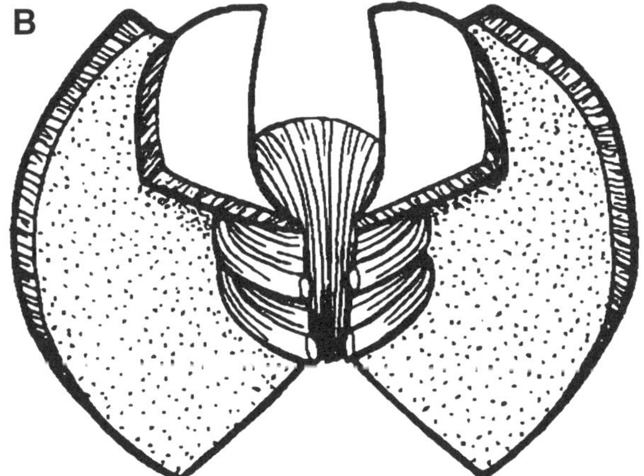


**FIGURE 3, B.**—The anterior tracheal wall is divided. (Courtesy of Campbell BH, Rubach BW, McAuliffe TL, et al: Tracheal advancement flap for postlaryngectomy stomal stenosis. *Head Neck* 19:211–215. Copyright 1997, reprinted by permission of John Wiley & Sons, Inc.)

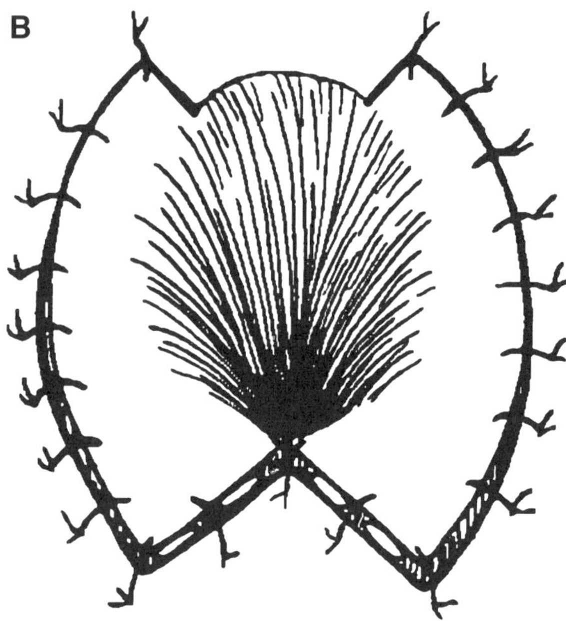

**FIGURE 4, B.**—The inverted V of skin is secured within the tracheal cut. The tracheal edge and membranous portion of the trachea are advanced out of the stoma and secured to the skin edges. (Courtesy of Campbell BH, Rubach BW, McAuliffe TL, et al: Tracheal advancement flap for postlaryngectomy stomal stenosis. *Head Neck* 19:211–215. Copyright 1997, reprinted by permission of John Wiley & Sons, Inc.)

*Conclusion.*—For the laryngectomy patient who has had or might have voice restoration, the tracheal advancement flap is a safe technique. A successful outcome occurred only in 1 of 4 patients who had complete postoperative tracheocutaneous separation. Failure usually occurred in patients with irritated peristomal skin. A wider excision of peristomal skin was needed in obese patients or those with redundant skin.

▶ This procedure appears to be neat and easily performed. The problem of stomal stenosis is very difficult, and any new solution is welcome. I also (frequently) find that if a wide-field laryngectomy has been performed, and the sternal attachments of the sternocleidomastoid muscle are still present, then their release might facilitate widening of the stoma. I usually will suture these sternal heads laterally, overlapping the clavicular heads.

**G.R. Holt, M.D., M.S.E., M.P.H.**

# 13 Comprehensive Otolaryngology

**Projected Societal Needs in Pediatric Otolaryngology**
Zalzal GH (George Washington Univ, Washington, DC)
*Laryngoscope* 106:1176–1179, 1996

13–1

*Background.*—The recent increase in pediatric otolaryngology fellowships has resulted in the training of record numbers of fellows. Concerns have been raised that the supply of these physicians will soon exceed society's needs. The number of fellowship-trained pediatric otolaryngologists that will be needed in the future was estimated.

*Methods and Findings.*—Data were obtained from national organizations and from a survey of fellowship training programs. A hospital-based practitioner model was used to predict the need for pediatric otolaryngologists, based on the anticipated changes in patient care, primarily managed-care capitated systems. The projected need was 382, which will be met in just over 7 years if current fellowship training levels continue (Tables 1 and 2).

*Conclusion.*—Using the hospital-based practitioner model, it is estimated that the societal need for pediatric otolaryngologists will be met in about 7 years (considering current fellowship training rates and assuming that all graduates will be hospital based). Many possible scenarios exist, depending on the number of accredited programs, the percentage of trainees working in children's hospitals, the residency programs, and children's hospital requirement. When the need for pediatric otolaryngologists will

TABLE 1.—Societal Needs for Pediatric Otolaryngologists

| | | | |
|---|---|---|---|
| Number of Free-Standing Children's Hospitals (1992) | 147 | | |
| Number of Otolaryngology Residency Programs | 88 | | |
| Number of pediatric otolaryngologists needed per children's hospital | 1 | 2 | 3 |
|   Total number of pediatric otolaryngologists needed | 235 | 382 | 529 |
|   Total number of pediatric otolaryngologists needed if only 67% take full-time staff positions in academic and children's hospitals | 351 | 570 | 790 |

TABLE 2.—Pediatric Otolyngology Manpower Projection at Current Production Rates

| Age (y) | 1995 | 2000 | 2005 | 2010 | 2015 |
|---|---|---|---|---|---|
| 31–35 | 54 | 135 | 135 | 135 | 135 |
| 36–45 | 66 | 87 | 178 | 225 | 249 |
| 46–55 | 46 | 55 | 70 | 122 | 170 |
| >56 | 12 | 29 | 41 | 54 | 87 |
| Total | 178 | 306 | 424 | 536 | 641 |

(Courtesy of Zalzal GH: Projected societal needs in pediatric otolaryngology. *Laryngoscope* 106:1176–1179, 1996. Copyright Triological Society.)

be met ranges from 2 to more than 20 years, depending on the scenario used.

▶ Probably more than any subspecialty in otolaryngology, pediatric otolaryngology has struggled in recent years to project its unique identity. I believe its "envelope" of practice is becoming better defined. Clearly, these fellowship-trained or experienced senior individuals have a well-accepted role in children's hospitals throughout the country. There has been more controversy regarding refining their roles in community-based hospitals where comprehensive otolaryngologists believe that they have been fulfilling that role adequately. However, I do not believe that many will dispute the expertise of the pediatric otolaryngologists in laryngotracheal disorders. This paper helps us better understand the evolving role of the pediatric subspecialist as well as the projected manpower requirements for the near and intermediate future.

**G.R. Holt, M.D., M.S.E., M.P.H.**

**Upper Airway Obstruction in Children With Down Syndrome**
Jacobs IN, Gray RF, Todd NW (Emory Univ, Atlanta, Ga)
*Arch Otolaryngol Head Neck Surg* 122:945–950, 1996          13–2

*Background.*—Children with Down syndrome commonly have obstructive airway problems. The complex nature of upper airway obstruction (UAO) and surgical outcomes in this patient population were analyzed.

*Methods.*—Seventy-one children with Down syndrome and significant UAO were included in the retrospective review. Thirty-four had pulmonary artery hypertension, and 44 had multiple sites of airway obstruction. Problems included lymphoid hyperplasia, macroglossia, narrow nasopharynx, laryngomalacia, congenital subglottic stenosis, tracheobronchomalacia, and tracheal stenosis. Surgical procedures included tonsillectomy, adenoidectomy, tonsillar pillar plication, uvulopalatopharyngoplasty, anterior tongue reduction, tongue-hyoid suspension, laryngotracheoplasty, and tracheotomy.

*Findings.*—Obstructive symptoms were mild in 27 of the 55 patients undergoing surgery. Most children with mild symptoms improved after tonsil and/or adenoid surgery. However, significant residual symptoms occurred postoperatively in 39% of the remaining patients. The patients with residual symptoms were younger and had more severe symptoms, multiple sites of obstruction, and a high incidence of cardiac disease. Four children are currently dependent on a tracheotomy. Five children have died, 3 from upper airway causes.

*Conclusion.*—In children with Down syndrome, UAO is often complex, with multifocal causes. Residual symptoms of airway obstruction postoperatively are common. The management of UAO in children with Down syndrome requires a comprehensive, individualized approach.

▶ Although this was not a prospective study, it does highlight some of the concerns we must have regarding children with Down syndrome who have major UAO. Remember, too, that in addition to enlarged tissue in the oropharynx, these patients have grossly enlarged tongues. These abnormalities give rise to increased risk of postoperatively UAO. It is wise to plan admission to a pediatric ICU after surgery for close airway monitoring. If an elective tracheotomy is not performed, a surgical tray with appropriate tubes, suction, headlight, etc. should be available in the patient's room to be used in an emergency or at a point where its use becomes indicated.

**G.R. Holt, M.D., M.S.E., M.P.H.**

## Management of Children With von Willebrand Disease Undergoing Adenotonsillectomy

Derkay CS, Werner E, Plotnick E (Eastern Virginia Med School, Norfolk; Children's Hosp of the Kings Daughters, Norfolk, Va)
*Am J Otolaryngol* 17:172–177, 1996         13–3

*Introduction.*—Patients with von Willebrand disease (vWD) are at increased risk of postoperative hemorrhage. Adenoidectomy or tonsillectomy in a child with a known bleeding dyscrasia can pose challenging problems for the surgeon and hematologist alike. The authors report a new transfusion-avoiding protocol for the management of children with vWD undergoing adenotonsillectomy.

*Methods.*—A careful bleeding history was obtained in all patients being evaluated for adenotonsillectomy. Laboratory studies, included measurement of von Willebrand factor, were performed in patients with a positive history (Table 1). Patients with abnormal laboratory results or a strong bleeding history were referred to a hematologist. The diagnosis of vWD was based on the history and the level of von Willebrand factor or antigen. A confirmatory trial dose of desmopressin also was given (Fig 1). At surgery, patients with vWD were managed with careful local control, preoperative and postoperative administration of desmopressin, and antifibrinolytic agents (Table 2).

*Results.*—Twelve patients with type I vWD were managed on the prospective protocol. Blood loss was estimated at 5 to 40 mL. The use of scissor or electrocautery technique had no effect on outcome. There were

---

**TABLE 1.**—Preoperative Historical Screening for Bleeding Dyscrasias

---

Patient or Immediate Family Member With:

| Easy bruising | Menorrhagia |
| Epistaxis | Excessive circumcision bleeding |
| Oral bleeding | Postoperative or dental hemorrhage |
| Post-trauma bleeding | Hemarthrosis |
| | Perinatal bleeding |

(Reprinted by permission of the publisher from Derkay CS: Management of Children With von Willebrand Disease Undergoing Adenotonsillectomy: *Am J Otolaryngol* 17:172–177, 1996.)

---

2 cases of late postoperative tonsillectomy hemorrhage (1 managed operatively and 1 with electrocautery). Patients managed later in the series were sent home with outpatient IV desmopressin therapy by postoperative day 4.

*Conclusions.*—A screening algorithm and treatment protocol proposed for the management of children with vWD undergoing adenotonsillectomy is described. The authors' experience shows the value of careful intraop-

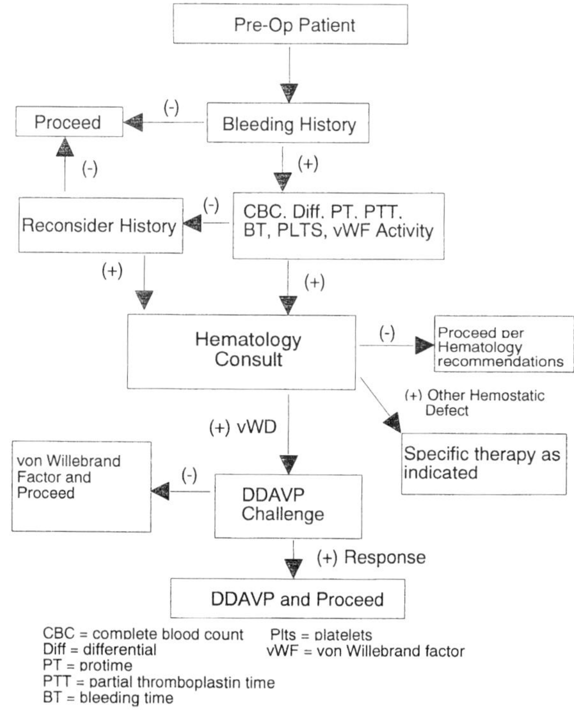


**FIGURE 1.**—Algorithm for Pre-Operative Hematologic Screening. (Courtesy of Derkay CS, Werner E, Plotnick E: Management of Children With von Willebrand Disease Undergoing Adenotonsillectomy. *Am J Otolaryngol* 17:172–177, 1996.)

---

TABLE 2.—Guideline for Tonsillectomy and Adenoidectomy in Patients
with vWD Who Are Desmopression Responsive

---

1. Preoperatively document adequate response to desmopressin
   (Rise in vWF and Factor VII $\geq 100\%$).
2. Document adequate hemoglobin.
3. No aspirin, glycerol guiacolate, ibuprofen, or other
   nonsteroidal antiinflammatory agents.
4. Preoperatively administer desmopressin 0.3 µg/kg IV
   over 30 minutes, repeat in 12 hours, 24 hours, then
   every 24 hours until eschar comes off.
5. Administer amicar 200 mg/kg loading dose preoperatively then 100 mg/kg orally every 6 hours or administer Tranexamic acid mouthwash 4.8%, 10 mL swish
   for 2 minutes and spit, three times a day.
6. Limit total fluids to maintenance plus losses and use
   $D_5LR$ for IV fluid.
7. Check serum sodium ($Na^+$) preoperatively and before
   each dose of desmopressin, if sodium <132 do not
   give desmopressin.
8. If bleeding develops use intermediate purity factor VIII
   containing high molecular weight vWF or cryoprecipi-
   tate at dosage calculated to bring Factor VIII >100%.

---

(Reprinted by permission of the publisher from Derkay CS: Management of Children With von
Willebrand Disease Undergoing Adenotosillectomy: *AM J Otolaryngol* 17:172–177, 1996.)

---

erative and postoperative management in reducing morbidity and exposure to blood products. The new protocol, including preoperative and
postoperative desmopressin, is recommended for use in this challenging
group of patients.

▶ Several interesting concepts arise from this article. It appears that a von
Willebrand activity level in addition to the bleeding time and activated partial
thromboplastic time have a significant chance of identifying this disorder
preoperatively. A comprehensive *patient* and *family* history also are of ut-
most importance. How many physicians actually take a detailed history in a
patient who will undergo adenotonsillectomy beyond the standard, "Are
there any bleeding problems in the family?" A major problem is that the child
may not have had clinical-level challenges to the clotting system yet to allow
vWD to be suspected. That places additional responsibility on the surgeon to
focus on that aspect of the history and to obtain pertinent laboratory support
if a problem is suspected. A preparation/treatment protocol is presented by
the authors. A final word of philosophy—such disorders as this force us as
surgeons to be super-responsible in following accepted and standard clinical
indicators for tonsillectomy and adenoidectomy in children. It can be a long
walk from the operating suite to the family waiting room in a case of
unpredicted and poorly prepared surgical bleeding in a child with borderline
indications.

**G.R. Holt, M.D., M.S.E., M.P.H.**

## Otolaryngologic Clinical Patterns in Pediatric Infectious Mononucleosis

Ganzel TM, Goldman JL, Padhya TA (Univ of Louisville, Ky)
*Am J Otolaryngol* 17:397–400, 1996

13–4

*Objective.*—Infectious mononucleosis (IM), caused by Epstein-Barr virus, is usually a disease found in older adolescents and young adults. The symptoms are characteristic (Table 1). Diagnosis is based on clinical features (Table 2). The occurrence in younger children is rare but it can result in severe pharyngotonsillitis. Results of a retrospective study evaluating the incidence of IM in a consecutive series of pediatric patients with pharyngotonsillitis and determining the patient demographics, clinical features (laboratory and serologic), and management and treatment outcomes are presented.

*Methods.*—Between 1989 and 1994, 109 consecutive patients with IM were admitted to Kosair Children's Hospital.

*Results.*—Sixty (55%, 27 girls), aged 1–17, had severe pharyngotonsillitis. Patients had symptoms for an average of 6 days prior to hospitalization. All had dysphagia and odynophagia, and 36 had moderate to severe airway obstruction. The 29 children with severe upper airway obstruction were treated with high-dose parenteral steroids, and 43 received antibiotics. Tonsillar hypertrophy was diagnosed in 87% of patients. All had cervical adenopathy, fever (101.6°F), elevated white cell count (14,900/mm$^3$), absolute lymphocytosis, and a positive heterophile antibody test. Three patients did not improve significantly with medical therapy and received a tonsillectomy for dysphagia (1) or peritonsillar abscess (2). Patients were hospitalized for an average of 3.7 days. All patients recovered.

*Conclusion.*—There was a high incidence of severe pharyngotonsillitis among patients hospitalized for IM. Treatment with parenteral steroids decreased the need for surgery.

▶ This article serves to remind us that infectious mononucleosis should be considered in the differential diagnosis of children with severe pharygotonsillitis and lymphadenopathy. It also reminded me of when I took my then three-year-old daughter to a respected emergency room in the middle of the night (it was 1980) with some stridor and huge tonsils. When I told the emergency department physician that I suspected mono he merely laughed at me and said that "three-year-olds don't get mono." I sat up with her all night back at home fretting about her airway until her regular pediatrician

TABLE 1.—General Clinical Features of IM

| | |
|---|---|
| Fever, malaise, lymphadenopathy, and pharyngitis | 90% |
| Splenomegaly | 50% |
| Mild hepatitis or hepatomegaly | 20% |

(Courtesy of Ganzel TM, Goldman JL, Padhya TA: Otolaryngologic clinical patterns in pediatric infectious mononucleosis. *Am J Otolaryngol* 17:397–400, 1996.)

|  |
|---|
| **TABLE 2.**—Diagnosis of IM |
| Clinical features<br>Lymphocytosis (>50% in differential) with atypical fraction<br>  being greater than 10%<br>Positive heterophile antibody assay (Monospot) |
| (Courtesy of Ganzel TM, Goldman JL, Padhya TA: Otolaryngologic clinical patterns in pediatric infectious mononucleosis. *Am J Otolaryngol* 17:397–400, 1996.) |

called the following morning and informed me that the chest radiograph taken the night before showed an enlarged spleen. A short course of steroids alleviated a repeat of the previous night's airway concerns. All turned out well, and I guess I should thank the ER physician because I have never forgotten what was learned and regularly use it in teaching.

**G.R. Holt, M.D., M.S.E., M.P.H.**

## Chronic Aspiration in Children: When Are Bilateral Submandibular Gland Excision and Parotid Duct Ligation Indicated?

Gerber ME, Gaugler MD, Myer CM III, et al (Univ of Cincinnati, Ohio)
*Arch Otolaryngol Head Neck Surg* 122:1368–1371, 1996          13–5

*Introduction.*—There is an increased risk of aspiration when congenital or postsurgical structural abnormalities of the upper aerodigestive tract or neuromuscular disorders result in discoordination of the swallow. Caring for the severely neurologically impaired child with chronic aspiration involves a multidisciplinary approach to reduce the number of episodes of aspiration pneumonia, to prevent acute and chronic bronchopulmonary complications, to decrease hospitalization and nursing care requirements, and to improve the overall quality of life for the patient and the family. The efficacy of bilateral submandibular gland excision and bilateral parotid duct ligation in decreasing the episodes of pneumonia and hospitalization, and improving the quality of life for the children, was retrospectively assessed.

*Methods.*—There were 16 patients, aged 16 months to 18 year who had bilateral submandibular gland excision and bilateral parotid duct ligation and at least 1 episode of aspiration pneumonia in the year before surgery. The change in the number of hospitalizations for pneumonia and the total number of lower respiratory tract infections in the year before surgery and the year after surgery were determined. Families were contacted by phone to determine parental satisfaction, effect on quality of life, care requirements, amount of suctioning, and use of voice.

*Results.*—There was a significant decrease in the mean number of pneumonias (2.3 before surgery, 0.9 after surgery) and hospitalizations (1.2 before surgery, 0.4 after surgery) after surgical intervention. At the time of surgery, 6 patients required a tracheostomy, and 2 years after surgery 1 patient required a tracheostomy. Laryngotracheal separation was not required by any patient. The telephone interviews revealed that quality of life was improved and care requirements decreased in 8 of the 11 patients who were contacted. For at least some degree of communication, 7 patients were able to use their voices. Postoperative complications involving the parotid glands occurred in 3 patients but had resolved after further therapy.

*Conclusion.*—In a select group of neurologically impaired children, the incidence of aspiration pneumonias and hospitalization is reduced and the overall care requirements are decreased after bilateral submandibular gland excision and bilateral parotid duct ligation. These procedure should be considered before laryngotracheal separation or tracheoesophageal diversion because they are voice sparing, have a low morbidity, and are efficacious.

▶ I suspect that each of us has seen at least 1 patient with excessive salivation, poor mouth closure, and chronic aspiration during our careers. Usually the result of neurologic trauma, these problems can be a constant source of frustration for the caregivers. The authors tell us of their experience with "desalivating" the oral cavity in a small group of these unfortunate patients. Their results are impressive, with only a few complications. Technically, we can do these operations—the big question is—when and on whom?

**G.R. Holt, M.D., M.S.E., M.P.H.**

---

**Local Injection Therapy in 107 Patients With Myofascial Pain Syndrome of the Head and Neck**
Tschopp KP, Gysin C (Univ Hosp, Basel, Switzerland)
*ORL J Otorhinolaryngol Relat Spec* 58:306–310, 1996                    13–6

---

*Introduction.*—It is difficult to determine the cause and appropriate treatment of myofascial pain syndromes. Treatments include correction of occlusional disturbances; reduction of muscular hypertonus; relaxation techniques such as biofeedback or hypnotherapy; and deactivation of trigger points by stretching the muscles with physical therapy, injection therapy of local anesthetics, or acupuncture. Pain can be relieved with local injection therapy, but it is unclear whether the pharmacologic effect can be enhanced by long-acting substances or whether there is an activation of reflex mechanisms. In patients with myofascial pain syndrome, lignocaine 1%, bupivacaine 0.25%, and saline solution 0.9% were injected.

*Methods.*—In double-blind study, 107 patients with myofascial pain syndrome of the head and neck received 1 of 3 solutions injected at the trigger points. The efficacy of bupivacaine 0.25%, lignocaine 1%, and saline 0.9% was compared.

*Results.*—Among the 3 groups, there was no significant difference with respect to reduction of pain and overall rating by patients of the therapeutic benefits. After treatment, 53 patients (49%) were free of symptoms,

48 patients (38%) reported substantial relief, and 14 patients (13%) had symptoms that remained unchanged. An average of 2.5 trigger points were found in each patient, and the most frequent trigger point was found at the dorsal insertion of the lateral pterygoid muscle (40%).

*Conclusion.*—Rather than pharmacologic effects of the injected solutions causing relief of pain, these findings suggest that reflex mechanisms cause relief of pain. For use in local injection therapy, physiologic saline solution is recommended. One hypothesis that accounts for the clinical observations at myofascial trigger points is that calcium ions are released from disrupted sarcoplasmic reticulum because of microtrauma, leading to a chain of biochemical reactions that induce uncontrolled muscular contraction, local ischemia, and excessive metabolites sensitizing neural muscle nociceptors. Therefore, injection of any liquid would wash out these nerve-sensitizing substances and the released calcium. However, plain placebo effects caused by the painful act of injection are not possible to exclude.

▶ Whereas many patients with myofascial pain syndromes have a specific muscular disorder, I suspect that many have an occupational origin—long hours at the computer, or desk, or some other nonergonomically designed workstation. Although these patients may not seek an otolaryngology consultation directly, we may be asked to see them before a pain management referral. This study notwithstanding, I would find it difficult to inject only saline into a patient without their knowledge. Perhaps it is the volume expansion alone that breaks the spasm, I don't know. Remember that torticollis may present initially as a tight, painful neck disorder.

**G.R. Holt, M.D., M.S.E., M.P.H.**

---

## Dexamethasone Decreases Vomiting by Children After Tonsillectomy

Splinter WM, Roberts DJ (Univ of Ottawa, Ont, Canada)
*Anesth Analg* 83:913–916, 1996                                    13–7

---

*Introduction.*—Nearly 73% of children vomit after undergoing general anesthesia for tonsillectomy. Prophylactic antiemetics can dramatically affect the incidence of vomiting after tonsillectomy in children. Dexamethasone is a corticosteroid with prolonged antiemetic effects in patients treated for cancer. Its effect on vomiting in the perioperative period is not known. The effect of dexamethasone on vomiting after elective tonsillectomy was assessed in 133 healthy children in a randomized, stratified, blocked, double-blind, placebo-controlled trial.

*Methods.*—Children aged 2 to 12 years were stratified according to use of premedication and anesthesia induction technique, and were randomly assigned to placebo or dexamethasone groups. Children underwent induction and maintenance of general anesthesia with inhalation of nitrous oxide and halothane or IV propofol. Before surgery, patients received either IV dexamethasone, 150 µg/kg up to a maximum dose of 8 mg, or placebo. Codeine, 1.5 mg/kg IM, was administered intraoperatively.

*Results.*—The overall incidence of vomiting (inpatient and after discharge) was 72% in patients receiving dexamethasone, compared with 40% in patients receiving placebo. Hospital discharge was prolonged by a mean of 13 minutes with each episode of inhospital vomiting.

*Conclusion.*—Vomiting in an ambulatory hospital setting was markedly diminished in healthy children after elective tonsillectomy with administration of dexamethasone. The effect on vomiting was significant after hospital discharge.

▶ The authors do not postulate the chemical basis for the reduction in vomiting after tonsillectomy utilizing dexamethasone. Perhaps the exact mechanism of action is not known. Each surgeon should discuss the implications of the study for his or her own practice with their anesthesiologist. As an aside, I find that introducing an orogastric tube just before awakening the patient will evacuate blood and irrigation fluids from the child's stomach and reduce vomiting on that basis. I always cringe to see children testing the integrity of the tonsillar fossa hemostasis with retching, even though I have routinely used suture ligatures for 25 years.

**G.R. Holt, M.D., M.S.E., M.P.H.**

## Contemporary Management of Deep Neck Space Infections

Gidley PW, Ghorayeb BY, Stiernberg CM (Univ of Texas, Houston)
*Otolaryngol Head Neck Surg* 116:16–22, 1997                    13–8

*Introduction.*—Deep neck infections remain a problem, despite availability of antibiotics to treat early infections of the head and neck. These infections follow along the facial planes of the neck and can create deep neck space abscesses. Understanding the anatomy of neck fascial planes and spaces, bacteriology, and potential complications helps in the successful management of these serious infections. The clinical management of deep neck space infections in 24 patients is described.

*Methods.*—Medical records of 24 patients admitted between 1988 and 1993 with a diagnosis of deep neck space abscess were reviewed for data regarding age, sex, racial group, symptoms and their duration, radiographic tests performed, precipitating causes, anatomic location of abscesses, and culture results.

*Results.*—The average age of 11 male and 13 female patients was 25.5 years (range, 7 months to 78 years). There were 12 black, 6 Hispanic, and 6 white patients. The most commonly involved area was the parapharyngeal space, then the retroparapharyngeal, submandibular, and parotid spaces (n - 10, 7, 6, and 1, respectively). Half of the patients received some form of antibiotic treatment of the ear, nose, or throat before being seen because of the abscess. Thirty-five organisms were isolated in 18 patients (1.9 isolates per person). Organisms cultured were *Streptococcus (n - 13),*

*Staphylococcus (n - 6)*, *Bacteroides (n - 5)*, *Micrococcus (n - 2)*, *Neisseria (n - 2)*, and *Candida, Enterobacter, Enterococcus, Peptostreptococcus, Proteus, Proprionobacter*, and *Pseudomonas (n - 1 each)*. There was no growth on culture in 6 patients, but organisms were found on Gram stain. Penicillin was regarded as the drug of choice at one time, but the emergence of β-lactamase-producing organisms necessitates choosing antibiotics on the basis of culture and sensitivity results. Major complications were jugular vein thrombosis, carotid artery rupture, mediastinitis, and meningitis.

*Conclusion.*—The infecting organisms of deep neck infections remain the same. The emergence of antibiotic-resistant strains may explain why these infections continue to occur, despite widespread use of antibiotics therapy for infections of the head and neck. Complications of deep neck abscesses require vigilance for prevention and treatment.

▶ The surgical treatment of deep neck abscesses is well reviewed in this article. I have always held that when a patient develops a deep neck abscess while on antibiotics (or having been previously treated) one or more of the following factors is at play: inadequate dosage, improper antibiotic, poor patient compliance, decreased local host (tissue) factors, altered absorption of the antibiotic, or bad luck. Since many of these patients will present to an after-hours medical clinic or an emergency room early in the course of developing the deep neck component, attention should be given to the education of their physician staff on the pathogenesis of this disorder.

**G.R. Holt, M.D., M.S.E., M.P.H.**

## Optimal Concentration of Epinephrine for Vasoconstriction in Neck Surgery

Dunlevy TM, O'Malley TP, Postma GN (Naval Med Ctr, Portsmouth, Va; Naval Hosp, Camp Pendleton, Calif)
*Laryngoscope* 106:1412–1414, 1996                                    13–9

*Background.*—Adding epinephrine to local anesthetics reduces bleeding and systemic toxicity and increases the duration of action. However, significant adverse effects are associated with epinephrine. Four concentrations of epinephrine are compared to determine the minimum concentration needed for maximal vasoconstriction.

*Methods and Results.*—Eighty-one patients scheduled for surgery with general anesthesia were studied. Solutions of 1% lidocaine containing varying concentrations of epinephrine were injected. Blood flow was measured once a minute for 10 minutes using a laser Doppler flowmeter. Blood flow reduction did not differ among groups receiving epinephrine concentrations of 1:100,000, 1:200,000, and 1:400,000. However, a concentration of 1:800,000 produced significantly less vasoconstriction.

*Conclusion.*—Although the higher concentrations of epinephrine used in this study did not produce toxic effects, the authors recommend a

1:200,000 or 1:400,000 solution to provide hemostasis and minimize the potential adverse effects. This is especially important in patients with cardiovascular disease and in children.

▶ The authors give us evidence that a 1:200,000 concentration of epinephrine may give adequate vasoconstriction with a safety factor suitable for use in children and older adults. They also acknowledge that their study did not address duration of action, which might have some practical significance. If the surgeon has to inject a second bolus of anesthetic with epinephrine, the benefits of a more dilute concentration would not be as apparent. Discuss the issue with your anesthesiologist for clarification.

**G.R. Holt, M.D., M.S.E., M.P.H.**

## CT Findings in General Practice Patients With Suspected Acute Sinusitis

Lindbæk M, Johnsen UL-H, Kaastad E, et al (Univ of Oslo, Norway; Larvik Hosp, Norway)

*Acta Radiol* 37:708–713, 1996

13–10

*Background.*—Acute sinusitis is often seen in general practice. Diagnosis usually based on clinical symptoms and signs, is usually not accurate. CT can be used as a noninvasive diagnostic tool for acute sinusitis. A large group of general practice patients with clinically diagnosed acute sinusitis were examined by CT to describe the range of findings and to evaluate interobserver variation in interpretation of CT images.

*Study Design.*—The study population consisted of 137 women and 64 men, aged at least 15 years, from Larvik, Norway with diagnoses of acute sinusitis during the winter of 1983. All patients were examined by CT within 2 days of diagnosis, and the images were independently interpreted by 2 radiologists.

*Findings.*—Of the 201 patients who participated in this study, 127 had fluid or total opacification in at least one of the sinus regions. CT signs of sinusitis were detected in the ethmoid region in 115, in the maxillary in 84, in the frontal in 18, and in the sphenoid in 10 patients. CT findings were negative in 49 patients. The overall interobserver agreement on assessment of CT findings had a κ value of 0.70.

*Conclusions.*—This study found great variation in the CT results of general practice patients with suspected acute sinusitis. Many of these patients had little change, or even had negative CT findings. Most patients with sinusitis confirmed by CT had infection in more than one sinus. The most commonly infected sinuses were the ethmoid and the maxillary. There were many cases of generalized sinus disease. The interobserver agreement on interpretation of the CT findings was considerable.

▶ I quote the authors, "Clinical diagnosis of acute sinusitis is not accurate." Although they were speaking of patients of general practitioners, I would also guess that otolaryngologists are not correct more than 80% of the time. What else could mask as acute sinusitis? Turbinate engorgement, nasal mucosal inflammation, trigeminal irritation, and pressure blockage with air absorption are examples. Clearly, an expensive CT scan does not need to be performed when a good history and physical examination should suffice. Symptomatic therapy is indicated, as well as antibiotics when signs of mucopurulence or toxicity are present.

**G.R. Holt, M.D., M.S.E., M.P.H.**

**Necrotizing Fasciitis of the Head and Neck: Role of CT in Diagnosis and Management**
Becker M, Zbären P, Hermans R, et al (Univ Hosp of Geneva; Univ Hosp of Berne, Switzerland; Univ Hosps of Leuven, Belgium)
*Radiology* 202:471–476, 1997                                                     13–11

*Background.*—Necrotizing fasciitis is a severe, acute and potentially life-threatening condition caused by bacterial infection of the soft tissues. The clinical course is characterized by septic complications that develop within hours and by a mortality rate as great as 73%. Antibiotic treatment alone is insufficient, and prompt aggressive surgical treatment is the only way to prevent death. Necrotizing fasciitis of the head and neck is uncommon and usually first seen with nonspecific swelling, erythema, and fever. Without immediate surgical treatment, it proceeds rapidly to mediastinitis and fatal sepsis. Therefore, it is essential to rapidly establish the correct diagnosis. To define the diagnostic features of necrotizing fasciitis, the CT scans of 14 patients with proven necrotizing fasciitis of the head and neck were retrospectively examined.

*Methods.*—In 6 years, 16 patients with a diagnosis of necrotizing fasciitis of the head and neck were seen at 3 institutions. Fourteen patients, 8 to 79, underwent CT at admission, and 11 of these underwent follow-up CT scans. Although 5 patients had compromised immune systems, the remaining 9 were young and otherwise healthy. Twelve patients initially were seen with nonspecific signs of inflammation and 2 had signs of sepsis. The initial neck palpation indicated induration and severe edema in all patients. Within 2 hours of admission, all patients became dyspneic and 9 required mechanical ventilation. The initial organisms isolated included staphylococci, β-hemolytic streptococci, and anaerobes. All patients were examined by CT within 2 hours of admission, and the findings were used as a guide to surgery. In patients who underwent follow-up CT, these findings were used as a guide to additional care. The CT images were independently reviewed by 2 radiologists and then correlated with clinical findings at admission, initial surgery, and outcome.

*Findings.*—The CT features that were always associated with necrotizing fasciitis of the head and neck were cellulitis defined as diffuse thickening and infiltration of the cutis and subcutis; fasciitis defined as diffuse enhancement and thickening of the cervical fascia; myositis defined as enhancement and thickening of the platysma, sternocleidomastoid, or strap muscles; and fluid in multiple neck compartments. Gas collection, mediastinitis, and pleural or pericardial effusions were also detected in some patients. All patients underwent extensive surgical débridement on the basis of their CT findings. Follow-up CT in 11 of these patients revealed clinically unsuspected progression of inflammation in previously unaffected areas. Additional surgery was performed in 9 of these patients on the basis of follow-up CT findings. Of the 14 patients in this series, 12 survived and 2 died of septic shock despite intensive treatment.

*Conclusions.*—This study examined the role of CT imaging in the diagnosis and treatment of necrotizing fasciitis of the head and neck. CT was useful in establishing a diagnosis at an early stage and in detecting continuing tissue necrosis after initial surgical débridement, which required further treatment. Necrotizing fasciitis should be suspected if CT inflammatory signs are not limited to cellulitis, but include fasciitis, myositis, and multiple fluid collections in neck compartments. CT examination should always include the chest.

▶ Recent media focus on necrotizing fasciitis has been beneficial, in that both physicians and patients are aware of its existence and deadly potential. If not diagnosed early and considered to be instead only a cellulitis, this infection can rapidly get out of control. The authors recommend that certain CT findings can support a presumptive diagnosis of necrotizing fasciitis, and that serial scans can uncover "hidden" infection or progression of the fasciitis into new locations.

**G.R. Holt, M.D.**

---

**Transnasal Butorphanol: Pain Relief in the Head and Neck Patient**
Cannon CR (Head & Neck Surgical Group, Jackson, Miss)
*Otolaryngol Head Neck Surg* 116:197–200, 1997                                    13–12

---

*Objective.*—Pain management in head and neck surgery patients is problematic because swallowing is frequently difficult or impossible and narcotic addiction can develop. Efficacy of the transnasal route of butorphanol tartrate, a nonnarcotic agonist-antagonist analgesic agent was prospectively evaluated in head and neck surgery patients.

*Methods.*—Transnasal butorphanol (1 mg) was administered to 28 patients (8 men), average age 40, after surgery at the patients' request using 1 puff of butorphanol in 1 nostril. The dose could be repeated after 1 hour and the dosage sequence could be repeated every 3–4 hours. Patients were observed and asked to rate their pain on a 0 to 3 scale (from no relief) to complete relief, at 15, 30, 60, 120, 180, and 240 minutes. Side effects were recorded.

*Results.*—Patients underwent a total of 20 head and neck procedures and 8 tonsillectomies. One tonsillectomy patient was removed from the study because of incomplete data. Of the 107 doses evaluated, 35% of head and neck surgery patients had complete relief at 15 minutes and 30% had no relief. At 4 hours, 70% of these patients still had adequate pain relief and 30% had no relief. The highest degree of pain relief was reported at 2 hours. In tonsillectomy patients, 10% had complete relief at 15 minutes, 30% had no relief, 60% reported some or moderate pain relief. At 4 hours, 10% of this group had complete relief and 5% had no relief. At 30, 60, and 120 minutes, 40%, 59%, and 75% (respectively) reported complete pain relief. There were no side effects. Patients were more ready to accept this method of analgesia delivery if they were aware of side effects at the beginning.

*Conclusion.*—Transnasal administration of butorphanol delivers safe and effective pain relief without side effects to patients after head and neck surgery.

▶ Dr. Cannon gives us some suggestions about pain control postoperatively, particularly in patients who are dependency risks. The intranasal route of delivery for butorphanol may also appeal to some patients who do not like shots. Obviously, if the medication is not effective, another analgesic must be made available to that patient, provided excessive sedation is watched for. Apparently, it is not necessary to "sniff" the medication during spraying the nose to be effective; that maneuver is not an option for the patient after laryngectomy.

**G.R. Holt, M.D., M.S.E., M.P.H.**

---

**Sleep-related Myocardial Ischemia and Sleep Structure in Patients With Obstructive Sleep Apnea and Coronary Heart Disease**
Schäfer H, Koehler U, Ploch T, et al (Univ of Bonn, Germany; Univ of Marburg, Germany)
*Chest* 111:387–393, 1997                                    13–13

---

*Background.*—Obstructive sleep apnea is a condition in which frequent arousals occur during noctunal sleep. It is common among middle-aged men and is associated with cardiovascular death. Patients with a combination of coronary heart disease (CHD) and obstructive sleep apnea may be at increased cardiac risk as a result of apnea-induced hypoxemia. Their sleep quality may be compromised by both apnea-associated arousals and ischemia-associated arousals. This study examined the association between nocturnal myocardial ischemia and sleep apnea in patients with CHD.

*Methods.*—Fourteen male patients with both obstructive sleep apnea and CHD and 7 male patients with obstructive sleep apnea alone were analyzed for 6 consecutive nights in the sleep laboratory, with standard sleep and cardiorespiratory measurements plus 6-lead ECG monitoring. Cardiac patients did not take any cardiovascular medications for 48 hours before sleep testing. All patients received a single dose of a sustained-release high-dose nitrate or placebo on nights 3, 4, 5 and 6 in a double-blind crossover, placebo-controlled design to test the effects of nitrate therapy on nocturnal ischemia.

*Results.*—During 3 nights of recordings, 144 episodes of nocturnal myocardial ischemia were detected in 6 participants. Of these 6 study participants, 5 had underlying CHD and 1 had diffuse coronary artery wall defects. During 85.4% of the ischemic episodes, there were concomitant apneas with greater than 3% oxygen desaturation. Although rapid eye movement sleep accounted for only 18% of total sleep time, 77.8% of ischemic episodes occurred during rapid eye movement sleep. The mean oxygen saturation was significantly lower during apnea-associated ischemic periods than during ischemic periods without associated apnea. Nitrate administration had no effect on ischemia. Sleep periods with myocardial ischemia were associated with significantly more frequent and severe arousals than those without ischemia. The microstructure of sleep was also disturbed by myocardial ischemia in the absence of apnea.

*Conclusion.*—Patients with both CHD and obstructive sleep apnea should be considered to be at cardiovascular risk, because apnea-associated oxygen desaturation can lead to nocturnal myocardial ischemia. Nocturnal myocardial ischemia may cause arousal, which in turn may result in increased daytime sleepiness. Patients with nocturnal ischemia should be screened for underlying sleep apnea, even if have no response to nitrate therapy.

▶ I'm not sure how you would know that a patient had nocturnal ischemia without a sleep study for apnea. But the main lesson from this article is, in my view, that sleep apnea and CHD are ominous partners, and all effort should be made to diagnose the extent of the cardiac disease. CHD is a two-edged sword here; one needs to improve the sleep apnea, but the CHD makes the patient a poor surgical risk. Continuous positive airway pressure should definitely be tried first and its results documented. If surgery for sleep apnea is performed in the patient with CHD, then the patient should clearly be placed in the ICU—possibly the surgical ICU, not the medical ICU—afterward, with his or her cardiologist in close contact.

**G.R. Holt, M.D., M.S.E., M.P.H.**

---

**Quality of Life Consequences of Sleep-Disordered Breathing**
Flemons WW, Tsai W (Univ of Calgary, Alta, Canada)
*J Allergy Clin Immunol* 99:S750–S756, 1997                13–14

---

*Introduction.*—Sleep-disordered breathing encompasses a broad spectrum of conditions in which individuals have apnea, a complete cessation of breathing, or hypopnea, a marked reduction in airflow. This occurs in up to 4% of the adult population. Hypoxemia and hypercarbia can occur with apnea or hypopnea. Little is known about how the quality of life is affected by sleep apnea.

*Symptoms.*—Symptoms of sleep apnea are restless sleep, nocturnal enuresis, snoring, excessive daytime somnolence, depression, irritability, inability to concentrate, memory deficits, and decreased alertness. These symptoms lead to impairment in work efficiency, decrements in quality of life, and increased automobile accident rates.

*Treatment.*—Continuous positive airway pressure is the main treatment for sleep apnea. It reduces sleepiness and improves mood disturbances, performance, and neurocognition. Continuous positive airway pressure effectively prevents upper airway collapse, resulting desaturations, and arousals from sleep. Current tests and scales used to quantify alterations in alertness, performance, sleepiness, or quality of life do not correlate well with traditional measurements of sleep apnea severity. After patient and physician interviews and literature reviews, a disease-specific quality-of-life scale has been developed. Aspects of quality of life important to sleep apnea patients will be captured in the Calgary Sleep Apnea Quality of Life Index, which can measure mood, cognitive function, and performance.

*Conclusions.*—Appropriate treatment of sleep-disordered breathing can improve cognitive function, mood, and performance. The lack of information on how sleep apnea affects the quality of life makes it difficult to help guide treatment. For patients with sleep-disordered breathing, further investigation in areas of cognitive functioning, performance, and quality of life is necessary.

► When my family accuses me of a waning memory, I blame it on the fact that I must have sleep-disordered breathing at night. However, they're having none of that; they're convinced it is my age. At any rate, we do have evidence that poor sleep can cause a number of problems, all of which can potentially interfere with our daily activities. As we learn more about sleep disorders, we must be aware of how they might contribute to some of the symptomatology in patients we encounter everyday. Even children may be victims of such problems, manifested by poor school performance and behavior abnormalities. We need to maintain a high index of suspicion, yet not go overboard on blaming this for too many symptoms.

**G.R. Holt, M.D., M.S.E., M.P.H.**

---

**Uvulopalatopharyngoplasty versus Laser-assisted Uvulopalatoplasty for the Treatment of Obstructive Sleep Apnea**
Walker RP, Grigg-Damberger MM, Gopalsami C (Loyola Univ Chicago)
*Laryngoscope* 107:76–82, 1997                                     13 16

---

*Objective.*—Uvulopalatopharyngoplasty (UPPP) is the first and still the most commonly performed surgery to correct the palatal abnormalities in adults with obstructive sleep apnea syndrome (OSAS). The new cost-effective laser-assisted uvulopalatoplasty (LAUP) can be performed under local anesthesia in an office setting. The surgical results of 79 patients with

OSAS, 38 treated with LAUP and 41 treated with UPPP, were reviewed for patient selection criteria, preoperative evaluation, surgical techniques, postoperative complications, and polysomnographic findings.

*Methods.*—Successful surgical response was defined as >50% reduction in preoperative respiratory distress index (RDI). Sex, age, BMI, RDI, average number of apneas/hr of sleep (AI), average number of hypopneas/hr of sleep (HI), lowest oxyhemoglobin saturation ($LS_{aO_2}$) were compared between groups.

*Results.*—Compared with LAUP patients, UPPP patients were significantly younger, had a higher mean BMI, and had a higher mean preoperative RDI, AI, HI, and a lower $LS_{aO_2}$. After surgery, the successful surgical response rate was 51.2% in UPPP patients and 47.4% in LAUP patients. RDI decreased from a mean preoperative value of 30.3 in LAUP patients and 52.1 in UPPP patients to a mean postoperative value of 22.2 and 25.5 respectively. $LS_{aO_2}$ values increased in UPPP patients from a mean of 72.8 to 80.9. $LS_{aO_2}$ values were unchanged in LAUP patients. Postoperative complications in LAUP patients included bleeding in 2, oral candidiasis in 2, and temporary velopalatal insufficiency in 1. Postoperative complications in UPPP patients included bleeding in 2, temporary velopalatal insufficiency in 3, and lower extremity deep venous thrombosis in 1.

*Conclusion.*—LAUP is as effective as UPPP for treatment of OSAS, but is safer and less expensive.

▶ The controversy regarding UPPP vs. LAUP for obstructive sleep apnea continues. The authors contend that LAUP is more cost effective than UPPP because it requires only local anesthesia in the office. However, I have commonly heard of surgeons charging $3,000 to $4,000 for multiple treatments of LAUP—I'm not sure how cost effective that really is. The authors also did not address the role of intranasal surgery as an adjunct to a soft palate procedure. Septoplasty with or without turbinoplasty may be required in patients with concomitant nasal obstructive signs and symptoms because of uncertainty about a multifactorial etiology. This study doesn't solve the sleep apnea controversy but it is nicely done and deserves consideration.

**G.R. Holt, M.D., M.S.E., M.P.H.**

---

**Objective Assessment of Snoring Before and After Laser-assisted Uvulopalatoplasty**

Walker RP, Gatti WM, Poirier N, et al (Loyola Univ, Maywood, Ill; Condell Hosp Med Ctr, Libertyville, Ill)
*Laryngoscope* 106:1372–1377, 1996                                    13–16

---

*Background.*—Laser-assisted uvulopalatoplasty (LAUP), an outpatient staged surgical treatment for snoring, has been performed in the United States since 1993. In most cases, the end point evaluated is patient satisfaction. The frequency, pattern, and volume of snoring in patients before and after each LAUP procedure were assessed objectively.

*Methods.*—Twenty-seven patients were assessed at home using a sonographic device that records oronasal respiration. Snoring parameters were then analyzed digitally.

*Findings.*—The sound of snoring was altered after each LAUP procedure. There were significant reductions in the maximum, average, and velumlike respiratory noise loudness. The fundamental frequency of snoring was found to increase significantly after each procedure. Treatments did not affect snoring index. These objective findings were well correlated with the subjective assessments of the patients and their bed partners.

*Conclusion.*—Objective data as well as subjective accounts show that the LAUP procedure favorably affects snoring. Further research is needed, however, including studies of the long-term efficacy of this relatively new procedure.

▶ It is heartening to see an objective study on the issue of snoring improvement after LAUP. Although subjective information is quite important (i.e., what the bed partner thinks about the outcome), we like to correlate that with data from an objective study. "Snoring science" is becoming more sophisticated, and we in medicine must insist that clinical decisions be based on outcomes research. I know of no disorder that needs more objective data at this time than snoring.

**G.R. Holt, M.D., M.S.E., M.P.H.**

---

**Direct Hypoglossal Nerve Stimulation in Obstructive Sleep Apnea**
Eisele DW, Smith PL, Alam DS, et al (Johns Hopkins Univ, Baltimore, Md)
*Arch Otolaryngol Head Neck Surg* 123:57–61, 1997　　　　　　　　13–17

---

*Background.*—Previous researchers have reported various methods for electrically stimulating the genioglossus muscle to improve pharyngeal patency in patients with obstructive sleep apnea (OSA). However, favorable outcomes have not been proved. In these studies, it is unclear whether the genioglossus muscle was selectively stimulated by the techniques used. The motor responses resulting from direct electric stimulation of the hypoglossal (HG) nerve were determined, and these responses were correlated with upper airway patency changes during sleep.

*Methods.*—Fifteen patients undergoing neck surgery that exposed the HG nerve were studied. The motor effects of direct electric stimulation of the main trunk of the HG nerve and branch supplying the genioglossus muscle during anesthesia and wakefulness were determined visually. In addition, 5 patients with OSA were studied. The main trunk or genioglossus branch of the HG nerve was stimulated electrically in these patients with a half-cuff tripolar electrode.

*Findings.*—Stimulating the HG nerve branch that innervates the genioglossus muscle resulted in protrusion and contralateral deviation of the tongue. Stimulating the main trunk of the HG nerve produced slight ipsilateral deviation and retrusion of the tongue. The mean arousal threshold for stimulation was 0.8 V greater than the motor recruitment threshold. In all patients, stimulation increased inspiratory airflow by 184.5 mL/sec.

*Conclusion.*—The motor responses occurring during electric stimulation of the HG nerve are site specific. Analysis of the motor effects and airflow responses in the patients in this study suggests that activation of the genioglossus muscle by HG nerve stimulation opened the airway, whether or not the tongue retrusor muscles were also involved. Direct stimulation of the HG nerve below the arousal threshold can improve airflow in patients with OSA.

▶ It is interesting that new ideas are being evaluated for the treatment of OSA. Most physicians would likely agree that the best treatment of OSA has not yet been developed. We see sleep studies postoperatively that do not demonstrate significant improvement, although the patients are usually clinically improved. Electroneural muscular stimulation is an intriguing notion which deserves further evaluation. How transcutaneous stimulation at night would affect the airway is unknown, but it has some basis, according to the authors.

**G.R. Holt, M.D., M.S.E., M.P.H.**

## Efficacy of Cold-Steel Uvulopalatoplasty

Casiano RR, Sheth S (Univ of Miami, Fla)
*Otolaryngol Head Neck Surg* 115:471–473, 1996                    13–18

*Introduction.*—Laser-assisted uvulopalatoplasty (LAUP) is considered a cost-effective technique for treating snoring in the outpatient setting. Proponents claim LAUP is easy to use, well-tolerated by patients, and inexpensive. Opponents point out additional costs associated with education of personnel and clinic alterations needed for appropriate laser safety and the potential risk of inadvertent laser injury to patients or personnel. The efficacy of the uvulopalatoplasty technique for snoring performed with LAUP is compared with more conventional instruments that are easily accessible and inexpensive.

*Methods.*—Seven patients underwent cold-steel uvulopalatoplasty (CUP) for snoring. Patients were given questionnaires postoperatively to determine the degree of improvement in snoring and sleep quality. Pain, length of time for resolution of pain, return to work, and ability to tolerate a regular solid food diet were also assessed.

> *Surgical Technique.*—The procedure can be performed under local anesthesia in the office setting. After tongue retraction, vertical cuts are made with back-biting endoscopic through-cut forceps. A forceps is used to clasp the uvula, which is then reshaped to a smaller size or completely removed. Suction cautery may be needed

to achieve hemostasis. The whole procedure usually takes less than 5 minutes.

*Results.*—Six of 7 patients underwent only 1 CUP procedure. One patient underwent 2 procedures. One patient had mild postoperative bleeding, which was resolved with silver nitrate. Three, 3, and 1 patient, respectively, had marked, moderate, and slight improvement in snoring postoperatively. On a 0 to 10 scale, average pain was 5.3 and lasted an average of 13 days. Patients returned to work at an average of 4 days and required an average of 6 days to tolerate a regular diet.

*Conclusion.*—Findings in this small patient series suggest that CUP is as efficacious as LAUP in treating snoring. The cost of CUP is negligible because it can be performed with available instrumentation in a typical otolaryngology practice.

▶ This is not a comparison study between cohorts. It either reinforces your belief that surgical uvulopalatoplasty is good, or you discount it based on the study design. However, the authors showed how to do it under local anesthesia, in the office, using nasal endoscopic instruments. Although costs are not detailed, there is the investment in endoscopic instruments (probably already purchased for nasal surgery) vs. the lease or purchase of a laser (one does not have to be a rocket scientist there). Also, don't forget that "cold-steel" warms up once it has been in the mouth a short time. "Warm steel" surgery, anyone?

**G.R. Holt, M.D., M.S.E., M.P.H.**

# 14 Environmental Health and Epidemiology

**Military Use of Nasopharyngeal Irradiation With Radium During World War II**
Warlick SR (Naval Med Ctr, Portsmouth, Va)
*Otolaryngol Head Neck Surg* 115:391–394, 1996

14–1

*Introduction.*—In May 1944, the Army surgeon called a conference of 10 otologists to address the problem of barotrauma to the middle ear (aerotitis media). Rapid pressurization of the middle ear during descent in combat aircraft and hyperplastic lymphoid tissue around the eustachian tube caused by upper respiratory tract infections in certain overseas locations resulted in airmen with chronically recurring aerotitis who were not available for combat one third of the time. Nasopharyngeal irradiation was used to treat children with chronic serous otitis media and enlarged adenoids at Columbia and Johns Hopkins universities and was adapted at Johns Hopkins for field use.

*Radon Applicator Use.*—The applicator was passed through the nares to the opening of the eustachian tube in the posterior nasopharynx. Treatments lasted about 8.5 minutes and were repeated at monthly intervals for 3–4 treatments. Besides this condition in airmen, aerotitis media was also common (incidence greater than 30%) in submarine trainees because of their exposure to hyperbaric conditions. After the radon applicators were adapted for field use and approved by the expert panel of air surgeons, a total of 8,170 United States military personnel were treated with nasopharyngeal irradiation. It has been estimated that a total of 25,000 treatments were given during World War II. Follow-up lasted only a few weeks to months after treatment

*Military Use After World War II.*—There is no record of military use of nasopharyngeal irradiation to treat aerotitis media after World War II. After returning to private practice, some of the military physicians continued to use nasopharyngeal irradiation in private practices into the 1960s.

*Conclusion.*—Over 8,000 United States servicemen with aerotitis media were treated with radium irradiation of the nasopharynx. There were no reported adverse effects of this therapy. Its efficacy in preventing recurrent barotrauma was high. At the same time, it was used widely in the United States to prevent deafness in children with hypertrophic adenoid tissue.

▶ I found this report fascinating as well as troubling. In recent times, we have heard disclosures from the United States Department of Energy about radioactive fallout from atomic testing in the 1950s. I do not fault the government for conducting the tests, nor for using the radium implants, as the available knowledge at that time did not contraindicate such use. However, it is disconcerting that medical professionals did not maintain a medical surveillance nationwide, or at least a high index of suspicion which would have led to medical examinations on the irradiated servicemen (or civilian children). We need to be more vigilant about such issues; witness Agent Orange and Gulf War syndrome.

**G.R. Holt, M.D., M.S.E., M.P.H.**

---

**Nasopharyngeal Radium Irradiation: Fundamental Considerations**
Royal HD (Washington Univ, St Louis)
*Otolaryngol Head Neck Surg* 115:399–402, 1996           14–2

---

*Introduction.*—Nasopharyngeal radium irradiation (NRI) was commonly used in the peri–World War II era to treat 2 major groups of patients. The first group included submariners and airplane crews who were vulnerable to barotrauma of the middle ear. The second group consisted of children with evidence of high-tone deafness because of chronic middle ear effusions. Concerns regarding use of this treatment approach were reported.

*Concerns About Nasopharyngeal Radium Irradiation.*—The possible effects of radiation exposure to the pituitary gland are of concern. The pituitary gland was exposed to 10 to 100 rems during NRI. Radiation therapy for tumors exposes the pituitary gland to greater doses (2,000 to 12,000 rems). No clinically significant hormonal insufficiencies are reported for the larger doses of radiation therapy, so none are expected for patients treated with NRI. The greatest long-term concern regarding the effect of NRI is a potential carcinogenic effect. The volume of tissue exposed to a large radiation dose was very small because of the type of radiation emitted from the radium applicator. The probability of cancer induction was small because (1) very high doses of radiation ($\gamma$-particles) cause cell death and dead cells cannot become cancerous and (2) the volume of tissue exposed to $\beta$-particles was not large enough to kill the cell, but the potential to cause cancer was small.

*Qualitative Risk Assessment of Nasopharyngeal Radium Irradiation.*— The Advisory Committee on Human Radiation Experiments calculated the risk of cancer development from NRI. The lifetime risk of brain cancer development was calculated to be about 3 per 1,000 persons. The lifetime risk of a fatal cancer was estimated to be 5.6 per 1,000 persons.

*Conclusion.*—There are 2 reasons for medical follow-up of persons who received NRI and are asymptomatic: (1) a program of medical follow-up would provide greater benefit than harm and (2) it would advance scientific knowledge. When any kind of screening is recommended, patients should be advised regarding the potential harm and benefits of screening so that they can chose whether or not to participate.

▶ This is a companion article to Warlick and Mellinger-Birdsong. The latter suggested that over 2.5 million Americans of all ages might have received NRI. This article addresses the medical benefits of screening asymptomatic patients vs. the costs in time and resources. I understand the arguments; however, I also believe we have *some* obligation to those patients to make them aware of the potential problem. The best way might be a news release from the medical profession to all news agencies asking them to apprise the public of the risks, the means for their own self-evaluation, and how they could be screened for a problem. We owe them no less.

**G.R. Holt, M.D., M.S.E., M.P.H.**

---

**Estimates of Numbers of Civilians Treated With Nasopharyngeal Radium Irradiation in the United States**
Mellinger-Birdsong AK (Natl Ctr for Enviromental Health, Atlanta, Ga)
*Otolaryngol Head Neck Surg* 115:429–432, 1996                                    14–3

---

*Introduction.*—Nasopharyngeal radium irradiation (NRI) was used 35 to 50 years ago to treat hearing loss, chronic ear infections, asthma, and other conditions. Most treatments were performed in the offices of private physicians, so it is not easy to estimate the number of patients who received these treatments. An estimate was made of the number of civilians treated with NRI in the United States.

*Background Information.*—Treatments were performed in several states of the United States, according to medical literature. It is likely that NRI was used in more states than those mentioned in the literature. Reports of 17 investigations in 12 different cities were found. In studies alone, 8,000–13,000 patients were reported to have been treated with NRI.

*Estimate of Use.*—Two estimates of physician use of NRI were used: a high estimate of 25 patients per week and a low estimate of 5 patients per week. Estimates were based on use of the radium applicators 50 weeks per year. The usual treatment involved 2 applicators at a time (one for each nostril) over 3 appointments. An estimate was made of the number of children who may have been treated with NRI using a formula that reflected the number of applicators in use, the number of patients a physician would treat each week, the number of weeks in a year an applicator would be used, and the number of applicators and sessions per patient. It is possible that 500,000 to 2.5 million patients were treated with NRI.

*Conclusion.*—A large number of assumptions were used to estimate the numbers of civilians treated with NRI in the United States. It is roughly estimated that 500,000 to 2.5 million civilians were treated 3 to 5 decades ago, before this modality lost favor.

▶ In addition to the estimated high number of individuals who were treated with NRI, there were also those who underwent external beam irradiation therapy for acne of the face and for "enlarged thymus glands" (I was in the latter group) in the 1950s and 1960s. We do know that carcinogenesis has occurred in some of these patients, but we have no firm handle on the statistics, partly because younger physicians caring for these patients may not be aware of what happened nearly 50 years ago. Education is the answer—for both physicians and the public.

**G.R. Holt, M.D., M.S.E., M.P.H.**

## Head and Neck Radiation Carcinogenesis: Epidemiologic Evidence

Ron E, Saftlas AF (Natl Cancer Inst, Bethesda, Md; Yale Univ, New Haven, Conn)
*Otolaryngol Head Neck Surg* 115:403–408, 1996                    14–4

*Introduction.*—The organs most likely to be affected by radium treatment to the nasopharynx are the pituitary glands, salivary glands, brain, and parathyroid and thyroid glands. The highest radiation dose from this treatment is to the pituitary gland. Little is understood regarding the role of radiation in the development of pituitary gland malignancies. This article gives an overview of the long-term carcinogenic effects of head and neck radiation, with an emphasis on trials that provide risk quantification.

*Thyroid Gland.*—The thyroid gland in children is particularly sensitive to the tumorigenic effects of external radiation for several years after exposure. The risk of thyroid cancer diminishes with increasing age at exposure. There is little, if any, risk among patients exposed to radiation as adults.

*Neural Tumors.*—High risk of neural tumors has been reported after moderate- to high-dose radiation in childhood. The magnitude of risk at low doses of radiation is not known for children or adults.

*Salivary Glands.*—Numerous reports have shown a correlation between radiation exposure and salivary gland tumors, but little is known about the magnitude of risk, the influence of host factors, or pathologic features. Salivary gland tumors are rare, so information is not easy to assess. Survival is high, making mortality data hard to calculate.

*Parathyroid Gland.*—Some data indicate increased risk of hyperparathyroidism in persons with childhood radiation exposure, particularly females.

*Pituitary Gland.*—The pituitary gland is irradiated during whole-body radiation, head and neck radiation, or radiation directly to the pituitary gland for treatment of pituitary adenoma or infertility. Infertility was treated with radiation to the ovaries and pituitary gland from around 1920 through 1960. Pituitary tumors are extremely rare and do not seem to be associated with increased risk in patients who have received radiation.

*Conclusion.*—Radiation exposure to the head and neck can cause tumors of the thyroid, salivary and parathyroid glands; the brain; and the CNS. Risks seem to be higher for childhood exposures and seem to continue long after exposure.

▶ Two issues are raised for me by this article. First, there is a clear risk for "baby boomers" who underwent head and neck irradiation 50 years ago that needs to be addressed with a public awareness campaign. Second, we have to think about the long-term risks in children and young adults who are undergoing chemotherapy/radiation therapy for head and neck tumors at this time, and what their chances are of developing a second primary tumor because of the radiation. As we are able to cure or provide long-term survival for many childhood tumors of the head and neck, the "down-the-road" impact must be studied.

**G.R. Holt, M.D., M.S.E., M.P.H.**

---

**Head and Neck Cancer Screening Among 4611 Tobacco Users Older Than Forty Years**
Prout MN, Sidari JN, Witzburg RA, et al (Boston Univ; Tufts Univ, Boston)
*Otolaryngol Head Neck Surg* 116:201–208, 1997                    14–5

---

*Background.*—Tobacco users are at high risk of upper aerodigestive tract malignancies. More han 4,500 smokers were screened to determine the prevalence, signs, and symptoms of head and neck cancers among this population.

*Methods.*—Primary care practitioners screened 4,611 patients 40 years of age and older (42% men and 58% women, mean age 59.8 years) who had used any kind of tobacco, past or present. Screening consisted of a risk factor assessment (smoking, alcohol use) and an examination of the oral mucosa for signs of lesions or patches that raised the examiner's suspicion. The vocal cords were not visualized, but any hoarseness was noted. On the basis of these preliminary findings, 313 patients were referred to an otolaryngologist for follow-up.

*Findings.*—The most common findings in the entire group were hoarseness (510 patients, or 11.1%), red patches (242, or 5.2%), mucosal lesions (204, or 4.4%), and white patches (144, or 3.1%). The most common reasons for referrals were white patches (112 of 144, or 78%), mucosal lesions (84 of 204, or 41%), red patches (78 of 242, or 32%), and hoarseness (134 of 510, or 26%). Of the 208 patients who completed a referral visit (67% of those referred), more than 70% had abnormal findings. The most common abnormal findings in these patients were mucosal lesions (76%), hoarseness (76%), white patches (71%), and red patches (66%). Six cancers were diagnosed (2.8% of those completing a referral visit).

*Conclusions.*—Although hoarseness and mucosal lesions are not specific for head and neck cancer, in this high-risk population of older tobacco users, the presence of these symptoms prompted a referral in two thirds of patients. Furthermore, compared with literature reports of oral mucosal lesions in 6.7% of the general population, the risk of oral mucosal lesions in this at-risk population was almost twice that of normal adults (12.7%). Thus, a screening program can help identify tobacco users 40 years of age and older who are most likely to have head and neck cancers.

▶ I fully support the author's call to consider head and neck cancer screening for high-risk individuals in a community. Small group screening could be performed by head and neck surgeons, but larger groups would require trained primary caregivers or nonphysician professionals who have been prepared for the screening by the specialists. Greater yield for screening would be to target workers at factories and industrial plants where smoking and exposure to toxic materials might cause a cumulative deleterious effect. I urge readers to assess their community needs in this area and work to develop a high-risk screening program where appropriate.

**G.R. Holt, M.D., M.S.E., M.P.H.**

---

**Laryngeal Carcinoma in Patients Without a History of Tobacco and Alcohol Use**
Agudelo D, Quer M, León X, et al (Hosp de la Santa Creu i Sant Pau, Barcelona)
*Head Neck* 19:200–204, 1997
14–6

---

*Introduction.*—The use of tobacco and alcohol are clearly related to squamous carcinomas of the larynx; however, about 5% of patients with this type of cancer have not used tobacco or alcohol. Little is known about patients without a history of tobacco and alcohol use who have squamous carcinomas of the larynx, and whether their characteristics and outcomes differ from tobacco and alcohol users. The existence of differences between laryngeal cancer patients who use tobacco and alcohol and those who do not was examined.

*Methods.*—There were 933 patients with laryngeal carcinomas who were treated with radiotherapy, total laryngectomy, or chemotherapy of the glottis, supraglottis, or subglottis. Patients were divided into those who used tobacco and alcohol and those who did not. Patients were then analyzed for age, sex, associated disease, degree of differentiation of tumor, localizations, treatment, and survival rates.

*Results.*—No history of tobacco and alcohol use was seen in 31 patients (3.3%) with laryngeal carcinomas. In the nonsmoker/nonalcohol users, the distribution between sexes was similar, whereas in the tobacco and alcohol users, there was a predominance of males. The mean age of patients who didn't use alcohol and tobacco was 70 years compared with 63 years in those with a history of tobacco and alcohol use. In those who didn't use tobacco and alcohol, the survival rate was also better. The 5-year survival rate for those who did not use tobacco and alcohol was 87%, for those who smoked fewer than 20 cigarettes a day and consumed less than 100 g of alcohol a day it was 68%, and for those who smoked more than 20 cigarettes a day and consumed more than 100 g of alcohol a day it was 58%.

*Conclusions.*—Different characteristics were found in patients without a history of tobacco and alcohol use who had laryngeal cancer when they were compared with smokers or drinkers. The nonsmokers showed no male predominance, were an average of 10 years older, and had lesions that were mainly located in the glottis, which allowed for earlier diagnosis and a higher survival rate.

▶ Although infrequently seen in my experience, patients who do not smoke or drink *do* get laryngeal carcinoma. The authors tell us that these patients may have different personal characteristics than smokers/drinkers and may have a more favorable prognosis. At least it is likely that they might be better risks for surgery, with possibly healthier lungs, livers, and immune systems. As to why their larynges undergo carcinogenesis, I would suggest that a detailed environmental exposure to toxicants be explored.

**G.R. Holt, M.D., M.S.E., M.P.H.**

---

**The Influence of Alcohol Consumption on Worldwide Trends in Mortality From Upper Aerodigestive Tract Cancers in Men**
Macfarlane GJ, Macfarlane TV, Lowenfels AB (Univ of Manchester, England; Univ Dental Hosp of Manchester, England; New York Med College)
*J Epidemiol Community Health* 50:636–639, 1996          14–7

---

*Introduction.*—The combination of alcohol intake and smoking in men may be responsible for as many as three fourths of cancers of the oral cavity, pharynx, esophagus, and larynx. The rate of upper aerodigestive tract tumors in men is increasing worldwide, despite a decrease in smoking in many countries. Current trends in mortality from upper aerodigestive tract cancers worldwide were reviewed and related to national alcohol and tobacco habits. Estimates of the future burden of mortality from these cancers were calculated.

*Methods.*—The World Health Organization mortality database was used to determine mortality data for cancers of the oral cavity/pharynx, esophagus, and larynx from 1955 to 1989 in 25 countries in North America, Australia, Europe, and Japan. Information on past and current alcohol consumption was extracted. Current national lung cancer rates were used as a proxy measure of past tobacco use.

*Results.*—Considered together, the national death rates from cancers of the oral cavity/pharynx, esophagus, and larynx are increasing among men.

These rates are most strongly associated with the level of per capita consumption of alcohol 20 years previously, less strongly associated with the level of alcohol consumption 10 years previously, and weakly correlated with the current level of lung cancer mortality. The national rate of upper aerodigestive tract cancer was estimated using information on past alcohol consumption and an interaction term between alcohol consumption and current lung cancer rates. The substantial increase in alcohol consumption, from 5 to 10 L per capita each year in some countries during the 1960s and 1970s, means increases of about 5 per 100,000 in the death rate from these cancers can be expected in these countries in the next decades.

*Conclusion.*—Previous alcohol consumption in the 1960s and 1970s can be related to current deaths from cancers of the upper aerodigestive tract in men. If the decrease in smoking that is already occurring in some countries could be coupled with a decrease in alcohol consumption, the incidence of these cancers could be significantly influenced.

▶ It is commonly held that the development of carcinogenesis in smokers is enhanced by heavy alcohol use. This long-term review confirms that belief and correlates mortality with periods of increased alcohol intake in the countries studied. It should be stressed that the higher the alcohol intake, the greater the risk. However, light intake of alcohol, say in the form of a glass of red wine each evening, may indeed have a salutary effect on the cardiovascular system, so such low intake need not be discouraged in patients, according to current thinking.

**G.R. Holt, M.D., M.S.E., M.P.H.**

---

**Sinonasal Cancer and Occupation: Results From the Reanalysis of Twelve Case-Control Studies**
Leclerc A, Luce D, Demers PA, et al (INSERM, Paris; Univ of British Columbia, Vancouver, Canada; Internatl Agency for Research on Cancer, Lyon, France; et al)
*Am J Ind Med* 31:153–165, 1997                                        14–8

---

*Introduction.*—The relationship between employment in wood- and leather-related occupations and the risk for sinonasal carcinoma are well documented. Associations with sinonasal carcinoma have been made with several other occupational groups, but few of these cohort trials have the power required to demonstrate correlations. Reported are pooled reanalyses of 12 case-control trials on sinonasal cancer and occupation from 7 countries that include a total of 930 research subjects and 3,136 controls. The analysis was restricted to workers never employed in wood or leather occupations.

*Methods.*—All trials included a detailed occupational history for research subjects and controls. All jobs were coded, using the same classifications for occupation and industry.

*Results.*—There were associations between squamous cell carcinoma among female and male agricultural workers with >10 years of employment. For textile workers, associations were observed between adenocarcinoma among women and squamous cell carcinoma among men. Among men, food manufacturing was associated with elevated risk for adenocarcinoma, and food preservers and cooks had increased risk for squamous cell carcinoma. There was a positive association between squamous cell carcinoma among male transport equipment drivers and adenocarcinoma for male motor-vehicle drivers.

*Conclusion.*—This reanalysis was able to make associations between sinonasal carcinoma and occupations and industries for which there was an a priori suspicion. Findings indicate excesses for squamous cell carcinoma among male and female workers and adenocarcinoma among male workers. The results of this reanalysis are more informative than the sum of results from individual trials.

▶ I personally feel it is mandatory for otolaryngologists, as the medical caretakers of the upper aerodigestive tract, to be quite familiar with the epidemiology of occupational neoplasia in this region. We also have a fiduciary responsibility to our community of patients to become proactively involved in the medical surveillance of high-risk occupational sites, to detect—or even better, decrease—the risk of carcinogenesis. Few of us practice in an area where agriculture, textile, food manufacturing, and transport industries are not present. Look around your community for high-risk sites, and get involved in surveillance.

**G.R. Holt, M.D., M.S.E., M.P.H.**

---

**Is There an Occupational Etiology of Inverted Papilloma of the Nose and Sinuses?**
Deitmer T, Weiner C (Westfälische Wilhelms Univ, Münster, Germany)
*Acta Otolaryngol (Stockh)* 116:762–765, 1996                    14–9

---

*Background.*—The etiology of inverted papilloma is thought to be viral. Because the nose is the first line of defense for the respiratory tract, the etiology may also include airborne pollutants, especially occupational pollutants. A pilot study tested this hypothesis.

*Methods and Findings.*—Forty-seven patients with nasal inverted papilloma seen at 1 center were studied. Lifelong professional history and occupational exposures were elicited. A control group of patients with nonmalignant diseases was studied for comparison. The patients with nasal inverted papilloma were found to have a significantly greater degree of occupational exposure to various smokes, dusts, and aerosols compared with the control group.

*Conclusion.*—Noxious occupational exposures appear to promote the pathogenesis of inverted papilloma of the nose and sinuses. Further studies are necessary to verify these novel findings.

▶ I have been calling for years in these commentaries and in other publications for the otolaryngologist to accept a role in closely monitoring those high risk occupations in the community that might result in neoplastic disorders of the upper aerodigestive tract. If we, as a specialty, will not search for epidemiologic connections, then we have failed to serve our patients. This is the first publication, to my knowledge, linking inverting papilloma to occupational toxic exposures. A detailed environmental exposure questionnaire for use with patients might shed light on these associations. My last patient with inverting papilloma was a painter and a nonsmoker who was exposed to paints and solvents for 30 years. A coincidence? I think not.

**G.R. Holt, M.D., M.S.E., M.P.H.**

## Crack Cocaine Smoking and Oral Scores in Three Inner-City Neighborhoods

Faruque S, Edlin BR, McCoy CB, et al (Ctrs for Disease Control and Prevention, Atlanta, Ga; Univ of Miami, Fla; Bayview-Hunter's Point Found, San Francisco; et al)
*J Acquir Immune Defic Syndr Hum Retrovirol* 13:87–92, 1996          14–10

*Background.*—Smoking crack cocaine causes blisters, sores, and cuts on the lips and in the mouth. Such sores may facilitate the oral transmission of HIV. This possibility was explored in a study of young adults in 3 innercity neighborhoods in New York, Miami, and San Francisco.

*Methods.*—A total of 2,323 persons between the ages of 18 and 29 years were recruited for the study. Sixty percent smoked crack cocaine. The participants were interviewed about HIV risk behaviors and a history of recent oral sores. They were also tested for HIV, syphilis, and herpes simplex virus.

*Findings.*—Ten percent of crack smokers and 4.5% of crack nonsmokers reported having oral sores in the preceding 30 days, for a prevalence odds ratio of 2.4. In addition, sores were more common among participants who had ever injected drugs than among those who had not (14.3% and 6.7%, respectively) and among those with HIV infection compared with uninfected participants (14.3% and 8%, respectively). Of the 429 participants reporting receipt of oral sex, those with oral sores were more likely to be infected with HIV than those without oral sores, after adjustment for other HIV risk factors.

*Conclusion.*—Smokers of crack cocaine have a high prevalence of oral sores. These data suggest that these sores may infrequently facilitate the oral transmission of HIV infection.

▶ Dentists and otolaryngologists may be among those health care workers who are in a position to diagnose the oral sores associated with crack cocaine smoking. Although it is important to identify the cause, the more worrisome problem is the association with HIV positivity. Testing for HIV should be encouraged, and universal precautions used in the office and the emergency room. These patients should be sent for drug counseling and/or AIDS counseling, as appropriate.

**G.R. Holt, M.D., M.S.E., M.P.H.**

**Social Ties and Susceptibility to the Common Cold**
Cohen S, Doyle WJ, Skoner DP, et al (Carnegie Mellon Univ, Pittsburgh, Pa; Univ of Pittsburgh Pa; Univ of Virginia, Charlottesville)
*JAMA* 277:1940–1944, 1997                                            14–11

*Background.*—Evidence suggests that susceptibility to common colds is increased among smokers and reduced among moderate drinkers. However, little is known about the role of other health practices, levels of catecholamines, cortisol, or normal variations in cellular immune function. The current study investigated the importance of network diversity for susceptibility, the importance of these behavioral and biological markers for susceptibility, and the possible role of these markers in linking social network diversity to common colds.

*Methods.*—One hundred fifty-one women and 125 men in good health participated in the study. None of the subjects was pregnant or HIV-seropositive. Data on 12 types of social ties (e.g., spouse, parent, friend, co-worker, member of social group) were elicited. The subjects were then given nasal drops containing 1 of 2 rhinoviruses and monitored for the development of a cold.

*Findings.*—Participants with more types of social ties were less susceptible to common colds, produced less mucus, were more effective in ciliary clearance of their nasal passages, and shed less virus. These findings were unaffected by controlling statistically for prechallenge virus-specific antibody, virus type, age, sex, season, body mass index, education, and race. Susceptibility to colds declined in a dose-response fashion with increasing diversity of the social network. Persons with the fewest types of social ties (1 to 3) had an adjusted relative risk of 4.2 compared to those with the most types of social ties (6 or more). Although smoking, poor sleep quality, alcohol abstinence, low dietary vitamin C intake, increased catecholamine levels, and being introverted were all associated with a greater susceptibility, they only partially explained the relationship between social network diversity and incidence of colds.

*Conclusion.*—Persons participating in more types of social relationships have less susceptibility to rhinovirus-induced colds. This association persists even after adjustment for the number of people in the social network, indicating that it is network diversity—having many types of relationships—that is important, not the sheer number of members in the network.

▶ This article gives an interesting perspective on some potential elements influencing susceptibility to colds. It seems that the more social and outgoing, the less the risk for contracting a cold after exposure to the virus. I find this fascinating because it is counter intuitive to the notion that the fewer individuals one comes in contact with, the less one's total risk of exposure. However, pediatricians and otolaryngologists may be examples of how increased exposure to acute upper respiratory infections eventually leads to the possession of a large number of viral-specific antibodies. Additionally, I believe that plenty of exercise; adequate intake of vitamins (especially vitamin C); and a positive, loving, stress-managed outlook on life are critical to the maintenance of our immune systems. A good gene pool also helps, along with clean living.

**G.R. Holt, M.D., M.S.E., M.P.H.**

## Molecular Epidemiology and Retinoid Chemoprevention of Head and Neck Cancer

Khuri FR, Lippman SM, Spitz MR, et al (Univ of Texas, Houston)
*J Natl Cancer Inst* 89:199–211, 1997                                             14–12

*Background.*—Head and neck cancer is a major health problem, affecting perhaps 900,000 people worldwide each year. Surgery and/or radiation therapy is generally the treatment of choice, and it is often successful in patients with early-stage squamous cell carcinoma of the head and neck. However, second primary tumors develop at a rate of 4% to 7% per year. The problem of second primary tumors is expected to increase together with advances in diagnostic and treatment procedures, raising the need for chemoprevention and other new approaches. Current evidence regarding the epidemiology and retinoid chemoprevention of head and neck cancers was reviewed.

*Epidemiology and Chemoprevention.*—Through molecular studies of premalignant and malignant tissues, there is now considerable evidence to suggest that clonal genetic alterations play a key role in the early development of aerodigestive tract carcinomas. Epidemiologic studies have clearly established the role of tobacco and diet in the carcinogenesis of head and neck cancers. This research provides the groundwork for integrating information from epidemiologic and genetic susceptibility studies into comprehensive models of risk for head and neck cancer. Future research will help our understanding of the interaction between mutagen sensitivity and other forms of genetic susceptibility and environmental risk factors, particularly cigarette smoke.

Combined, the molecular and epidemiologic data pave the way for clinical trials of retinoids and other compounds for the reversal of premalignant lesions and the prevention of second primary tumors. The active retinoid 13cRA is the subject of a current multicenter phase III trial, and may one day be the standard of adjuvant therapy for patients who have been successfully treated for head and neck cancer. Translational approaches have allowed studies of the nuclear retinoic acid receptors and other intermediate end-point markers in chemoprevention. Ongoing research advances may soon provide ways of identifying patients at greatest risk of head and neck cancer and, thus, most likely to benefit from chemoprevention.

*Conclusion.*—Epidemiologic and molecular studies have moved us much closer to the ability to provide effective chemoprevention for head and neck cancer. Further advances in prevention and treatment seem likely to arise from translational chemoprevention trials of retinoids. This may pave the way for newer agents—such as α-tocopherol, interferon-α, and retinamides—which can be usefully integrated into combined-modality approaches.

▶ This is a "must read" article for all who are involved in the care of patients with head and neck cancer. Its excellent review of pertinent studies and its prediction of future developments in treatment and prevention are comprehensive. If one believes that free radicals are threats to DNA, the use of antioxidants (through dietary or supplemental intake) makes sense. A better understanding of the complex relationship between genetic susceptibility and environmental influences will advance our ability to reduce the risk of cancer development.

**G.R. Holt, M.D., M.S.E., M.P.H.**

## Warthin's Tumor and Cigarette Smoking

Vories AA, Ramirez SG (Brooke Army Med Ctr, San Antonio, Tex)
*South Med J* 90:416–418, 1997                                                   14–13

*Introduction.*—The most common type of salivary gland neoplasm is the parotid gland neoplasm, accounting for up to 80% of salivary gland tumors. Previous studies showed a predominance of Warthin's tumors in men, but recent studies have shown more women having this tumor. It was determined whether there was a relationship between smoking and Warthin's tumor.

*Methods.*—A retrospective review was conducted of 82 patients with parotid tumor during a 20-year period. They were evaluated for sex, age, and history of tobacco use. To test for significance when comparing the incidence of smoking inpatients with Warthin's tumor versus those with other tumor types, Chi-square analysis was done.

*Results.*—Earlier reports were similar to this review in relative percentages of benign and malignant disease, as well as the frequency of individual tumor types. There was a high proportion of Warthin's tumor identified, or 23% of all tumors. Women accounted for more than one third of patients with Warthin's tumor. A history of tobacco use was found in 94%

of patients with Warthin's tumor. Only 60% of patients had a history of tobacco use for all other tumor types combined.

*Conclusion.*—The correlation between cigarette smoking and Warthin's tumor was supported. The mechanism by which smoking predisposes patients to Warthin's tumor is still unknown. Further research should be conducted.

▶ I was intrigued by the demonstration that 23% of a 20-year series of parotid tumors were Warthin's tumors and fully a third of those who had them were women. Of additional note, the high association of smoking or other tobacco use (94%) raises the specter of this disease being induced and/or influenced by tobacco. It would be interesting to also look at secondary smoke as an associated factor. The clinician should seek detailed environmental pollutant exposure for *all* patients with irritative, inflammatory, and neoplastic disorders of the head and neck if we are to better understand the effect of pollutants on the upper aeordigestive tract.

**G.R. Holt, M.D., M.S.E., M.P.H.**

## A Cost of Illness Study of Allergic Rhinitis in the United States

Malone DC, Lawson KA, Smith DH, et al (Univ of Colorado, Denver; Univ of Texas, Austin; Univ of Washington, Seattle; et al)
*J Allergy Clin Immunol* 99:22–27, 1997                                  14–14

*Objective.*—Although the direct and indirect costs of treating allergic rhinitis are believed to be substantial, no studies have been conducted to quantify those costs. Estimates of those costs are presented and their impact on the U.S. economy is discussed.

*Methods.*—Data from the 1987 National Medical Expenditure Survey of 36,259 individuals were used to determine prevalence of allergic rhinitis and estimate direct medical costs and value lost productivity resulting from infection.

*Results.*—There were 26.7 million adults and 12.3 million children who reported having allergic rhinitis in 1987, 1.3 million who lost school or work days, and 4.7 million who sought medical treatment. Approximately 16.7 million made physician visits. An estimated 11.5 million prescriptions, costing $184 million, were written. Individuals who made between 734,000 and 101,000 outpatient and emergency department visits incurred $96.3 million of hospital outpatient expenditures and $10 million of emergency department costs. Indirect costs as a result of lost work productivity (811,000 days) amounted to $37 million. School absenteeism (824,000 days) was calculated at $13 million in terms of caretaker lost productivity. Restricted activity days (4,230,000), valued at 25% of a full day's wages, totaled $17 million of lost productivity. Total costs were $775 million in 1987 and $1.23 billion in 1994 dollars (Consumer Index, $846 million to 1.62 billion). These costs, small compared with other medical conditions, represent 0.2% of the nation's healthcare budget (Table 4).

TABLE 4.—Medical Expenditures by Disease Group

| Diagnostic category | Medical expenditures (billions) | Percent of total costs |
|---|---|---|
| Cardiovascular | 79.6 | 13.9 |
| Injury and long-term effects | 69.1 | 12.1 |
| Neoplasm | 49.6 | 8.7 |
| Genitourinary | 49.3 | 8.7 |
| Pregnancy/birth-related | 39.7 | 6.9 |
| Respiratory | 38.3 | 6.7 |
| Allergic rhinitis* | 1.2 | 0.2 |
| Digestive | 35.9 | 6.3 |
| Musculoskeletal | 27.7 | 4.8 |
| Other circulatory diagnosis | 20.2 | 3.5 |
| Mental health | 19.3 | 3.4 |
| Well care | 17.4 | 3.0 |
| Congenital anomalies | 8.7 | 1.5 |
| Medical misadventure | 6.9 | 1.2 |
| Miscellaneous | 110.6 | 19.3 |
| Total | 572.3 | 100.0 |

*Note:* Source (except for allergic rhinitis): Miller TR, Lestina DC, Galbraith MS, et al: Medical care spending—United States. *MMWR* 43:583, 1994.

*Allergic rhinitis is a subcategory of respiratory.

(Courtesy of Malone DC, Lawson KA, Smith DH, et al: A cost of illness study of allergic rhinitis in the United States. *J Allergy Clin Imunol* 99:22–27, 1997.)

*Conclusion.*—Allergic rhinitis consumes a substantial amount of health-care dollars and results in lost productivity for a large number of sufferers and caretakers. Most allergic rhinitis sufferers apparently do not seek medical attention.

▶ The figure of $1.23 billion of estimated health costs of allergic rhinitis was staggering. While the prescribed medical costs may have been $300 million, the amount of over-the-counter expenditures for self-medication may be triple that amount. It is noteworthy that self-reported medical visits for nasal allergies included only 3.9% made to otolaryngologists. In my view, such data make a very strong case for including the study of allergic disorders in the residency curriculum in otolaryngology programs—a major deficiency in many programs.

**G.R. Holt, M.D., M.S.E., M.P.H.**

## Risk of Cancer and Exposure to Gasoline Vapors

Lynge E, Andersen A, Nilsson R, et al (Danish Cancer Society, Copenhagen, Norsk Kreftregister, Oslo, Norway; Sahlgrenska Univ Hosp, Gothenburg, Sweden; et al)

*Am J Epidemiol* 145:449–458, 1997

14–15

*Objective.*—Service station attendants in Nordic countries were exposed to benzene in gasoline vapors until about 1970 when self service became popular. In 1993, the International Agency for Research on Cancer decided to investigate the cancer risk in these workers exposed to an 8-hour time-weighted average of 0.5–1 mg/m³ benzene.

*Methods.*—From the 1970 census 16,524 service station workers (2,445 women), aged 20–64, from Norway, Sweden, Finland, and Denmark were identified and followed through November 1987. Incident cancer sites diagnosed during this period were recorded and compared with national incidence rates.

*Results.*—The observed cancer incidence was 1,130 in males and 179 in women. An excess of leukemia was not observed. The risks for kidney cancer (standard incidence ratio [SIR] = 1.3) and lung cancer (SIR = 1.3) were slightly elevated. The risks for laryngeal cancer (SIR = 1.5) and pharyngeal cancer (SIR = 1.7) were increased. A previously unnoticed excess risk for nasal cancer (SIR = 3.5) was found.

*Conclusion.*—Whereas studies in Nordic service station workers exposed to benzene concentrations of 0.5–1 mg/m³ show no increased risk of leukemia, particularly acute myeloid leukemia the risks for lung, laryngeal, and pharyngeal cancer were increased by 20%, 40%, and 60%, respectively. The risk for nasal cancer was elevated by a factor of 3.5.

▶ This large, well-constructed study showed increased risks of upper aerodigestive tract cancers to persons exposed chronically to gasoline vapors— 60% for pharyngeal and 40% for laryngeal. additionally, there was a 3.5-fold excess risk for nasal cancer. Since chronic exposure to gasoline vapors affects a large segment of our workforce across many occupations, both epidemiologists and otolaryngologists should be aware of the association. This is particularly true when evaluating patients for upper respiratory complaints—an environmental hazard exposure history should be obtained. We need to be sensitive to any suspicious sites of occupational exposures which may need to be placed under surveillance.

**G.R. Holt, M.D., M.S.E., M.P.H.**

# Subject Index

## A

# Author Index